Holistic Health and Healing

Mary Anne Bright, RN, CS, EdD

Associate Professor
School of Nursing
University of Massachusetts
Amherst, Massachusetts

F. A. DAVIS COMPANY • Philadelphia

F. A. Davis Company
1915 Arch Street
Philadelphia, PA 19103
www.fadavis.com

Printed in the United States of America

Last digit indicates print number: 10 9 8 7 6 5 4 3 2 1

Acquisitions Editor: Melanie Freely
Developmental Editor: Marilyn Kochman
Production Editor: Nwakaego Fletcher-Perry
Cover Designer: Louis Forgione

As new scientific information becomes available through basic and clinical research, recommended treatments and drug therapies undergo changes. The author(s) and publisher have done everything possible
to make this book accurate, up to date, and in accord with accepted standards at the time of publication.
The author(s), editors, and publisher are not responsible for errors or omissions or for consequences from
application of the book, and make no warranty, expressed or implied, in regard to the contents of the
book. Any practice described in this book should be applied by the reader in accordance with professional
standards of care used in regard to the unique circumstances that may apply in each situation. The
reader is advised always to check product information (package inserts) for changes and new information
regarding dose and contraindications before administering any drug. Caution is especially urged when
using new or infrequently ordered drugs.

Library of Congress Cataloging-in-Publication Data

Bright, Mary Anne, 1947-
 Holistic Health and Healing / Mary Anne Bright.
  p. cm.
 Includes bibliographical references and index.
 ISBN 0-8036-0796-2 (pbk.)
 1. Holistic medicine. 2. Alternative medicine. 3. Health. 4. Healing.   I. Title.

R733 .B823 2001
615.5—dc21   2001042157

To my wonderful children, Julie and Mike,
and to the memory of Michael Perlman.

Foreword

Healing is not so much about something that happens to us, as it is about how we live our lives and how we are in the world. Holistic healing is ultimately a way of living, a way of being in the world that recognizes our innate wholeness, holiness, and connectedness with all that is. Healing has to do with being in the right relationship—within ourselves, with others, with our earth, world, environment, and with the Sacred Source (however we may name this Source).

My conscious journey toward understanding healing and wholeness began 30 years ago when I was privileged to work as a field health nurse with the Navajo people. Although the Navajo people appropriately utilize the Western health-care system, their tradition recognizes that healing requires more than the curative interventions of biomedicine. Healing in this tradition implies a return to balance or harmony within the person, and with the family, community, nature, and the realm of Spirit. The interconnectedness of all of life is a basic teaching of both indigenous and mystical spiritual traditions. Rather than seeing ourselves as the weavers of the web of life, these traditions show us that we are each a strand in an intricately woven tapestry. Our life, our relationships, our actions, our priorities, and our decisions affect every part of the web, and what we do to the web we ultimately are doing to ourselves. Within this understanding we recognize that our health is intricately connected with the health of the physical, emotional, social, and spiritual environments in which we live.

Nursing's heritage is rooted in a holistic framework. In her early instructions to nurses, Florence Nightingale espoused care of the whole body-mind-spirit person, and taught nurses to appreciate the importance of nutrition, water and air quality, noise, sanitation, and other environmental factors that affect health and healing. Nightingale understood that, ultimately, it is nature that heals, and that our role is to help the person to be in the best condition for the natural processes of healing to work. Through the efforts of many visionary nurses, particularly in the American Holistic Nurses Association, the concept and practice of holistic healing has become increasingly reintegrated into nursing over the past 30 years.

Mary Anne Bright's book is part of this visionary process. It offers support and encouragement to nurses and other health-care professionals as they attempt to understand the essential concepts of holistic healing and to incorporate these concepts into caring for the people whom they serve. Interest in holistic healing and complementary and alternative therapies (CAM) continues to expand among health-care professionals and among the public. Many of the books now available on CAM emphasize particular therapies and their application within conventional medicine. In contrast, Mary Anne Bright grounds this book with a sound philosophical basis for holistic healing, while providing needed information about various healing modalities.

General exploration of CAM usually begins with healing practices in other cultures and traditions. Often, a technique or therapy is presented as an entity unto itself rather than in relationship to a larger system. This practice tends to "medicalize" the therapy, treating it as if it were a new drug or procedure and associating healing solely with the technique or modality. Although particular complementary or alternative modalities or therapies can contribute to a person's healing, this book helps us to appreciate how holistic healing is more than incorporation of one or more CAM therapies into our health-care practices.

By providing pertinent descriptions of the explanatory models from which various therapies and modalities derive, this book offers insight into how healing is understood within these models and how particular therapies relate to this healing. This provides a basis for understanding how various systems of healing can be incorporated into holistic health-care planning.

Mary Anne Bright and the contributors to this book offer nurses and other health-care professionals a view of holistic healing that is grounded in an appreciation of the sacred, relational perspective of the universe. They describe the necessary paradigm shift that is occurring in Western health care: from an illness-oriented, biomedically dominated perspective to a model that encompasses health, quality of life, and recognition of the primacy of relationship or 'interbeing' among all living things. This shift implies a reawakened awareness of what it means to be human in the context of a living world—one in which we are in a relationship with all the life energy within and around us, contrasted with an attitude toward the world as an inanimate object. This book helps us to understand at all levels of our being that individual health cannot be considered apart from our relationships with our world, with others, and with the Sacred in all of life. Indeed our survival depends on our relationship with all life on this planet (and beyond). This book reminds us that holistic healing is needed in nursing and health care now more than ever, and is a valuable resource for reintegrating this healing into our personal and professional lives and care.

Peggy Burkhardt PhD, RN, CS, HNC
Author of *Spirituality: Living Our Connectedness*
Delmar Publishers, 2002

Preface

Americans today are asking more from health-care practitioners than ever before. They are dissatisfied with the fragmentation of care that has resulted from profound political, economic, and technological shifts in health-care delivery. In the past two decades, there has been an unprecedented trend in the use of complementary and alternative modalities (CAM) that reflects preferences for natural health-care options that promote health and well-being, as well as treat illness.

On July 13, 2000, President Clinton announced the appointment of the chair of the White House Commission on Complementary and Alternative Medicine Policy. President Clinton commented on the need to do more to integrate CAM into the current health-care system: "We need to be able to use information about alternative therapies to set the national agenda for the education and training of health-care practitioners in this field and provide recommendations for advisable coverage policies for alternative therapies."[1]

The public's interest has been driving the current trend toward expanding the mainstream biomedical system to include more choices for health and healing. Clients are becoming more verbal about the importance of egalitarian, caring relationships with practitioners that foster engaged coparticipation in treatment. Environmental activism has raised public consciousness about the innate interconnectedness of all life and about the undeniable link between environmental and human health.

This book presents an overview of 16 commonly used CAM therapeutics in the United States today. They are organized into three categories: holistic healing modalities, such as imagery and massage; Western complementary healing practices, such as naturopathy and homeopathy; and Eastern healing systems, including Chinese medicine and Ayurveda. For each modality discussed, clinical examples and current research on efficacy are included to facilitate the practitioners' evidence-based CAM treatment, referral, and counseling interventions with clients.

Holistic Health and Healing also includes chapters on topics that are essential to the practitioners' understanding of effective CAM utilization. There is a comprehensive overview of the sociopolitical and scientific-technological evolutionary influences that bring us to this moment in the health-care history of the United States, and the paradigm shifts that are moving us toward the future. The philosophy and theory of holism are presented as the basis for understanding healing, and as a model of professional relating that differentiates professional from technical health-care providers. Health and healing are considered not only from the perspective of individual biology, but also within cultural and environmental contexts, which influence the experience of health and illness.

The text is intended for use in college nursing and health courses, and as a resource for practicing professional nurses and health-care providers. It is a source book for all health-care professionals who want to ensure that their clinical practice is current and is responsive to the influences of the burgeoning CAM movement, while also creating a holistic relational environment that supports healing.

---

[1] Muscat M: James Gordon Selected to Chair White House CAM Policy Commission. Alternative Therapies 6(24), 2000.

Acknowledgements

This book emerged from the song of many voices and from the work of many hands. First and foremost, I am deeply grateful to each contributor, whose visionary work now extends through the pages of this book to inspire a larger audience.

Special thanks to my F.A. Davis Company editorial staff: To Marilyn Kochman, for superb editorial assistance, to Nwaka Fletcher-Perry, for patient attention to the editing details, and to Melanie Freely and Alan Sorkowitz, for believing in this book. This work would not have come into existence without my own transformative experiences of "complementary and alternative" treatment, which began 25 years ago with the chiropractic care of Howard Ewert, DC, and Joanne Ehret's practice of Chinese medicine. Thank you both for your part in my walking down this path, and for the excellent health care. I am also grateful to the faculty and staff of the University of Massachusetts Amherst School of Nursing for valuing the course, *Holistic Health and Healing,* which inspired the need for this text.

To my circle of Loved Ones with whom I am privileged to share my life, I extend the heartfelt appreciation that transcends words: to Karen Plavin, for invaluable guidance; to the Monday night meditation group, for unfailing encouragement; to Vernon Turner Kitabu Roshi, for the new name and vision; to Byron Katie, for The Work; to Mother Meera, for The Presence; to Penny Mahoney, for the bubbling rock garden; to Mark Kosarick and Bruce Scofield, for the cosmic weather reports; to Jack Wideman, for the roses; to Patty Gates, for the transformational bodywork; to Mary Scott, for the bird's eye view; to Phil and Eileen Munning, Leslie Case and Phil Helfaer, for the new beginnings; and, to Paul Munning, Bev Flynn, Pete Munning, and Theresa Munning, for being there. A big hug to each of my wonderful children, Mike and Julie Stanitis, for the frequent reminders of what's important in life, and for walking Elmo when I needed to write. And, to John Reed Copen, a heartfelt smile for the joyful meditation that is our life together.

Contributors

Jayne Alexander, DO
Private Practice
Bridgewater, Massachusetts

Veda L. Andrus, RN, MSN, EdD, HNC
President/CEO
Seeds and Bridges Center for Holistic Nursing
  Education
Amherst, Massachusetts

Melissa Blacker, MA
Senior Instructor, Stress Reduction Program
Coordinator, Teacher Development Program
Center for Mindfulness
University of Massachusetts Medical School
Worcester, Massachusetts

Andrea Callanan, DC, FICPA
Private Practice
Gainesville, Virginia

Edward Chapman, MD, DHt, FAAFP
Private Practice
Clinical Instructor
Harvard University School of Medicine
Cambridge, Massachusetts

Joanne Ehret, MA, Lic.Ac.
Licensed Acupuncturist
Northampton, Massachusetts

Dorothy Ann Gilbert, PhD
Associate Professor
University of Massachusetts
School of Nursing
Amherst, Massachusetts

Andrew M. Goldman, DO
Private Practice
Sharon, Connecticut

Philip M. Helfaer, PhD, CBT
International Institute for Bioenergetic
  Analysis
Private Practice
Boston, Massachusetts

Gary Holt, PhD, RPh
Medical Writer
Arlington, Texas

Stephen M. Koral, DMD
Private Practice
Boulder, Colorado

Samir A. Kouzi, PhD
Associate Professor
School of Pharmacy and Health Sciences
University of the Pacific
Stockton, California

Alicia Landman-Reiner, MD
Baystate Health Systems
Northampton, Massachusetts

James M. Lemkin, ND
Private Practice
Haydenville, Massachusetts

Robert Levine, BA
Instructor, Villa Julie College School of
  Nursing
Baltimore, Maryland

Director, The Balance Institute
Baltimore, Maryland

Elinor Levy, PhD
Associate Professor
Boston University School of Medicine
Boston, Massachusetts

Jane Yetter Lunt, MEd, BSN, RN, HNC
Vice President, General Program Director
Seeds and Bridges Center for Holistic Nursing
  Education
Amherst, Massachusetts

**Daniel Ogrydziak, certified T'ai Chi
  instructor, BS**
University of Massachusetts
Amherst, Massachusetts

Neil S. Orenstein, PhD, CNS
Private Practice
Lenox, Massachusetts

Abbas Qutab, MD, DC, PhD, DSc.
President/Founder
International Ayurvedic Institute
Worcester, Massachusetts

Vivian S. Roman, DC
Private Practice
Florence, Massachusetts

Lois Steinberg, PhD
Director
Yoga Institute of Champaign-Urbana
Urbana, Illiniois

R. Brooke Thomas, PhD
Professor
University of Massachusetts
Amherst, Massachusetts

Valerie Vaughan, MLS, MST
Professional Writer and Librarian
Amherst, Massachusetts

Rothlyn P. Zahourek, PhD(c), HNC, CS
Clinical Nurse Specialist
Private Practice
Amherst, Massachusetts

Consultants/Reviewers

Ivy Alexander, RN, PhD
Assistant Professor
Yale University School of Nursing
New Haven, Connecticut

Shiva Barton, ND
Wellspace Complementary Health Center
Cambridge, Massachusetts

Steve Baer, DDS
Executive Vice President
International Academy of Oral Medicine and
  Toxicology (IAOMT)
Sedona, Arizona

Michael Bassan, DC
Doctor of Chiropractic
Multi Specialty Health Care
Baltimore, Maryland

Randall S. Bradley, ND, DHANP
Private Practice
Omaha, Nebraska

Clare Collins, RN, MSN, PhD, FAAN
Professor
Michigan State University

Howard T. Ewert, DC
Private Practice
Amherst, Massachusetts

Peter Fernald, PhD
Professor
University of New Hampshire
Durham, New Hampshire

Robert Fishman, DO, FACP
Private Practice
South Hadley, Massachusetts

**Bob Floss, Diplomat of Acupuncture and
  Chinese Herbs**
Blue Poppy Seminars
Boulder, Colorado

Deborah Gingras, RN, MS
Women's Services
Baystate Medical Center
Springfield, Massachusetts

Robert Gorter, MD, PhD
Associate Professor
University of California
San Francisco Medical School

Also: Professor
Western Cape University, School of Pharmacy
Cape Town, Africa

Professor
University of St. Petersburg, School for Post-
  Graduate Training, Russia
Associate Professor
University of Witten/Herdecke, Germany

Bill Griffin, RN, MS, CS, PC
Director of Psychiatric Services
Heywood Hospital
Gardner, Massachusetts

Patricia A. C. Hildebrand, RN, MSN
Family Nurse Practitioner
Alternative Health Care
Beaumont, Texas

Lucia Kellar, PhD, CBT
Research Assistant Professor
New York University
Medical Center
New York, New York

Also: Senior Psychologist
Bellevue Hospital Center, New York

**Maggie McKivergin, RN, MS,
  CNS, HNC**
Program Coordinator
Center for Alternative Health
Charleston, West Virginia

Thom Namaya, MIA, MSN, FNP
Proprietor
Wellness Services
Brattleboro, Vermont

**Lynn Rew, RNC, EdD, FAAN,
  HNC**
Professor and Graduate Advisor
School of Nursing
University of Texas
Austin, Texas

Steven Rosenzweig, MD, FACEP
Director
Center for Integrative MedicineJefferson
  Medical College
Philadelphia, Pennsylvania

Josephine Ryan, RN, DnSc
Associate Professor
University of Massachusetts
Amherst, Massachusetts

Elizabeth Shannon, PhD (c), MSN, RN, CPNP
Assistant Professor
Simmons College
Boston, Massachusetts

Deborah Shelton, MSN, APRN, CNA, OCN
Assistant Professor
Northeastern State University
School of Nursing
Shreveport, Louisiana

Marilyn Smith-Stoner RN, MSN
Adjunct Faculty
University of Phoenix
Beaumont, California

Julie Tackenberg, RN, MA, MAOM, LMT, OBT
Clinical Supervisor
University Medical Center Home Health
Tucson, Arizona

Lucia Thornton, RN, MSN, HNC
California State University
Department of Nursing
Fresno, California

Patricia Wachter, LMT
Director
Stillpoint School of Massage
Amherst, Massachusetts

Jared Zeff, ND, LAc
Private Practice
Portland, Oregon

Contents

UNIT I
Health As Wholeness 1

1 *Paradigm Shifts 3*
Mary Anne Bright

2 *Health, Healing, and Holistic Nursing 31*
Mary Anne Bright

3 *The Bioenergetic Basis of Health 47*
Philip M. Helfaer and Mary Anne Bright

4 *Psychophysiology of Mind-Body Healing 55*
Elinor M. Levy

5 *Culture and Holistic Healing 71*
Dorothy Ann Gilbert

6 *Global Health Issues 81*
R. Brooke Thomas and Mary Anne Bright

UNIT II
Holistic Healing Modalities 103

7 *Meditation 105*
Melissa Blacker

8 *Imagery 113*
Rothlyn P. Zahourek

9 *Nutrition 121*
Neil S. Orenstein

10 *Herbs through the Ages 135*
Gary A. Holt and Samir Kouzi

11 *Therapeutic Massage 161*
Valerie Vaughan

12 *Therapeutic Touch 171*
Mary Anne Bright

UNIT III
Complementary Healing Practices 181

13 *Naturopathic Medicine—Vis Medicatrix Naturae: The Healing Power of Nature 183*
James M. Lemkin

14 *Homeopathic Medicine 197*
Edward H. Chapman

15   *Anthroposophic Medicine 213*
        Alicia Landman-Reiner

16   *Osteopathy 227*
        Jayne Alexander and Andrew Goldman

17   *Chiropractic 239*
        Vivian Roman and Andrea Callanan

18   *Holistic Dentistry 247*
        Stephen M. Koral

UNIT IV
Traditional Healing Systems 259

19   *Chinese Medicine 261*
        Joanne Ehret

20   *Ayurveda 273*
        Abbas Qutab

21   *Yoga 285*
        Lois Steinberg

22   *T'ai Chi 305*
        Dan Ogrydziak and Robert Levine

Index 312

Health as Wholeness

CHAPTER 1

Paradigm Shifts

Mary Anne Bright

Mary Anne Bright, RN, CS, EdD, the editor of this book, is associate professor at the University of Massachusetts–Amherst School of Nursing. She teaches courses in holistic health and mental health nursing, conducts research on Therapeutic Touch, and is a member of the International Institute of Bioenergetic Analysis and of the American Holistic Nurses Association.

"There is nothing permanent except change."

The Greek philosopher Heraclitus made this observation around 500 BC,[1] and the current state of flux in the U.S. health-care system tells us that it is still true today. The cost of health care is rising above a trillion dollars per year, making the U.S. system the most expensive in the industrialized world. Highly specialized and technologically advanced biomedicine is the capstone of this system and is a remarkable achievement of modern science.

Previously untreatable diseases can now be cured or ameliorated because of advances in pharmacologic knowledge and sophisticated surgical techniques. Developments in the fields of genetics, immunology, neurology, and organ transplantation are advancing the treatment and prevention of a wide range of diseases and disabilities. The practice of biomedicine emerged, along with the field of public health, as a significant solution to the health problems of the 19th century and has an impressive track record of success in reducing death from infection and life-threatening physical traumatic injury.[2]

Public support for lifesaving technological advances is strong. People demand access to sophisticated diagnostic technology, such as radiography and magnetic resonance imaging, high-tech care centers, medical specialists, and the most current treatment that medicine has to offer. However, U.S. health statistics indicate a consistent rise in chronic illness that is not ameliorated by exorbitant expenditures for medical care. The public has become aware that high-tech biomedical advances are only part of the solution to health problems. Modern medicine, most effective in the treatment of acute illness, is less successful in managing chronic diseases, the primary current health problem, which often requires greater health-care expenditures.[3] Our emphasis on expensive, high-tech cures has not advanced an understanding of health that serves the needs of all individuals and fosters collective well-being. What we call the "health-care system" in the United States is really a "disease-cure system." The medical model has met impressive challenges, but the rise of progressive chronic and stress-related diseases has added a burden to the Western quality of life not mitigated by biomedicine. The effects of cumulative environmental pollution and degradation have undermined health worldwide and have threatened the integrity of the ecosystems on which all planetary life depends.

Although biomedicine is a remarkable achievement, it is a relatively new arrival on the world scene: the conventional medical profession, riding on the wave of scientific and technological innovations, has enjoyed exponential growth as an influential social force over the past hundred years. But other systems of health care that have existed for thousands of years continue to address the health needs of millions of people on the planet very effectively.

Westerners who have been acculturated into the medical model may not appreciate its comparative uniqueness and its idiosyncratic limits. Cassidy[4] identified the unusual characteristics of biomedicine when compared to a worldwide viewpoint:

1. Its intense attachment to materialist interpretative models
2. Its focus on the physical body, almost to the exclusion of other possibilities
3. Its focus on the disease, often to the virtual exclusion of the person
4. Its vast development of disease types
5. Its highly technological delivery system
6. Its invasive curative interventions
7. Its emphasis on acute disease, trauma, and end-stage malfunction, with relatively little emphasis on prevention or wellness
8. Its high cost

Health-care-reform activist John Robbins[5] questions whether the Western medical approach is the best answer to the world's health problems:

> In our society, the medical myth has led to an emphasis on intervention instead of prevention that has generated a crisis in health care of epic proportions. The current level of dissatisfaction and frustration with the U. S. medical system is enormous. Corporate health-care expenditures now exceed corporate profits. Doctors and patients alike feel depersonalized and used.
>
> Year after year, the difference between our system and that of other nations becomes more embarrassing and disturbing. We spend far more money for health care than any other country in the world, and yet we are the only nation in the industrialized world that does not guarantee minimum health care to every single citizen. Increasing numbers of Americans have no health coverage. We lead the world in malpractice suits, but continue to fall further behind in infant mortality rates, life expectancy, and the other indicators used to measure the health of a people. . . . We're seeing how false and destructive is the belief that the more money we spend and the more technology we have, the healthier we will be. We're seeing how alienating and harmful it can be to think that experts always know more than we do about our bodies and our lives.

What we have is a health-care crisis in an illness-care system. Tom Monte,[6] scholar and health activist, observed that "our medical system's inability to define health is at the very core of our health care crisis." Without a broad understanding of health, illness, or how the body heals itself, the prevailing medical science establishment has been unable to offer an integrated approach to disease prevention or health enhancement. Recent research has documented consumer dissatisfaction with the limits of the biomedical model.[7–10] Discontent seems to be growing, as demonstrated by estimates of the use of alternative and complementary therapy: up to one in three citizens in the United States, Europe, and Australia is seeking some form of unconventional care.[11]

Has Biomedicine Promised Too Much?

Recent trends in increased interest in, research on, and use of complementary and alternative health care reflect the public's desire for more than what conventional medicine can offer. As a model, biomedicine cannot adequately incorporate other perspectives and sustain itself in the face of new knowledge development. It is going the way of all scientific paradigms in a changing culture, with competitive battles taking place between old and new that will inevitably result in the development of more comprehensive models.[12,13]

A paradigm shift from biomedical dominance and illness orientation to a model that encompasses health and quality of life is in full progress. (See Table 1–1.) This shift is reflected in the remarkable rise of what has been come to be known as "complementary and alternative medicine" (CAM), one of the most significant changes in the medicine of Western postindustrial countries of the 20th century. A landmark research study in 1993 conducted by David Eisenberg and colleagues[14] revealed that many Americans desire more than biomedical treatment and are willing to pay for "alternative" care out of pocket. These researchers estimated that Americans made 425 million visits to alternative health-care providers in 1990, a figure that exceeded the number of visits to conventional primary care physicians during the same period. This study has had a major impact on the health-care industry and has led to other studies, which have outlined the demographics of the rise of complementary and alternative health care. Another study by Eisenberg[15] 5 years later showed that the trend of CAM use is increasing and is shifting the economic base of health care.

In 1997 an estimated 4 in 10 Americans used at least one alternative therapy, compared with 3 in 10 in 1990. Prevalence of use increased by 25 percent; total visits to alternative practitioners rose by 47 percent in 4 years. The most frequently used therapies included herbal medicine, massage, megavitamins, self-help groups, folk remedies, energy healing, and homeopathy. Use of herbal remedies increased 380 percent, and vitamin use increased 130 percent.

Approximately 60 percent of those seeing alternative practitioners paid out of pocket. Expenditures for alternative therapies rose from about $14.6 billion in 1990 to $22.6 billion in 1997. Fewer than 40 percent of those who used alternatives revealed this use to their physicians. CAM use was highest among adults aged 35 to 59, more prevalent among women (48.9 percent) than among men (37.8 percent), higher among people with a college education, highest among whites, and less common among African-Americans than members of other racial groups.

Other studies have described the same demographic characteristics. Astin's[16] national study, which surveyed a sample of 1035 Americans across the country, identified variables that emerged as predictors of using alternative health care: more education, poorer health status, a holistic orientation to health, having had a transformational experience that changed the person's worldview, a commitment to environmentalism and/or feminism, and interest in spirituality and personal-growth psychology. Dissatisfaction with conventional medicine did not predict use of alternative medicine; rather, users found health-care alternatives to be more congruent with their own values, beliefs, and philosophical orientations toward health and life. Although some people remain adamantly loyal to either a conventional or an alternative orientation to health care, many more prefer to receive the benefits of "the best of both worlds."

The implications of this trend toward increasing use of alternative health care are very significant: it is evident that attitudes and behaviors toward health and illness are changing. Advertising and marketing have risen to the occasion of this trend, flooding the popular press and the marketplace with CAM information and products. It is not uncommon to see an array of herbal, homeopathic preparations and vitamin supplements on supermarket shelves, products that a few years ago could be obtained only in specialty health food stores and by mail order. The Internet is now a source for easy access to the world of CAM products. People often use these products without telling their health-care practitioners.

People have less access to information about CAM in their primary care practitioners' offices than they do from popular women's magazines and in the recent proliferation of

TABLE 1–1   The Emergent Paradigm of Health

ASSUMPTIONS OF THE OLD PARADIGM OF MEDICINE	ASSUMPTIONS OF THE NEW PARADIGM OF HEALTH
Treatment of symptoms.	Search for patterns and causes, plus treatment of symptoms. Integrated, concerned with the whole patient.
Emphasis on efficiency.	Emphasis on human values.
Professional should be emotionally neutral.	Professional's caring is a component of healing.
Pain and disease are wholly negative.	Pain and disease are information about conflict, disharmony.
Primary intervention with drugs, surgery.	Minimal intervention with "appropriate technology," complemented with full armamentarium of noninvasive techniques (psychotherapies, diet, exercise).
Body seen as machine in good or bad repair.	Body seen as dynamic system, context, field of energy within other fields.
Disease or disability seen as thing, entity.	Disease or disability seen as process.
Emphasis on eliminating symptoms, disease.	Emphasis on achieving maximum wellness, "metahealth."
Patient is dependent.	Patient is (or should be) autonomous.
Professional is authority.	Professional is therapeutic partner.
Body and mind are separate; psychosomatic illness is mental, psychiatrist.	Body-mind perspective; psychosomatic illness is province of all health care be referred to professionals.
Mind is secondary factor in organic illness.	Mind is primary or coequal factor in all illness.
Placebo effect shows the power of suggestion.	Placebo effect shows the mind's role in disease and healing.
Primary reliance on quantitative information (charts, tests, dates).	Primary reliance on qualitative information, including patient's subjective reports and professional's intuition; quantitative data an adjunct.
"Prevention" largely environmental: vitamins, rest, goals, exercise, immunization, not smoking.	"Prevention" synonymous with wholeness, work, relationships, body-mind-spirit.

Source: Ferguson, M: The Aquarian Conspiracy. JP Tarcher, Los Angeles, 1976, with permission.

alternative health magazines. The quality of this mass-market information is variable and often unreliable, but in the absence of informed health-care practitioners, people are making self-care choices based on popular information sources. Sensing a lack of knowledge among and disapproval from conventional practitioners, many people are not including their primary providers in decisions for alternative care.

Cassidy[17] observed that, while biomedicine considers itself the conventional standard compared to which others methods are labeled "alternative," it is itself "unconventional" when compared to the larger number of traditional healing worldviews. She suggested that biomedicine is best considered "just one more alternative"; current consumer trends indicate that many people consider conventional medical care to be such.

Conventional practitioners are also participating in the expansion of CAM: referrals to CAM therapies are frequently made by such practitioners.[18] We can expect to see this trend in health care continue. Practitioners must assume the responsibility of becoming informed about complementary and alternative practices in which their clients engage, so that they can:

- Be credible and trustworthy sources of information and guidance
- Be alert to potential adverse interactions between conventional and CAM treatments
- Communicate with other health professionals and coordinate client care
- Facilitate an integration of all health-related activities in partnership with the client

The Rise of Complementary and Alternative Health Care

Terminology

The terms *complementary* and *alternative* are often used interchangeably, but they are not equivalent in meaning. The term *complementary* implies a therapy used *in conjunction* with a conventional one. An *alternative* therapy refers to one that is utilized *instead* of conventional treatment. Complementary/alternative medicine covers a broad range of healing philosophies, approaches, and therapies that conventional Western medicine does not commonly use, accept, study, understand, or make available.

Many, but not all, CAM therapies are called "holistic," which generally means they consider the whole person, including physical, mental, emotional, and spiritual aspects. Health insurance reimbursement for many of these therapies has been slowly evolving and changing, but their formal integration into current biomedical practice has not yet occurred.[19] Nursing, medical, and other professional schools have been including information about CAM in their curricula, but they are only beginning to teach CAM approaches as part of standard professional practice.

What is considered complementary and alternative depends on one's perspective and on who is doing the defining. The definition of the National Institutes of Health (NIH) is one of exclusion, made from the perspective of the prevailing biomedical paradigm. The definition of CAM changes as the perspective changes. In China, for example, biomedicine is complementary to traditional Chinese medicine. The passage of time can also alter the definition. Osteopathic practice, once considered outside of the prevailing medical establishment, now enjoys equal status in licensure and insurance reimbursement; its practice is often indistinguishable from MD practice in certain health-care settings. Chiropractors, once considered "quacks" by conventional critics, have become a more integral part of the health-care system because of research demonstrating their unique contribution to health and the enormous popularity they enjoy among their clientele. Today, doctors of osteopathy (DO) serve as primary providers and as medical specialists throughout the country, and chiropractors provide routine health maintenance, as well as care in acute and chronic illness, for tens of thousands of Americans.

History

The current paradigm shift toward CAM has its roots in early influences of unorthodox medicine. Cassidy[20] has described the rise and fall of the unorthodox medicine that flourished in the United States during the 19th and 20th centuries as well as the positive but unappreciated impact it made on orthodox thinking and practice.

Many of what we consider CAM methods today are not new; they are considered "alternative" primarily in relationship to the dominant biomedical paradigm. For example, practices that were available throughout the 1800s and into the 1900s included homeopathy; "nature cures" such as hydrotherapy, nutritional therapy, and herbs; manual manipulation; and midwifery.

Homeopathy, founded by the German physician Samuel Hahnemann (1755–1843), became popular in the United States in the 1830s as a safer and less violent alternative to the harsh orthodox practices of bloodletting, emetics, and cathartics. Constituting about 10 percent of the medical practitioners of the day, homeopaths endured rejection and ridicule for the premises on which their practice was based. Thompsonism, founded in the United States by Samuel Thompson during the same time period, advanced a therapy based on the use of botanicals and steam baths. Thompson thought that disease was caused by cold conditions in the body, which his treatments purported to eradicate by increasing body heat. Influenced by contemporary democratic values, Thompson challenged the status of medical experts and promoted the idea that people could be their own doctors. He sold herbal kits for self-care treatment, presaging the popular self-care movement that has grown into a contemporary industry. Naturopaths promoted hydrotherapy, or "water cures," along with natural food and hygiene practices, which contributed to what became known as the Popular Health Movement in the first half of the 19th century. Franz Mesmer's theory of "magnetic healing," which proposed that an imbalance of magnetic fluid in the body was the cause of disease, foreshadowed current discoveries in energy-based healing; it was also the basis for the practice of osteopathy and chiropractic, which focus on spinal and joint manipulation to restore and maintain the energetic forces that underlie physiologic functioning.

The discovery and use of antibiotics and vaccines dramatically changed medical practice and, along with the shifting trend in medical education and the organization of the American Medical Association, created the biomedical focus that became central in medical education, practice, and health care in the 20th century. The effects of this shift are seen today in the primacy of the biomedical industry and the ongoing, and sometimes not-so-subtle, competition for influence and resources between conventional and CAM practitioners.

Medical anthropology emerged as a distinct subdiscipline of anthropology, its development paralleled by escalating interest in "alternative and complementary" healing, specifically non-Western healing systems. The field of ethnomedicine emerged as an academic specialization focusing on traditional healing systems.[21] Along with the increasing use of alternative treatments in the 1970s and 1980s came growing opposition from the biomedical community to perceptions (some real, others false and politically motivated) of the "quackery" of alternative therapies.

More recently, this struggle has received attention at the national level. In 1990, the NIH and Office of Technology Assessment (OTA) published a report expressing the need for more clinical research evaluating alternative treatments for cancer. In 1991, funds to start the Office of Alternative Medicine (OAM) were appropriated by Congress in response to the general public's interest in expanding the range of available health treatment modalities, especially for conditions that sometimes were treated unsuccessfully by conventional medicine.[22] In 1998, Congress established the National Center for Complementary and Alternative Medicine (NCCAM) at the NIH to stimulate, develop, and support research on CAM for the benefit of the public. Since fiscal year (FY) 1993, the budget of NCCAM—which is located on the NIH campus in Bethesda, Maryland—has risen steadily from $2 million to $68.7 million in FY 2000. This funding increase reflects the public's growing need for CAM information that is based on rigorous scientific research. (See Box 1–1.)

Types of Complementary and Alternative Therapies

NCCAM organizes alternative therapies into seven categories:[23]

1. *Mind-body interventions.* These therapies are based on awareness of the unity of mind and body and on the ability of social, familial, and economic factors to affect all aspects of health and illness. Examples of mind-body interventions include biofeedback, relaxation therapies, meditation, hypnosis, and imagery.
2. *Bioelectromagnetic therapies.* Bioelectromagnetics is the study of interactions between living organisms and electromagnetic fields. Areas of study include the effects of exposure to strongly ionizing, nonionizing, and low-frequency electromagnetic radiation on health and the effects of electrical currents and magnetic fields on healing.
3. *Alternatives systems of medical practice.* These include systems used by hundreds of millions of people throughout the world, such as Indian Ayurveda and Chinese medicine as well as less well known indigenous healing practices.
4. *Manual healing methods.* These include osteopathic and chiropractic manipulation, physical therapy and massage, and a variety of hands-on healing techniques, such as Therapeutic Touch.
5. *Pharmacologic and biological treatments.* These include substances that are used like certain pharmaceuticals: for example, shark cartilage therapy for cancer and chelation therapy for coronary artery disease.
6. *Herbal medicine.* Herbs were most likely the first human healing system; their therapeutic uses, synergistic combinations, and side effects are studied.
7. *Diet and nutrition.* Hippocrates said that food should be used as medicine. This category includes research on the effects of diet and dietary supplements on the treatment and prevention of disease.

The Challenge of Integrating Different CAM Approaches

Diverse and dynamic, CAM includes a wide range of theory and practice, all of which undergo continuous modification and reinterpretation. Boundaries within CAM and between CAM and conventional treatment are not always sharp or fixed.[24] The millions of people who are using CAM bring a new set of challenges to their practitioners' offices: How do practitioners elicit from clients the information needed for managing the use of multiple therapies with safety, clinical effectiveness, and cost containment? What new relationships need to be established with clients and other practitioners to do so? One approach that has gained in popularity—and is the current preferred term among those who wish to bridge the separation between CAM and conventional health care—is referred to as "integrative care."

Integrative Care

The concept of "integrative," popularized by Andrew Weil, refers to care that includes communication among all health providers who share the responsibility in

BOX 1–1
Sociopolitical Evolution of the Holistic Perspective

Dissatisfaction with the limits of the current biomedical dominance of the health-care system fuels pressure for health-care reform and demands for relevant and effective alternative solutions. However, this dissatisfaction is only one aspect of the social forces that have ushered in the CAM health-care revolution. Profound shifts in culture, science, technology, and communication in this century have brought us to a level of consciousness that requires evolution to new understandings and approaches to living.

Civil Rights, Women's Rights Movements

Gordon[1] identified major cultural movements that have converged into the current holistic perspective. He credits the civil rights, women's rights, consumer rights, and ecology movements of the 1960s as the forebears of today's holistic movement. Beginning with the civil rights movement, reactions to forces of cruelty, injustice, inequality, fragmentation, and destructiveness in American culture began to unite groups to work toward their elimination. Both the civil rights and women's rights movements brought to American consciousness the deleterious effects of unequal personhood and citizenship that racism and sexism perpetuate. The success of these movements precipitated changes in the legal and social climate for groups with minority status: people of color, women, the elderly, homosexuals, and people with handicaps have more legally acknowledged rights as a result.

The Ecology Movement

The ecology movement emerged from a growing awareness of the damage that was being done worldwide to the health of humans, animals, and vegetation from unrestrained industrial growth, accumulation of toxic waste, and exploitation of natural resources. Protest began after scientific demonstration of the deleterious effects of pollutants to health over time; for example, higher cancer rates in populations downwind of nuclear weapons and power plants as well as the transgenerational effects of substances such as insecticides and herbicides (e.g., Agent Orange). Political action on behalf of survival of all life on the planet arose from various parts of social landscape—from grassroots organizations, such as Greenpeace and various citizen action groups; from representatives of the scientific community, such as the Union of Concerned Scientists; and from the health-care field, led by Physicians for Social Responsibility and others.

The ecology movement reflects a growing consciousness of the interconnectedness of all life, described as "interbeing" by the noted Buddhist monk Thich Nhat Hanh.[2] This concept acknowledges that what we do to the environment, we do to ourselves; what we dispose of recycles in the air, water, and ground to become part of what we and our children and their children are exposed to. The ecology movement, which has championed the holistic paradigm, acknowledges interconnectedness with, rather than on domination of, the natural world. Gordon observed that "ecologists told us that if we developed a new attitude toward nature—one of loving stewardship rather than of selfish exploitation—we might also create a new attitude toward ourselves."[3]

The Consumer Rights Movement

The consumer rights movement evolved more recently, built on the gains of the former movements, to extend fairness and legal protection to people in health care, the marketplace, and the workplace. In health care, the effects of this movement can be seen in the change in the values that affect the relationship between the health-care provider and the recipient of that care. For example, there has been a gradual process of renaming the recipient of health care. The term *patient*, which connotes a passive role fraught with the possibility of paternalistic exploitation, is being replaced in many health-care arenas with the term *client*, which implies an equal, co-participant relationship between the provider and receiver of health care. The term *consumer*, earlier used in marketing, advertising, and sales to indicate the passive acquirer of products and a unit of material consumption, is now used more generically to refer to that recipient of goods and services to whom the provider is responsible and accountable. Egalitarian partnerships between health-care provider and recipient are evolving as a direct result of these social forces, which also shaped the growth of the consumer movement.

continued

BOX 1–1 continued
Sociopolitical Evolution of the Holistic Perspective

The Wellness Movement

The wellness movement, which has been developing momentum since the 1970s, has paralleled the rise of the holistic movement. The concept of wellness was popularized by John Travis, who established the first "wellness center" in California in 1970s, where the focus was not on curing illness but rather on educating people to alter their attitudes, behaviors, and lifestyles to promote health.[4] The wellness industry goes beyond medical treatment to include nutritional therapies, stress management, spiritual development, health spas, exercise training, and lifestyle coaching and counseling. It might be said that biomedicine helps people to survive and wellness interventions help people to thrive.

The Holistic Movement

The concept of holism was first introduced in 1926 by South African statesman and biologist Jan Christiaan Smuts,[5] who viewed living things as more than the sum of their parts, not explainable either by vitalistic or mechanistic theories of biology. The philosophy of holism, discussed in Chapter 2, is an approach comprising humanistic, psychosocial, and/or systemic perspectives evolved as a reaction to the characteristics of modern medicine that dehumanized the individual and limited the scope of the health-care encounter to a materialist perspective, devoid of concern for anything but physical cure. The holistic paradigm fosters an integrated understanding of clients within the context of their life experiences, interpersonal relationships, perception of health-care needs, and the function and meaning of health-care issues within their value systems and life goals. This model sets the stage for a client-centered, egalitarian partnership between practitioner and client; that is, active client participation in the healing enterprise. The model includes in its view the environment and the relationship between human and other forms of life on earth. It gives credence to the interconnection of all life, includes the influence of consciousness, and acknowledges the larger mystery of the source of life, known by many names: Spirit, God, Tao, the Higher Self, to name just a few. And the model invites the practitioner to maintain professional credibility by "walking the walk and talking the talk" of a holistic lifestyle.

REFERENCES

1. Gordon, JS: Holistic Medicine. Chelsea, New York, 1988.
2. Hanh, TN: Interbeing: Fourteen Guidelines for Engaged Buddhism, ed. 3. Parallax Press, Mountain View, Calif., 1998.
3. Gordon: Holistic Medicine.
4. Ibid.
5. Smuts, JC: Holism and Evolution. Macmillan, New York, 1926.

coordinating the best possible treatment plan for a client, including the client's choices for care and the providers' expertise in understanding and managing the complexities of conventional–complementary treatment interactions. There is a great need for integrative care for clients who self-treat or who are using more than one type of therapy. The need for an integrative approach goes beyond the conventional-CAM mix; a client seeing two conventional practitioners is also at risk for complications caused by treatment interaction. CAM practitioners as well as conventional practitioners need to know what other therapies their clients are using. For instance, practitioners of Chinese medicine and of homeopathy prefer that the client not mix these approaches, because it then becomes difficult to know which treatment is effective or ineffective or to predict treatment interaction effects.

If It Is Integrated, Is It Holistic?

Integrative health care that is coordinated between conventional and alternative practitioners would certainly be an improvement over the fragmented care that prevails today. However, even effective integration of these two modalities will not be holistic unless practiced within a holistic perspective. For example, a practitioner might coordinate care with an herbalist to minimize the possibility of drug-herb interaction that could harm the client. No doubt the client would benefit from this proactive integration of treatments. However, simply increasing treatment benefit or reducing untoward side effects does not make the care holistic. It is not the treatment or the integration of treatments that determines whether the care is holistic. Rather, it is the practitioner's holistic perspective that makes all the difference.

Political Implications of CAM

From a political standpoint, the trend toward an integrative care model is an interesting one. The biomedical industry is struggling to maintain its dominance, both politically and economically, in a rapidly changing environment. Cost-containment trends have affected the provision and delivery of health care, and practitioners as well as consumers experience their effects:

Biomedical practitioners have felt the effects of health-care fiscal management in the restructuring of insurance reimbursements: the scope of biomedical practice and professional decision making is being regulated by the constraints of "managed care," which has become a euphemism for "managed cost."

Biomedical care, delivered in short time segments with little reimbursed "talking time" with the client, continues to be an inadequate response to a client's needs for care beyond diagnosis and treatment of illness. A growing number of people desire more from their health care, as demonstrated by increased use of CAM. As people learn to take more responsibility for their health, their dependence on medical personnel will shift. The public's growing interest in CAM, wellness, and self-care activities appears to be a trend that will extend far into the future.

Regulation and Appropriation: Control Strategies That Can Work against Holistic Care

Given the high economic stakes involved in the health-care gatekeeper role, which for the past century has been assumed by conventional medical practitioners, there is a clear possibility that efforts to "integrate" CAM will be done by subsuming it into the prevailing biomedical paradigm. This could happen in a number of ways, most likely through regulation and appropriation. Regulation strategies place limits on who can practice, who will be included in a referral network, and who will receive reimbursement. Appropriation strategies control what can be practiced and by whom. Some examples follow.

Regulation Strategies. Insurance case managers, whose primary responsibility is to the insurance company and its cost-containment requirements, could limit effective CAM treatment by superimposing cost-containment decisions on treatment protocols. For example, reimbursement for treatment might be curtailed at the first signs of symptomatic relief and might be discontinued before the full treatment effect is achieved. Interference in treatment based on economic expediency could very likely result in reduced treatment effects and rendering the CAM treatment ineffective.

State medical boards could influence legal definitions and the scope of medical and health practices, making the physician's role comprehensive and granting CAM practitioners only limited practice privileges. For example, the practice of nurse midwifery, which is considered complementary and alternative to conventional obstetric medical care, is defined and limited by state medical boards. It has only been the urgent needs of the medically underserved public that have loosened the medical bureaucracy's grip on the control of nursing practice, resulting in new professional roles for nurses, such as nurse-midwife, nurse–clinical specialist, and nurse-practitioner. CAM practitioners face similar challenges to the definition and regulation of their practice.

A more blatant example of interference in CAM practice is seen in the 1987 antitrust suit (*Wilk et al. v. AMA et al.*) won by chiropractors against the American Medical Association (AMA). U.S. District Court Judge Susan Getzendanner referred to "systematic, long-term wrongdoing" on the part of the AMA, which she said spearheaded a physicians' boycott designed to "contain and eliminate the chiropractic profession."[25] "Evidence in this case demonstrated that the AMA knew of scientific studies implying that chiropractic care was twice as effective as medical care in relieving many painful conditions of the neck and back as well as related to musculoskeletal problems."[26] The U.S. District Court for the Northeast District of Illinois, Eastern Division, ordered a permanent injunction against the AMA, to prevent further attempts at restriction of the chiropractic profession.

In fact, the efficacy and cost benefits of chiropractic care have been clearly established in both the United States and Canada. Based on clinical research studies over three decades, the U.S. Agency for Health Care Policy and Research[27] recommended chiropractic care as the most effective treatment for lower back pain. In Canada, the Ontario Ministry of Health funded a research study, conducted by Pran Manga and colleagues in 1993, to evaluate the evidence for the efficacy and economic efficiency of various treatments for lower back pain. The study concluded that the public would be assured access to chiropractic treatment only through the Canadian government's initiation of health policy reform.[28] More recently, the medical establishment's opposition to chiropractic services has been continued through bureaucratic efforts to limit chiropractors' treatment of Medicare patients and to restrict the flow of money to alternative health-care providers no matter how useful or popular their services are to the public.

Conventional practitioners can limit their clients' exposure to CAM by refusing to refer. Mainstream professional organizations that maintain legislative lobbies can support reimbursement strategies and legislation that limit the practice of CAM. Biased or naive researchers can advance an anti-CAM sentiment through research funding from special-interest groups with anti-CAM agendas. Professional publications have been known to include or exclude reports of CAM research for political purposes. Competition for control of the health-care dollar can result in greater concern about interprofessional competition than about benefit to the public.

Appropriation Strategies. It is possible for the medical bureaucracy not only to regulate CAM practitioners but also to designate aspects of CAM practice as its own—without fulfilling basic competency requirements in the CAM method. For example, the Massachusetts state statute for licensing acupuncturists includes the provision that medical doctors may legally practice acupuncture without the training and supervision required for licensed acupuncturists.[29] The benefit of this strategy to the public is unclear. How is client care improved by the legal empowerment of persons untrained in acupuncture to practice it? This appropriation strategy may benefit the state medical association and its members by expanding the scope of medical practice to include acupuncture, but it does not necessarily benefit the client, who may receive acupuncture from a physician who may be inadequately trained but legally empowered to practice the technique.

Health care is more likely to be safe, effective, and "integrative" when practitioners—both conventional and CAM—consider the welfare of the client above political advantage, professional turf building, and economic gain, and work together to coordinate care for optimal treatment outcomes. Nurses, other health-care professionals, and consumers would be wise to remain involved in the political processes that result in policies that regulate health care.

Who Is a Holistic Practitioner?

All CAM practitioners are not necessarily holistic; in fact, many CAM practitioners who consider themselves "holistic" are not. Any method can be applied symptomatically, without regard to the whole person, be it CAM or conventional. For example, an herbalist who prescribes botanicals or an acupuncturist who administers treatments without establishing a collaborative relationship with other health-care providers, and without an understanding the nature of the client's situation beyond symptom reduction, is not practicing holistically. Similarly, clients who seek "the magic bullet" in an herb, a vitamin, a chiropractic adjustment, or some other treatment are not requesting holistic care. Nurses, physicians, and other health-care practitioners who take the time to get to know the client and his or her family regard the client as an equal, respect the client's beliefs and desires, meet the client's needs within the scope of their practice, and refer when the client requests or could benefit from another perspective are demonstrating holistic practice.

Holism is a worldview or paradigm that guides the practitioner's relationship with the recipient of care. It does not describe certain interventions or techniques. A holistic approach, as delineated in Chapter 2, is based on an understanding of the client's experience, how it is embedded in complex internal and external dynamics and relationships, and how and where to intervene in a manner that best serves the whole of the client's life. Both CAM and conventional practitioners can offer care from a holistic perspective.

James S. Gordon[30] promoted the current usefulness of this approach: "The [holistic model] is, at least potentially, a corrective to the excesses of biomedicine, a supplement to its deficiencies, and an affirmation of its most enduring strengths. It sets out contemporary concern with the cure of diseases in the larger frame of health care . . . and provides a framework within which many techniques, old and new, Western and non-Western may be used."

Who Is a Holistic Client?

Certain characteristics are indicative of individuals who are likely to benefit from holistic care:[31]

you are thinking
way

- Those who have a high need for affiliation and who therefore want a relational style of health care
- Those who wish to alleviate symptoms gently or with fewer side effects
- Those who will not take "hopeless" for an answer
- Those who wish to prevent disease or enhance wellness
- Those who interpret the body-person as having more than a physical aspect and who want to be able to address the energetic, psychosocial, and spiritual bodies when receiving or delivering health care
- Those who are concerned with the end-stage focus and invasiveness of typical biomedical care

People who use CAM and those who do not act from different frameworks of perception and understanding. It is important to understand what motivates and influences people in making health-care choices, whether they are choosing conventional care or CAM. Three models are presented to illustrate the ways to understand and support clients' choices for health. These are the Health Belief Model, Personal Theories of Health Model, and the Theory of First- and Second-Order Change Model.

Choices for Health and Models of Change

Health Beliefs and the Health Belief Model

The Health Belief Model (HBM), developed in the 1950s by a group of U.S. Public Health Service social psychologists,[32] attempted to understand why certain people fail to take advantage of diagnostic procedures or disease prevention programs. Since Becker and Maimon's[33] application of the HBM to people's responses to illness and compliance with medical regimens, it has been one of the most influential and widely used psychosocial approaches to explaining health-related behavior.[34]

The model has five components that describe a person's perception of him- or herself in relation to health or illness and which aspects of these perceptions are involved in health-related behaviors. (See Table 1–2.) People are more likely to engage in health-related or medically compliant actions if they consider themselves vulnerable to a disease state, if they believe that the disease state is a serious one, if they believe that there are benefits to prevention or treatment of the condition, and if they believe that taking action outweighs the barriers to inaction.

A 10-year review of clinical intervention and research studies, both retrospective and prospective, based on the HBM demonstrated the model's efficacy, with perceived barriers identified as the most single influential predictor of all the HBM components. Both

---

TABLE 1–2 Components of the Health Belief Model

Perceived Susceptibility

One's subjective perception of the risk of contracting a health condition. In the case of medically established illness, acceptance of the diagnosis, personal estimates of resusceptibility, and susceptibility in general.

EXAMPLE: Kiesha is concerned about her breast cancer risk because her mother died of the illness.

Perceived Severity

Concerns about the seriousness of contracting an illness or of leaving it untreated. The seriousness of both physical consequences (e.g, pain, disability, death) and social consequences (e.g., effects of the condition on work, family life, and social relationships).

EXAMPLE: Sam decides to practice safe sex because he's learned that AIDS, which can be sexually transmitted, is currently incurable.

Perceived Benefits

The effectiveness of available actions that are likely to reduce the susceptibility or severity, or overall perceived threat, of the condition, and the perceived benefits of taking health action as feasible or efficacious.

EXAMPLE: Paul doesn't smoke because he thinks he will be more popular and attractive if he does not.

Perceived Barriers

The potentially negative aspects of a particular health action that may act as impediments to undertaking the recommended behavior. Barriers can include negative side effects— unpleasant, painful, upsetting, difficult, expensive, inconvenient, time-consuming, and so forth.

EXAMPLE: Janet, who is lesbian, doesn't take advantage of free clinics at her neighborhood health center because she is afraid that she will be stigmatized by the center staff because of her sexual orientation.

Source: Rosenstock, IM: The Health Belief Model: Explaining health behavior through expectancies. In Glanz, K, Lewis, F, and Rimer, B (eds): Health Behavior and Health Education. Jossey-Bass, San Francisco, 1991, p 39, with permission.

perceived susceptibility and perceived benefits were important overall; perceived suscep-tibility was a stronger predictor of preventive health behavior than sick-role behavior, and the reverse was true for perceived benefits. Perceived severity was the least powerful predictor but was strongly related to already diagnosed or actual illness states and sick-role behavior.[35]

Beliefs other than those identified in the HBM may have a strong influences in health behavior. For example, a German study by Furnham and Kirkcaldy[36] determined that persons who believed that their condition was caused by physiological factors were more likely to consult with orthodox physicians. By contrast, those who stressed the importance of psychological factors in causing illness were more likely to seek treatment from a complementary practitioner. In addition, factors that affect perceptions and beliefs also need to be understood, for example, gender, age, social class, educational level, and ethnicity.[37–39]

A singular focus on influencing perception and other aspects of inner life for every ailment of mind and body discounts the significance of social and environmental ecology in health and illness behavior.[40,41] As an individual-based focus, it places the burden of change on individuals, which can limit the attainment of desired outcomes when health problems are embedded in the socioenvironmental context.[42] For example, expecting people to act on perceptions of the superiority of organic food or of pure air and water when these are not locally available is to put them in impossible situations of conflict because a real choice for health is not possible.

Health behavior is influenced by more than perception, feelings, attitudes, and beliefs. A person's values are as much behavioral determinants as are perceptions of health and illness. For example, religious orientation may determine health and treatment decisions, as in the case of Jehovah's Witnesses who refuse blood transfusions on the basis of their relationship to God and the agreements established among those of their community of faith.

Some conditions, such as those with a physiological addictive base, may not be as responsive to the perceptual dimensions of the model. Some psychological factors may also influence decision making: the state of one's emotional balance, concurrent stresses, self-esteem, confidence, and identification with others are a few of the factors that need to be considered when assessing and advising about health and making treatment recom-mendations.

The HBM, though useful in understanding what motivates people to act on behalf of their health and in compliance with health-care treatment, has its limitations. The assumption that compliance with health advice or medical regimens is always beneficial needs to be challenged. For example, many medical practices that were strongly recom-mended in the past have subsequently been abandoned because of their harmful effects. Removal of the thymus in infancy, yearly chest x-rays for the diagnosis of tuberculosis, routine tonsillectomy, and prescription of thalidomide during pregnancy are just a few medical interventions that people were encouraged to accept as part of routine medical care. Health-care professionals may not always be right in their assessment of treatment benefit. In addition, judgmental attitudes toward clients who do not comply with what the practitioner thinks is best set up the client for negative perception and blame.[43] Paternalistic attitudes such as these, in which clients are viewed as manipulable objects of care, have no place in the holistic paradigm, in which clients and providers are considered full partners in healing.

Personal Theories of Health Model

While the HBM fosters understanding of how beliefs and behaviors relate to specific perceptions of health and illness states, it does not indicate patterns of thinking about health that influence general patterns of behaviors, such as the tendency to believe in and utilize alternative health practices. Individuals holding this view conducted research to illuminate how people learn about health in a complex and rapidly changing information environment and how individuals systematically think about health and wellness. Their research revealed that personal theories of health were reflected in four categories: the Conventionals, the New Conventionals, the Spirituals, and the Unconventionals.

The Conventionals. This group reflects the traditionally dominant or conventional perspective on health and wellness. Conventional thinkers express confidence in the scientific approach to health care and in drugs, vaccines, and other chemical treatments. They strongly believe in the primacy of the medical profession and in physicians' primary responsibility in clients' health. They believe that regular checkups at the doctor's office help to keep them well and that managing one's lifestyle leads to better health. They do not adhere to concepts of the body's self-healing capacities or the mind-body connection. They are indifferent to alternative health care, expressing neither favorable nor unfavorable attitudes toward it.

The New Conventionals. This group, like the Conventionals, strongly believes in conventional medicine and physicians' importance in maintaining good health; unlike the Conventionals, however, they see health as ultimately the client's responsibility. Although dismissing the spiritual aspects of health and healing, New Conventionals acknowledge the importance of uncovering the underlying cause of illness rather than relying only on treatment of symptoms. Alternative methods are rejected because they lack scientific proof and are considered appropriate only as a last resort. This viewpoint is associated with skepticism of alternative treatments.

The Spirituals. The members of this group see health as determined primarily within the person and his or her spiritual realm. A strong belief in personal responsibility for long-term health marks this group, as do certain alternative health assumptions: for example, that the body is self-healing and that remedies can be effective without scientific proof. Unlike the Unconventionals, this group respects conventional care, does not see one method as superior to the other, and sees a place for both types of practice.

The Unconventionals. This group has the most nonconformist perspective. Unconventionals value natural remedies for healing and self-responsibility for health; they have little concern for scientific proof—indeed, they have a wariness of conventional medicine, believing it is inadequate in meeting society's health-care needs. This perspective reflects a broad holistic orientation.

Kleine and Hughner's[44] research on personal theories indicates that multiple health belief systems exist in the United States. The Personal Theories of Health Model has its limits, because it neither identifies the relationship between personal theories of health and health behaviors nor addresses other important questions about the demographics of the different groups. Furthermore, the categories need to be refined in future research. Nevertheless, this research expands the either/or categorization of one's health beliefs as either conventional or as an alternative for a broader and more complex understanding of changing values and beliefs that influence peoples' health-care choices.

In a large nationwide study on what motivates the use of CAM, Astin[45] discovered that the majority of those who use alternative medicine do so not so much because they are dissatisfied with conventional medicine as because they find CAM to be more congruent with their own values, beliefs, and philosophical orientations toward health and life. Understanding clients' values and beliefs is critical in knowing how to anticipate their treatment preferences and how to support their health-care choices.

First- and Second-Order Change Model

Clients' perceptions, values, and beliefs about health and illness are only part of the larger picture of understanding health behavior. Another crucial component is understanding the level of the problem as well as the level of intervention that is most likely going to address the problem. This kind of understanding helps us to address questions raised by health educators Bates and Winder:[46] What is required to bring about changes in persistent behaviors of individuals, groups, and societies when those behaviors have become unproductive, problematic, or destructive? Or, more directly stated, what do we change? Whom do we target for change? How do we accomplish change? Should we focus our efforts on the environment, on access to health services, on the biology of the individual, or on the individual's lifestyle? In choosing targets, shall we direct our attention toward small units (individuals) or large units (organizations or society)? What strategies, or types of interventions, shall we use to accomplish change? The answer to the last question will depend both on whether our aim is first-order or second-order change and on which change strategies are appropriate in a given situation.

The theory of first- and second-order change was introduced by Watzlawick, Weakland, and Fisch,[47] who synthesized an approach to change that provided solutions to these problems. The theory is based on a systems perspective—one that takes into account the dynamics embedded in individual motivation, group behavior, and resistance to change. Units of change, levels of change, and intervention strategies are all part of this model, which advances a practical understanding of persistent problems that face us as individuals and as a society. Bates and Winder[48] synthesized this model and applied it to problems in health behavior, both on the individual and on the systems level.

In order to appreciate the complexity of this theory, it is important to understand how a problem formation occurs. Let's look at the nine-dot problem. (See Fig. 1–1.) The task is to solve the problem by connecting the nine dots with four straight lines, without lifting the pencil from the paper. Most people have difficulty solving the problem because they base their attempted solutions on the premise that they must stay inside the nine-dot square while connecting the dots. In fact, the only way all the dots can be connected, without lifting the pencil from the paper, is if the premise changes to allow one to go outside the square, beyond the dots. The solution to the problem then becomes possible.

FIGURE 1–1   The Nine-Dot Problem

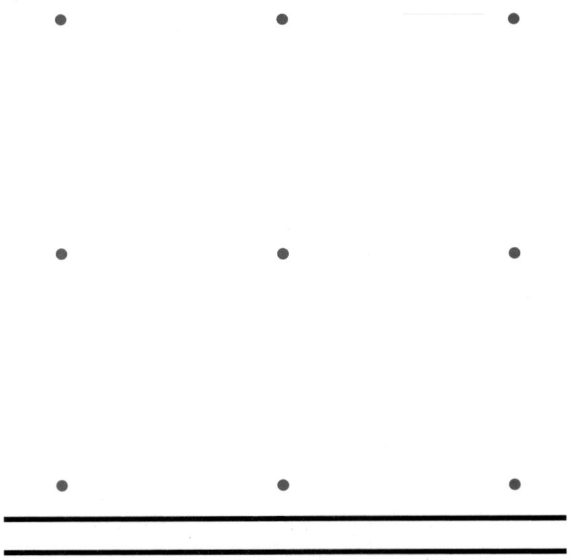

FIGURE 1–2   Solution to the Nine-Dot Problem

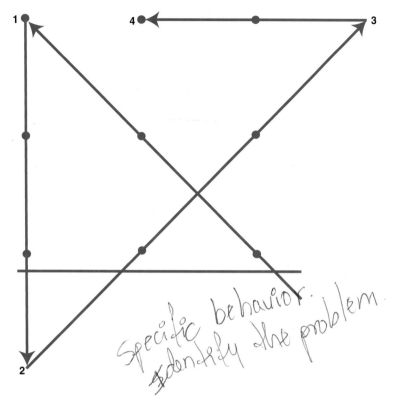

(See Fig. 1–2.) Repeated attempts to solve the problem from the wrong premise do not solve it! Rather, changes in perspective, assumptions, and rules are required to find resolution.

Attempts to solve the nine-dot problem from within the square are attempts at first-order change. First-order change is equivalent to attempts that are focused on specific problem behaviors rather than on the premises on which those behaviors are based. For example, a smoker who wishes to "kick the habit" but "cannot" has probably tried a myriad of strategies that do not break through his or her existing premises (this is like attempting to solve the nine-dot square within the structure of the dots). He or she may cut down on the number of cigarettes smoked or even go for long periods of time without a cigarette, but if the smoker's underlying values about his or relationship to smoking do not change, he or she will discover that cutting down or even cutting out cigarettes is not producing the desired result. Even external restrictions—such as anti-smoking workplace rules, friends' and family members' pleadings and threats, and even serious health problems caused by smoking—are usually not enough to inspire the "first-order change" smoker to abandon the habit for good.

Smokers who successfully quit change their lifestyle patterns and adopt behaviors that reflect their new health value. They find ways to keep their overall goal in mind—that is, to live a smoke-free life—rather than try to manipulate how many cigarettes they smoke in a day. Instead of smoking, they will organize their time away from the usual places with which smoking is associated.

Let's take a look at another example of first- and second-order change. The famous *Titanic* disaster is a useful illustration. When the ship hit the iceberg, the huge hole made in the hull caused the ship to start sinking. What saved some people's lives? Certainly not running in a panic, going from one part of the ship to the other, trying to find a solution to the problem within the ship itself. A solution unconnected to the ship itself—the lifeboats—saved some lives. What would have saved all the people's lives? Repair of the hole made by the iceberg, of course, which would have required a context of intervention beyond the boundaries of the ship itself. Or a preventive attitude on the part of the shipping line that would have resulted in provision of enough lifeboats for all passengers. All these interventions are examples of a second-order change: a change that requires a shift in perception and values, which in turn influences the situation. Using this disaster as an example, first-order change is equivalent to rearranging the deck chairs on the *Titanic*; second-order change is equivalent to being able to fix the hole in the ship, providing enough lifeboats, or better strategies to have prevented the disaster.

Let's look at a problem that plagues us currently: the incidence and prevalence of cancer. Although exciting advancements have been made in the treatment of certain cancers, allowing more cancer patients who receive treatment to enjoy a longer life span, the larger picture offers few reasons for optimism: cancer is on the rise worldwide. Although we are most certainly happy for those individuals who have survived cancer through the miracles of biomedicine, this situation is analogous to rearranging the deck chairs on the *Titanic* or getting just a few people into the lifeboats.

The theory of first- and second-order change helps us to understand why health care in the United States—even though we are spending more money on biomedical care—is substandard in many significant ways when compared to that in the majority of other industrialized nations. A common solution to this problem has been tried over and over; that is, spend *more* money on biomedicine to improve the nation's health. But increasing expenditures on illness care does not address the nation's most pressing health issues. The wrong solution is being applied to the problem. Second-order solutions require a change in premises that reflects a change in values toward health—and a movement away from the premise that health care is only about symptom relief and reduction of illness.

First-order solutions are about changes in single behaviors, and they reflect the premise structure of the problem: doing more or less of something, such as smoking cigarettes, taking painkillers for a headache, vomiting and purging to lose weight, taking steroids to gain weight, taking vitamins, buckling the seat belt. Long-term resolution of a problem will not be achieved if the value system of the individual does not also change and become reflected in lifestyle decisions and behavior.

It is important to realize that some health problems—if they are temporary or episodic—require only a first-order solution. For example, an accidental injury can be addressed at the first-order level and a complete healing achieved. However, a person whose life is unsettled by long-standing accident-prone behavior will benefit from assistance from outside the "box" of the problem—perhaps in the form of psychotherapy, which enables the person to examine and understand the dynamics of self-harm and self-defeat. A thorough understanding of a problem is a good first step toward knowing at which level change strategies and efforts are best targeted. A change in behavior will effect first-order change, but it takes a change in values to effect second-order change.

Table 1–3 illustrates how both first- and second-order change can occur on two levels; that is, the microlevel and the macrolevel of system organization. The individual, as a system, constitutes the microlevel, whereas groups, organizations, and societies make up the macrolevel. The only difference is the size of the system.

Change at the Individual Level

The effectiveness of a change at the appropriate level can be seen in the outcome—"the proof is in the pudding." If a smoker can quit by cutting down gradually, we know that smoking has not become a permanent lifestyle habit—part of the person's individual identity—and that a change in values was unnecessary. In this case, a first-order change will suffice.

TABLE 1–3   Types and Levels of Change

TYPE	MICROLEVEL	MACROLEVEL
First-order change	Individual change from one behavior to another	Organizational change from one behavior to another
Second-order change	Individual change in values and ways of behaving	Community/society change in values and ways of behaving

Source: Bates, I, and Winder, A: Introduction to Health Education. Mayfield Press, Mountain View, Calif., 1984, p. 79.

On the other hand, if a smoker who wants to quit is unable to do so, no matter what strategy is used, we know that this smoker (1) does not really want to quit smoking yet, because smoking is involved with self-identity or functioning, or (2) does not yet have a good enough reason that reflects an evolution of personal health values that would exclude smoking because of the harm it causes. There is a third, physiological possibility—the smoker is so addicted that a more comprehensive smoking-cessation strategy is required, and the person has not yet found the strategy that will make the difference. Participation in a smoking-cessation program is a second-order change—the smoker has elicited help beyond the individual level to support the decision to stop smoking.

Second-order change reflects a shift in consciousness, based on one's desire to be in relationship with oneself and others in a new way. Here are some examples of second-order shifts in values that influence smoking cessation:

- Wanting to live longer (rejection of self-destructive attitudes and behaviors; the desire for aliveness)
- Wanting to have more energy (rejection of self-defeating attitudes and behaviors; the desire for potency)
- Wanting to be healthy for other people (the awareness of one's importance to others; love for others)
- Wanting to overcome addiction to a substance (the desire for mastery)
- Wanting to be free of cultural and corporate manipulation (the desire for freedom)
- Wanting to be more appealing to others (the desire for love and connection)
- Wanting a personal identity of being a "nonsmoker" (the desire for self-respect)

First- and Second-Order Levels Coexist

Although two levels of change have been defined as different and discussed separately, they are not mutually exclusive. The individual will most likely use a combination of change strategies in the process of smoking cessation as well as in other decisions that support a healthier life. One level influences the other. For instance, the smoker whose values have shifted toward nonsmoking needs to operationalize the decision to quit in first-order behaviors, and attempts at these behaviors will reinforce the value change. Conversely, initial changes of the first order, such as not smoking for a period of time, can serve as encouragement for the smoker that quitting is possible and become part of the process of developing new health values.

Resistance to Change

This model of change includes the dynamic of resistance to change; that is, the force of the status quo in the system that maintains its identity and its current functioning. Resistance is the force that we feel when we experience change as difficult. Resistance maintains the status quo, even when the status quo is problematic and could benefit from an evolution to another level of functioning. A smoker may be resistant to quitting because smoking is associated with familiar and comforting people and activities. To stop smoking is to expose oneself to the potential loss of the pleasure associated with smoking behavior, and the desire for those pleasurable associations will energize resistance to the decision to quit.

Resistance to change occurs on the macrolevel of organizations and institutions as well. Resistance is easily identified in bureaucratic organizations. As complex systems, organizations move through the processes of change slowly, and impediments to evolution can be many. First-order organizational change appears as more or less of the same behavior that reflects the organization's current vision and mission as well as the nature of the organization's relationship to the larger world outside itself. Second-order organizational change will not occur until its vision and mission are reorganized to reflect new values and purpose.

Change at the Organizational Level

Let's look at another example—this time at a larger system, or the macrolevel—and examine the nature of resistance to change there. Public awareness of the environment's impact on health has grown in the last decade, but economic profit often conflicts with environmental protection and public health. Environmental research has demonstrated the relationship between industrial pollution and health. Industrial waste products are usually very toxic and have deleterious effects on human, animal, and plant health. Industries can respond to this growing body of research documentation by resisting change or by initiating first- or second-order change. An organization that resists behavior conducive to a healthy environment leaves itself potentially vulnerable to control by larger social regulatory forces, such as governmental agencies, negative public opinion, and grassroots opposition. Consider the following situation.

The incidence of cancer and other illnesses is rising in a small rural town in New England. Public health officials and concerned citizens suspect a connection between the rising illness rate with a local manufacturing firm's unrestrained dumping of industrial waste into the river and a landfill. The implications of this problem, if identified as the responsibility of the manufacturing firm, are enormous: the costs of environmental clean-up, redesigning and constructing a new waste disposal system, and insurance liability for related illness and disability are likely to be perceived as prohibitive by the firm. To reduce the possibility of liability, the firm resists attempts on the part of public health officials and concerned citizens to implicate its manufacturing processes and dumping activities in the rising incidence of illness in the community. For a while, corporate executives deny any claims made against the firm and pressure employees not to divulge the company's procedures for handling manufacturing waste. Meanwhile, people continue to get sick.

This scenario suggests that the manufacturing company is the "bad guy," heartlessly avoiding its responsibility to the community it serves and to whom it owes its base of operation. It is not this simple, however, because the manufacturing firm is a major contributor to the life of the community—it provides the major source of employment in the area. Community members receive their livelihood, health-care insurance, and pensions through their employment at the manufacturing company. Employed people support local businesses and services that are crucial to others not employed by the firm. In short, the manufacturing firm is central to the community's economic stability. It is made up of community people, caught in a major conflict of interest. What is it to be? Resisting change, maintenance of the economic status quo, or a value shift toward including the people's health as an issue in the firm's operating procedures?

First-order changes might include shipping the toxic waste elsewhere or reducing the amount produced. A public relations campaign might be initiated in the community to shore up the firm's failing image. The firm could take a first-order perspective by continuing to deny its health-threatening effect on the community while at the same time acknowledging the rising illness rate by making a major contribution to the building of a new hospital to accommodate the increasing need for the care of those made sick by the toxic waste in the river, groundwater, soil, and air. The firm's corporate leadership could also attempt to influence legislators to reduce its responsibility for its environmental impact by repealing environmental protection laws. In short, the firm's first-order efforts would give the impression that it was making a significant response to the public health problem when in fact it was not—rearranging the deck chairs.

Second-order change would look quite different; it would be based on a shift in values toward interconnectedness and accountability for the firm's impact on health. Corporate decision makers would listen to those concerned about the firm's role and its responsibility for maintaining a healthy environment. The firm's mission would be expanded to include its role in being a "good neighbor," not only in the economic sense but also as a co-inhabitor of the environment, another guest of Nature. The firm would acknowledge the importance of health and recognize that the health of its employees and their families is dependent on its environmental stewardship. The firm would work with community members, public health workers, and environmental agencies to identify and clean up sources of contamination for which it was responsible. Monies would be provided to compensate those who had suffered pollution-related illness.

The firm's public relations department would work toward healing the breach of trust that was violated by its irresponsible actions. The corporate structure could seek a relationship with legislators and the Environmental Protection Agency to establish an unprecedented, proactive industrial-environmental partnership that could serve as a model for the nation, even the world, demonstrating that both industry and the environment can benefit from a cooperative approach. Change on this level would result in a healthier environment, healthier people, and a new model of industrial responsibility that could have far-reaching, transformative effects toward the sustainability required for all life on the planet.

Understanding the importance of second-order strategies is crucial to the effective solution of the sociopolitical conditions that affect and maintain contexts for health and illness. All health problems are not the result of individual choice or behavior. For example, people living in a contaminated area who are not aware of the pollution to which they are exposed or who cannot move to a healthier environment are vulnerable to becoming sickened by the toxins they involuntarily ingest. Every human innovation that impacts on the environment also impacts on human health and the health of all living systems within it—including those interventions that are designed to protect humans.

Insecticide spraying to prevent cases of West Nile virus, carried by mosquitoes, is a current example. The insecticide kills not only mosquitoes but also birds and marine life. What effect will the insecticide have on human health, as well as the health of other species, beyond the prevention of the virus? Changes at the macrolevel have consequences that can either enhance or threaten the health of individuals and communities. Real and long-lasting changes for the health of the entire population, and for the life of our companion species and the plant life that sustains both, require conscious and complex interventions of the second order at the macrolevel.

Resolution of a problem as complex as industrial pollution may seem idealistic, even impossible. Chapter 6 will detail the numerous environmental issues that will require measures of second-order change if we are to approach health and illness from a truly holistic perspective. How are we to get beyond the madness of ecological destruction from which we now suffer so as to sustain life? If not health, then what? If not now, then when?

Metaparadigm Shift: Many Worldviews, One Medicine

Although it is important to explicate the myriad perceptions, beliefs, and values that influence health on both individual and institutional levels, as well as to appropriate strategies for change, our exploration is limited if it does not also include knowledge of worldviews from which social organization and personal experience emerge. A worldview is the overall interpretive paradigm on which perceptions of reality are based, and it changes over time. Worldviews are broader than a set of beliefs about singular topics such as health; rather, they provide the context for the entire human experience and coincidentally influence beliefs about health. For example, a worldview that includes interaction with the spirit realm will define health to include appropriate relationships with the unseen.

Is our contemporary relationship with the germ realm, which reflects a particular worldview that influences our health beliefs and practices, really much different from other worldviews, except in its sociocultural expression? All "isms" (racism, sexism, elitism, etc.) are based on a worldview that equates difference with inequality: How much suffering and ill health, on both the individual and social levels, has been perpetuated in the name of this worldview? A worldview that assumes humankind's superiority in the evolutionary chain of life has a dramatically different impact on earthly life than does the Eastern view of "interbeing" among all living things. What might it be like to live within the worldview of "interbeing" for a change?

What is real? What is true? How do things work? There are many ways to answer these questions, and the answers are embedded in worldviews. Questions that confront health-care practitioners and their clients include these: What is health? What is the nature of being human? How should we treat one another and ourselves in the search for health? Our health-care system is currently experiencing a clash of worldviews, which fuels the conflict and confusion inherent in the current paradigm shift. This state of conflict can be seen as a crisis—or an opportunity to reinvent the health-care system.

If health care is to become integrative and holistic, the health sciences need to evolve from their present state of specialization and fragmentation toward a synthesis that will enable practitioners to improve treatment efficacy and patient satisfaction, to reduce the economic cost of health care, and to create a comprehensive theory that integrates the wealth of seemingly disparate data and theories of health and illness into an organized whole. Schwartz and Russek[49] offer a model that provides a framework for this evolution toward what they call "One Medicine." This model expands on the work of Stephen C. Pepper,[50] who, in 1942, published *World Hypotheses*, which sought to explain how assumptions about the world affect people's understanding and actions. Schwartz and Russek's model expands on Pepper's original four hypotheses to include four others on which many complementary/alternative therapies, as well as traditional models of care, are based. (See Table 1–4.) The hypotheses, progressing from one to eight and becoming increasingly complex, describe the theoretical underpinning of attitudes that influence beliefs and behavior from each perspective.

This is a comprehensive model that provides a basis for understanding health beliefs and behavior, efficacy and limitations among levels of intervention, and the conflict that can arise from the clash of different worldviews. This model offers a method to make comparisons between and among levels of knowledge, and it also allows one to trace progression from older to newer ideas in scientific thought. Finally, it offers a framework to support the paradigm shift toward transdisciplinary integration that is occurring in the health-care system today.

TABLE 1–4   Eight World Hypotheses

WORLD HYPOTHESES	DESCRIPTION
WH 1: Formistic	All structures and functions exist as separate categories.
WH 2: Mechanistic	All effects have causes that precede them.
WH 3: Contextual	All structures and functions exist in context and are relative.
WH 4: Organismic	All structures and functions reflect organizations of relationships—parts interact and become whole systems.
WH 5: Implicit Process	All systems involve implicit processes of information/energy/matter that interact over time.
WH 6: Circular Causality	All systems involve the circulation of information/energy/matter that interact over time.
WH 7: Creative Unfolding	All systems reflect flexible orders, express plans, and serve multiple purposes.
WH 8: Integrative Diversity	All phenomena in nature reflect complex interconnected, integrated orders or harmonies of diverse processes.

Source: Schwartz, GE, and Russek, GL: The challenge of one medicine. ADVANCES: The Journal of Body-Mind Health 13:9, 1997, with permission.

World Hypothesis 1: Formistic Models

Formistic thinking assumes that nature consists of independent categories of structures and functions. Information is processed into discrete and mutually exclusive either/or categories. There is no gray area in this black-and-white view of the world. Information is used to answer the question "What category describes the phenomenon?"

Application to health. People are either sick or well. Health is the opposite of, or the absence of, disease. People can be classified into categories, such as personality typology (Type A, hypertensive, psychotic, etc.).

World Hypothesis 2: Mechanistic Models

The mechanistic hypothesis presumes cause and effect—and that cause precedes effect. It examines categories of processes over time. This view adds the dimension of time to categories: that events can cause effects and that chains of cause and effects exist in nature. The person who thinks mechanistically thinks beyond categorization to connect events with cause: television causes violence; an apple a day keeps the doctor away. If there is something wrong, there is a cause; the solution is to find the single cause. This model is the basis for classical Newtonian science, in which a causal relationship between the independent and dependent variables is assumed.

Application to health. Single causes are assumed to cause single diseases: HIV causes AIDS; high fat content causes arteriosclerosis. Mind and body are seen as influencing each other causally: a sound mind is (causes) a sound body; losing weight will increase self-esteem.

World Hypothesis 3: Contextual Models

The contextual hypothesis assumes that everything is relative, that it "depends on how you look at it." One's perspective is paramount in understanding the world. This view moves from a Newtonian scientific base to Einsteinian, quantum assumptions about understanding nature and the universe. Contextual thinking is implicit in traditional Eastern, Native-American, and contemporary Western biopsychosocial approaches to health and healing.

Application to health. Contextual information processing allows no one single way of understanding health or disease. The definition of either is relative to the context in which the person is considered. Health can be relative to the functioning of one's immune system (host resistance) or to the presence of pathogens (outside agent), to the state of one's emotional life, or to diet. Health can be different for different people, and value is placed on understanding a person's opinions about health in the context of his or her culture, beliefs, or personal experience.

World Hypothesis 4: Organismic and Relationship Models

This hypothesis postulates that all things reflect the interaction of multiple component structures and functions and that all things are simultaneously a part of larger entities. The systems notions that the whole is greater than the sum of its parts and that those systemic properties emerge from interaction among component parts are good examples of this hypothesis. These concepts are relatively new, having emerged from biology and engineering in the 1920s. Persons holding this view see things as interconnected and interdependent, with multiple causes and effects that have dynamic relationships within ongoing and unpredictable, synergistic processes.

Application to health. Health and disease involve combinations and interactions of factors. This model supports the view that health and disease can coexist in the same person—for example, a person with a cold or a broken bone can be considered healthy overall, even when living with a temporary subsystem limitation; a dying person can be healthy in the sense that he or she can experience optimal comfort, intimacy, happiness, and meaning up to the moment of death. Self-care in the presence of illness is considered a hallmark of overall health. The capacity to integrate physical, mental, and spiritual needs is a systems view of healthy integration. An organismic hypothesis supports the view that "health is a combination of the capacity to heal and the capacity to function optimally."

World Hypothesis 5: Implicit Process and Information Energy Models

This view advances the notion that nature contains invisible processes, such as energy and subatomic particles; although based on quantum physics, it is presaged by earlier theorists. For example, the notion of an intrinsic vital life force (*chi, ki,* or *prana*) dates back thousands of years; Newton spoke of gravity as a force, Mesmer of animal magnetism, Freud of the id, Reich of orgone, Native Americans of spirit energy, and so forth. In this model, inferences about implicit processes in nature that are not limited to the concrete or the visible underpin the worldview.

Application to health. The notion that good or bad "vibes" can be felt and can influence health exemplifies these models. Imagery or attitudinal interventions are based on theories of implicit process and energy as information.

World Hypothesis 6: Circular Causality and Circular Logic Models

This model adds the complex aspect of information circulation to the understanding of how the world works. The circular causality hypothesis, developed over the last hundred years, goes beyond interaction and explicitly includes the circulation of interacting information, energy, and matter—not only between parts of a system but also recursively between systems over time. The circular causality process allows the buildup of information and energy in a system. In order to understand health it is necessary to understand how the circulation of information is occurring. Circular causality applies to all physiological systems, for example, the cardiovascular, respiratory, and lymphatic systems in the body. It also applies to systems of information and can account for energy exchange between individuals.

Application to health. Ancient healing practices such as Qigong can be understood within this model. Circular causality may also help to explain the dynamic effects of energetic "memory" phenomena, such as homeopathy, kineosiology, and organ transplant memory.

World Hypothesis 7: Creative Unfolding and Intentional Models

Important concepts of this model are intentions, order, and growth. It explains the evolution of systems based on the assumption that systems do not arise from random or chance occurrences, but rather from a larger plan or design. Life itself is the expression of a deep invisible pattern, which is constantly being manifested. The genetic code is an example of an implicit plan in nature from which living systems evolve or unfold. Bohm's[51] theory of "implicate order" is a model of creative unfolding process. This theory postulates that the cosmos is a hologram, and asserts that every unit of the cosmos, including the human being, carries a representation of the whole.

Application to health. Health and illness are not dichotomous; rather, disease is important information for growth. Health is experienced as a way of living and evolving, not a static state. This model supports some of the most controversial perspectives on health, such as spiritual healing, prayer, and the power of love to heal.

World Hypothesis 8: Integrative Diversity and Interconnected Models

This model anticipates that processes and orders beyond those currently envisioned can be included in the ongoing understanding of the world in general and of health in particular. This hypothesis has been associated with searches for grand unifying theories (GUTs) and theories of everything (TOEs) in disciplines such as physics and astrophysics. This model asserts that agreement among hypotheses or worldviews is less valuable than understanding and utilizing their differences, an understanding from which new and useful information can emerge. It requires a synthesis of intuition and reason that will generate the wisdom necessary to bring the whole into balance and harmony. Competing perspectives, multiple sources of information, and the influence of time and change can be understood such that more integrated solutions to the serious, complex problems facing us today can emerge.

Application to health care. Health problems can be seen from multiple perspectives that are noncontradictory and that form the basis of cooperative, noncompetitive solutions. Examples include CAM and conventional health-care practitioners' creation of professional communities that, through conscious communication, seek new ways to meet their shared clients' needs—such as healing gardens, massage therapists, homelike atmospheres, and music in hospitals; insurance carriers that reimburse both conventional and CAM care; and expansion of locations where care is delivered, such as in school-based health-care clinics that serve the entire community. These are but a few examples of what is possible with a worldview that sees how all levels of human experience and interaction are connected.

Schwartz and Russek's extension of Pepper's World Hypothesis Model has contributed a creative and useful vision that can guide the health professions toward true integrative models of care. In particular, hypothesis 8 supports the inevitable discovery and development of new world models over time and their integration into the ongoing working models to date. This framework provides a map for collective transdisciplinary cooperation in health care. It asserts the value of creative integration of all approaches into an evolving understanding of how to promote health, alleviate suffering, and reconnect with the environmental context of life on which health and life is dependent. Hypothesis 8 encompasses the previous seven hypotheses and provides a base into which all appropriate models can be incorporated. Transdisciplinary convergence toward an integrative approach to health and illness is occurring more frequently in health-care settings throughout the country.

Conclusion: *Back to the Future*

Heraclitus, the Greek philosopher cited at the beginning of this chapter, made another observation about the constancy of change when he said, "You never step into the same river twice." Again, the current revolution in health care is a good example. The rise of complementary and alternative health therapies is the result of interaction among knowledge developments of the past, health-care needs of the present, and desired health goals for the future. Biomedical science has been, and will continue to be, central to the evolution of effective health care. Humankind's health problems are beyond the scope of the curative bias of mainstream medicine, and the current popularity of the holistic and CAM movements is evidence of this. The time has come for a true integration of knowledge and wisdom from all sources, both mainstream and unconventional, for the benefit of the public.

Personal values and beliefs reflect worldviews that influence culture, social interaction, and individual behavior, both conscious and unconscious. Health-care practitioners' effectiveness will depend on a working knowledge of varied worldviews, personal beliefs, and larger systems dynamics. "Think globally, act locally" is a good reminder of the connection between individual and larger systems levels. Support for individual health needs and preferences can coexist with advocacy for a healthy environment, health promotion, and disease prevention at the macrosystems level.

A fuller knowledge of health requires greater understanding of what it means to be human in the context of the living world of which we are a part. Individual health cannot be considered separately from our relationships with nature, with one another, and with the other species with which we share the planet. Conscious awareness of our "interbeing" is the most potent energy behind the current paradigm shift that is affecting not only health-care industries but also international relationships that are forming around a shared vision of sustainable living. The vision of sustainable interbeing is the only vision that will heal the deadly conflicts that separate us from one another, the natural world, and our own sense of inner wholeness, and that will ensure the possibility of health for all in the future. And not a moment too soon.

Resources

NCCAM Clearinghouse
P.O. Box 8218
Silver Springs, MD 20907-8218
Phone: (301) 589-5367
Toll-free, TTY/TDY, and fax-on-demand: (301) 495-4957
E-mail: *nccam-info@nccam.nih.gov*
Website: *http://nccam.nih.gov*

References

1. Oxford Book of Quotations. Oxford University Press, Oxford, England, 1979, p 274.
2. Garell, DC: Foreword. In Gordon, JS: Holistic Medicine. Chelsea, New York, 1988.
3. Pincus, T, and Callahan, LF: What explains the association between socioeconomic status and health: Primary access to medical care or mind-body variables? ADVANCES: The Journal of Mind–Body Health 1:4, 1995.
4. Cassidy, CM: Unraveling the ball of string: Reality, paradigms, and the study of alternative medicine. ADVANCES: The Journal of Mind–Body Health 10:6, 1994.
5. Robbins, J: Reclaiming Our Health. HJ Kramer, Tiburon, Calif., 1996, pp 3–4.
6. Monte, T: World Medicine: The East–West Guide to Healing Your Body. JP Tarcher, New York, 1993, p 56.
7. Eisenberg, DM, et al: Unconventional medicine in the United States: Prevalence, costs, and patterns of use. The New England Journal of Medicine 328: 246, 1993.
8. Eisenberg, DM, et al: Trends in alternative medicine use in the United States, 1990–1997: Results of a follow-up national survey. JAMA 280:1569, 1998.
9. Astin, JA: Why patients use alternative medicine: Results of a national study. JAMA 279:1548, 1998.
10. Reilly, D: CAM in Europe: Reflections and Trends. Paper presented at: Alternative Medicine: Implications for Practice and State of the Science Symposium; Harvard Medical School; March 12, 2000: Boston.
11. Ibid.
12. Kuhn, TS: The Structure of Scientific Revolutions. University of Chicago Press, Chicago, 1970.
13. Dasher, ES: A systems theory approach to an expanded medical model: A challenge for biomedicine. Journal of Complementary and Alternative Therapies 1:187, 1995.
14. Eisenberg et al: Unconventional medicine.
15. Eisenberg et al: Trends in alternative medicine use.
16. Astin: Why patients use alternative medicine.
17. Cassidy: Unraveling the ball of string, p 6.
18. Hayes, KM, and Alexander, IM: Alternative therapies and nurse practitioners: Knowledge, professional experience, and personal use. Holistic Nursing Practice 12:49, 2000.
19. Spencer, JW, and Jacobs, JJ: Complementary/Alternative Medicine: An Evidence-Based Approach. Mosby, St. Louis, 1999.
20. Cassidy: Unraveling the ball of string.
21. Foster, GM: Medical Anthropology. Wiley, New York, 1978.
22. Spencer and Jacobs: Complementary/Alternative Medicine.
23. Gordon, JS: Alternative medicine and the family physician. Am Fam Physician 54:7, 1996.
24. Panel on Definition and Description, CAM Research Methodology Conference, April 1995. Defining and describing complementary and alternative medicine. Alternative Therapies 3:49, 1995.
25. Associated Press. Judge: AMA conspired against chiropractors. Daily Hampshire Gazette, August 29, 1987, p 3.
26. Summaries of Opinion and Order and Permanent Injunction Order and Complete Copy of Opinion and Order and Permanent Injunction Order in *Wilk et al. v. AMA et al.* U.S. District Court for the Northeastern District of Illinois, Eastern Division, August 25 and September 25, 1987.

27. Agency for Health Care Policy and Research: Acute Pain Management: Operative or Medical Procedures and Trauma, 1992 Publication No. AHCPR 92-0032.

28. Manga, P, et al: The Effectiveness and Cost-Effectiveness of Chiropractic Management of Low Back Pain. Kenilworth Publishing, Richmond Hill, Ontario, 1993, p 80.

29. An Act Relative to the Practice of Acupuncture. The Commonwealth of Massachusetts. Chapter 114, H4642. 1998.

30. Gordon, JS: The paradigm of holistic medicine. In Hastings J, et al (eds): Health for the Whole Person, Westview Press, Boulder, 1980.

31. Cassidy: Unraveling the ball of string, p 6.

32. Becker, MH (ed): The health belief model and personal health behavior. Health Education Monographs 2:324, 1974.

33. Becker, MH, and Maimon, LA: Strategies for enhancing patient compliance. Journal of Community Health 6:113, 1980.

34. Becker, MH: A belief model: A decade later. Health Education Quarterly 11:1, 1984.

35. Rosenstock, IM: The Health Belief Model: Explaining health behavior through expectancies. In Glanz, K, et al (eds): Health Behavior and Health Education: Theory, Research and Practice. Jossey-Bass, San Francisco, 1991.

36. Furnham, A, and Kirkcaldy, B: The health beliefs and behaviors of orthodox and complementary medicine clients. British Journal of Clinical Psychology 35:49, 1996.

37. Lantz, M, et al: Socioeconomic factors, health behaviors, and mortality. JAMA 279:1703, 1998.

38. Ruberman, W: We need to know the pathways by which mind–body interactions could link socioeconomic status and health. ADVANCES: The Journal of Mind–Body Health 11:21, 1995.

39. Williams, RB: Conditions of low socioeconomic status increase the likelihood of the biological bases underlying psychosocial factors that contribute to health. ADVANCES: The Journal of Mind–Body Health 11:24, 1995.

40. Dreher, H: The social perspective in mind–body studies: missing in action? ADVANCES:The Journal of Mind–Body Health 11:39, 1995.

41. Chooproian, TJ: Reconceptualizing the environment. In Moccia, P (ed): New Approaches to Theory Development. National League for Nursing, New York, 1986, p 39.

42. Winkleby, M: Environmental influences underlying the mind–body hypothesis. ADVANCES: The Journal of Mind–Body Health 11:26, 1995.

43. Stanitis (Bright), MA, and Ryan, J: Non-compliance: An illegitimate nursing diagnosis? Am J Nurs 6:941, 1982.

44. Kleine, SS, and Hughner, RS: Paradigm shifts in health care: Consumers' personal theories of health. Alternative Health Practitioner 5:187, 1999.

45. Astin: Why patients use alternative medicine.

46. Bates, I, and Winder, A: Introduction to Health Education. Mayfield, Mountain View, Calif., 1984.

47. Watzlawick, P, et al: Change: Principles of Problem Formation and Problem Resolution. WW Norton, New York, 1974.

48. Bates and Winder: Introduction to Health Education.

49. Schwartz, GE, and Russek, GL: The challenge of one medicine. ADVANCES: The Journal of Mind-Body Health 13:9, 1997.

50. Pepper, SC: World Hypotheses: A Study in Evidence. University of California Press, Berkeley, 1961 (reprint).

51. Bohm, D: Wholeness and the Implicate Order. Routledge & Kegan, London, 1980.

CHAPTER 2

Health, Healing, and Holistic Nursing

Mary Anne Bright, Veda Andrus, and Jane Yetter Lunt

Mary Anne Bright, RN, CS, EdD, the editor of this book, is an associate professor at the University of Massachusetts–Amherst School of Nursing. She teaches courses in holistic health and mental health nursing, conducts research on Therapeutic Touch, and is a member of the International Institute of Bioenergetic Analysis and of the American Holistic Nurses Association.

Veda Andrus, EdD, MSN, RN, HNC, is the president and CEO of Seeds and Bridges Center for Holistic Nursing Education. She is also the former president and international director of the American Holistic Nurses Association.

Jane Yetter Lunt, BSN, MEd, RN, HNC, is the executive vice president and general program director for Seeds and Bridges Center for Holistic Nursing Education.

Gina awakens to the sound of her alarm clock. It is 6:30 AM and still dark outside. Is it already time to get up for school? she wonders as she shifts to a sitting position and thinks of the day ahead of her. Gina is not looking forward to her day: three midterms, two boring classes, demanding teachers, and terrible dining commons food. To make matters worse, she hasn't had time to study for the exams, between working four nights a week and losing sleep over the breakup with her boyfriend, Ben.

Gina's head, heavy with fatigue and worry, begins to throb and a cold sweat beads her face. A deep ache erupts in her chest, and she feels sick to her stomach. "I can't handle all this," she thinks to herself. Her roommate, Jennifer, asks when she'll be ready to leave. "I'm sick," Gina replies. "I can't go to school today." Jennifer knocks on her door and looks in. "You were fine before you went to bed last night, and you look fine now," Jennifer says.

"I wish I *felt* fine," Gina replies, pulling the covers over her head. "I can't take any more. Life is too much."

This example illustrates the many factors that affect health. What is health? Does it go beyond physical experience? Is it the absence of disease? What does health have to do with the way we think? How is it related to our relationships with others and with the environment? Is health in the eyes of the experiencer or in the eyes of the beholder?

Gina and her friend reached different conclusions about the state of Gina's health. Even though Jennifer did not see signs of what she called "being sick," Gina's lack of well-being was real. Gina's perception of her life had a real impact on her experience—the headache, the heartache, the queasy stomach, and the cold sweat were her body's responses to what was happening in her life. Her mental distress was heightened by the pressures of school.

Gina's conclusion about her inability to cope expressed a disruption of her self-respect and her spiritual balance. Gina felt "dis-eased" in body/ mind/spirit. This was manifested in her inability to meet the day's demands.

"Health" has eluded a single, definitive description. If we fully understood the meaning of health, we would better understand what it means to be human, understand our human potential, and see where we are headed in our evolution.[1]

Holism and Health

The words *holism* and *health* come from the same Anglo-Saxon root as *heal, whole,* and *holy.* To be healthy means to be whole; to heal is to recognize innate wholeness. The word *holism* implies a sacred, relational perspective on the universe. Holism encompasses a person's relationship with the environment, with other people, and with the ongoing process of understanding the meaning and purpose of life. The holistic model asserts that health cannot be understood if the health of the earth, or the integrity of human relationships, or spiritual meaning is not also taken into consideration.

Holism suggests a wholeness that is a fundamental completeness, an integration within a larger environmental context of energy and matter. Einstein understood this innate connectedness. He once said:

> A human being is part of a whole that we call "Universe," a part limited in time and space. He experiences himself, his thoughts and feelings as something separated from the rest, a kind of optical delusion of his consciousness. This delusion is a kind of prison for us, restricting us to our personal desires and to affection for a few persons nearest to us. Our task must be to free ourselves from this prison by widening our circle of compassion to embrace all living creatures and the whole nature in its beauty. Nobody is able to achieve this completely, but the striving for such achievement is in itself a part of the liberation, and a foundation for inner security.[2]

Philosophical and Theoretical Basis of Holism

The philosophy of holism evolved from the rich work of scientific theorists and philosophers who created a worldview of interconnectedness, one that will serve human/ planetary health. Among these contributors are Faraday, Einstein, de Chardin, Pribam, Prigogine, Bohm, Swimme and Berry, and Sheldrake. These great thinkers helped bring contemporary science from the mechanistic Newtonian perspective to an understanding of the universe as an energetically connected, whole, living system. "Nothing rests; everything moves; everything vibrates," states the hermetic philosophy in the principle of vibration.[3]

Scientific understanding of a universe made of energy is a relatively new perspective in the human story. In the last few centuries science has discovered the dynamics that govern the earth and the cosmos. Whereas 17th-century mechanistic scientists viewed the building blocks of life as solid, permanent, and separate particles of matter, by the middle of the 19th century, scientists were perceiving the world as a dynamic and integral dance of energy. By the late 1890s, physicists were claiming that energy, expressed as physical matter, was the soul's real substance in nature.

Faraday's early conceptualization of field theory, in which energy fields were seen as invisible regions of influence or force patterns, is instrumental to this shift in awareness. Science describes electromagnetic, gravitational, morphic, and biological fields. Like waves in the ocean, each of these spheres of influence is seen to exist in a greater universal energy field—fields within the field. The interconnected, vibrational effect of one field on another is comparable to movement being felt in each fiber of a spider's web. Energy fields are a concept that unifies and relates all kinds of force, flow, and activity. Field theory provides a view of how all life is vibrationally connected.

In his famous equation of $E = mc^2$ (energy = mass × the velocity of light squared), Einstein states that all matter is a manifestation of energy. This idea provides the basis for understanding humans, all other living creatures, and the natural world as dynamic energy systems. A vital force of energy breathes life into the biomechanics of living systems, constantly building and transforming their cellular expression. The physical body interfaces with complex subtle energy structures and networks that mediate the flow of this life force as well as consciousness into it, maintaining and nurturing its existence.[4] Einstein's physics underpins the holistic view that health is a vibrational spiritual/mental/physical phenomenon. Focus of care expands from "fixing" physical solutions to considering the existence, purpose, and dynamics of organizing energy patterns. This new view approaches health and healing from an understanding that matter emerges from universal energy, which brings life to the physical experience. Holistic practitioners acknowledge the relationship between the physical body and the subtle energies that some call spirit in the experience of health.

Einstein's proposition that energy and matter are dual expressions of the same universal substance supports a unitary worldview. Theoretical physicist David Bohm calls this *substance* the "implicate order." This "primary reality" is a key concept in the work on holographic theory by Bohm and Stanford neurophysiologist Karl Pribam. Pribam observed:

> A hologram is a photographic image produced by laser light. The image is stored on the holographic plate, then retrieved by shining a laser beam through the plate to create a three-dimensional projection. Curiously, if a piece of the holographic plate is broken off and the laser beam is passed through it, the whole image still appears, though it is somewhat fuzzy. In other words, "each part has implicitly retained information about the whole.[5]

One might imagine a broken mirror. The reflected image of the room that is seen in the whole mirror is seen in the pieces as well. The concept that information is distributed throughout a system, each piece encoded with information of the whole, relates not only to how the human brain functions but also to the actual nature of the universe. "Our brains mathematically construct 'concrete reality' by interpreting frequencies from another dimension, a realm of meaningful, patterned primary reality that transcends time and space. The brain is a hologram, interpreting a holographic universe."[6]

The capacity of the human mind to create a perceptual (or virtual) map of the world, and to act as if this virtual creation were real, was observed by Bohm.[7] The human intellectual capacity to perceive oneself as autonomous from nature has made it possible to imagine that there is an actual separation and then to act as if that separation were real. This split in perception, which is entrenched in decades of what is called "progress," results in a fragmentary self-world view and is manifested by overspecialization and a way of living that ignores the fundamental connectedness that sustains all living things. The holistic paradigm has as its goal the healing of this fragmented perception, which perpetuates a false view of the world, the self, and the states of personal and environmental "dis-ease" that result.

The holographic view that "the macrocosm is present in the microcosm" and that "the microcosm is present in the macrocosm" is reflected in the hermetic principle of correspondence: "as above, so below; as below, so above."[8] Everything in the universe emanates from the same source. The same principles and characteristics apply to people or activities as each manifests its own individual expression. All forms of physical matter unfold (to open or to evolve) and enfold (to surround or to contain) higher energy vibrations. The familiar view of reality has been to focus on physical, or unfolded, aspects of things, not their source. The hologram demonstrates that what appears to be real is actually a temporary appearance; what is physical has "unfolded" from an invisible substance of inseparable connectedness, the web of life.

Holographic theory includes humans integrated with an innately whole universe and the potential for participation in the ongoing transformation of life. We contain not only the information of the whole but also the power of the whole, though in slightly "fuzzy" form. Holographic theory reveals that patterns of universal energy may be accessed, understood, and purposefully transformed. As an energy pattern, the human body can be comprehended as a teacher about the true nature of oneself, one's larger world, and even the nature of the universe itself. In exploring our inner nature, we access the fundamental power of the universe. By tapping into our own power, we empower the part of the universe for which we are responsible—ourselves.

These holistic premises have important implications for individuals' ability to affect their life and reality. As a fundamental expression of life energy, human consciousness is experienced as thought, imagination, insight, and inspiration. In discussing evidence of the way the mind and consciousness penetrate all matter, Bohm states that matter emerges out of consciousness. There is mind even down at the quantum level.[9] In *The Kybalion*, the hermetic principle of mentalism states: "All is mind; the Universe is Mental."[10]

The "all," or underlying reality, is Spirit: an unknowable, indefinable, universal, infinite, living mind. As a microcosm, a holographic piece of the whole, the human mind is an expression of the mind of Spirit. The human mind is recognized as perhaps the most powerful of all healing forces. Bohm asserts that it is the higher spiritual impetus that drives the biological process itself.[11]

Love Makes the World Go 'Round

Visionary paleontologist and Jesuit priest Teilhard de Chardin recognized that love is the essential energy of the universe. He saw love not as a sentimental or romantic human feeling but as "a universal form of attraction linked to the inwardness of things: It is the fundamental impulse of Life . . . the blood of spiritual evolution."[12] This "within-ness" of the universe is neither lifeless nor stationary: It is a passionate power that reconciles, heals, and unifies. It is a power inherent in every cell of the universe and as close as our own being.[13]

This alluring attraction of life is life. Attracting activity is a powerful and mysterious force of existence that propels life to continue and to evolve. Life is a *unitary reality* based not on the emotional power but the ontological power of love that is the essence of life itself.[14] To feel love for oneself, for others, for other living things, and for the planet is the natural experience of connectedness with life. In this time of great environmental, social, and spiritual upheaval, the holistic perspective holds out hopeful methods for sustainable health and continuity of life on earth. Awareness of our connectedness, which is the power of love, is literally the key to our survival.

Health

Two holistic thinkers, Rudolph Steiner and George Vithoulkas, developed perspectives on health that transcend the fragmented materialistic view of it as a collective of chemical reactions responding to physical laws. Both take the meaning of health beyond conventional understanding. Steiner (1861–1925), an Austrian-born scientist and philosopher, intuited that the individual comprises not one but four interrelated "bodies." These bodies are the physical, etheric, astral, and spiritual; health is reflected in a state of dynamic balance that is constantly created and re-created, and can be observed in the unitary functioning of these four bodies. Illness is manifested in symptoms that reveal imbalance. Some healers are able to "see," through clairvoyant means, the bodies other than the physical that are invisible to most people.[15–17]

TABLE 2–1 Stages of the Life Cycle: Aurobindo Model

1. Sensorimotor (physical, sensory, and locomotive aspects)
2. Vital-emotional-sexual (prana, libido, or bioenergy)
3. Will-mind (simple representational and intentional thought)
4. Sense-mind (thought operations performed on sensory or concrete objects)
5. Reasoning mind (thought operations performed on abstract objects)
6. Higher mind (synthetic-integrative thought operations; "sees truth as a whole")
7. Illumined mind (transcends thought and "sees truth at a glance"; psychic or inner illumination and vision)
8. Intuitive mind (transcendental-archetypal awareness; subtle cognition and perception)
9. Overmind (unobstructed, unbound spiritual awareness)
10. Supermind (absolute identity with and as spirit; this is not really a separate level, but rather the "ground" of all levels)

Source: Wilber, K, Engler, J, and Brown, DP: Transformations of Consciousness: Conventional and Contemplative Perspectives on Development. Shambala, Boston, 1988.

What Steiner called "bodies," Vithoulkas calls "levels," "states," or "spheres." Vithoulkas, one of the world's leading teachers and practitioners of homeopathy, describes health in a framework of freedom. Health is present to the extent that the person is "free from" certain constraints on each of three levels, which enables a certain "freedom to" experience the fullness of the level's expression. Health on the physical level is freedom from physical pain or any sense of negative awareness in the body as well as freedom to experience a state of well-being.

Emotional health is a state of freedom from being enslaved by human emotions and the capability to feel a full range of emotions that is experienced as dynamic serenity. Mental health is freedom from selfishness, in which the person is in a state of complete unification with the divine or with truth and in which actions are dedicated to creative service. To the question, "How do we measure the comparative degree of health of an individual at any given moment?" Vithoulkas asserts: "The parameter which enables such measurement of health is creativity. By creativity, I mean all those acts and functions which promote for the individual himself and for others their main goal in life: continuous and unconditional happiness. To the extent that an individual is limited in the exercise of his creativity, to that degree he is "ill.""[18] These two perspectives on health show that the values of holism extend beyond a body that is symptom-free.

Health has a developmental component, seen in the process of maturation to more complex levels of awareness, functioning, and integration. The holistic perspective integrates models of development that extend beyond our own Western conventional psychoanalytic and cognitive theories. Wilber, Engler, and Brown[19] observed that there are Eastern models from contemplative orientations that go beyond stages that Western developmental theorists suggest are possible.

Aurobindo, one of India's most revered sages, created a model that included stages of development beyond those described by Western developmental theorists such as Piaget, Loevinger, and Kohlberg. Aurobindo's model (see Table 2–1) offers a description of human potential that describes the experience of highly evolved persons, such as sages and saints, whose advanced development is seen as the natural unfolding of human maturation and individual examples of the evolution of humankind.

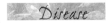 *Disease*

Dis-ease, according to Laurence Bendit, a psychiatrist and author on subjects of health and spirit, is not only ill health within the body but all forms of unease between oneself and one's environment, in social relations and everything else that is uncomfortable. Richard

Gerber, a physician who researches the vibrational aspects of healing, says that disease is a multifactorial condition. In addition to the negative effects of unbalanced internal and external factors, illness is often a symbolic reflection of our own internal states of emotional unrest, spiritual blockage, and dis-ease.[20] Disease is a healing crisis, requiring release of that which has prevented the person from healing himself or herself.[21]

From the perspective of holism, health is not a static state that can be "achieved" and held onto; rather, it is an ongoing process that embraces the ease that is wellness and the dis-ease that is illness. Newman's[22] definition of health as expanding consciousness transcends the dichotomy of health and disease, instead viewing both wellness and illness as expressions of the life process in its totality. Disease is not considered an "enemy" in the holistic perspective, as it is in the biomedical model, where cure is success and lack of cure is failure. Rather, disorder or disease is disequilibrium, which stimulates the person toward growth and regaining wholeness.[23] From a holistic perspective, disease, which is an inevitable part of the human condition, is actually necessary and beneficial to growth, adaptation, and maturation.[24]

Barbara Dossey,[25] a visionary leader in the field of holistic nursing, emphasizes the importance of understanding the centrality of meaning in wellness and illness. She asserts that the meanings attached to disease and its symptoms are central to the healing process. Meanings are individual constructions that reflect a person's values, belief systems, expectations, and the unique way in which health and illness are experienced. In addition, the context of an illness, which involves a person's perceptions of the present and the past as well as hopes and beliefs about the future, directly affects its meaning. Meaning is directly linked with all the body systems that influence states of health, wellness, disease, and illness, and as such, is a point of intervention in a plan of holistic care. The holistic practitioner embarks on a journey with the client, respecting and working with the meaning that the client has given to the illness and his or her vision of healing, in service to the client's life context and goals. (See Box 2–1.)

Death

The holistic view regards death in a very different light than does the cure-based conventional health-care model. In this perspective, death is part of the natural cycle of life. When cure is the goal, death is seen as failure, either of the person's resistance or will, or of the practitioner's skill. But healing can occur even unto death. A holistic perspective allows for a "good death," one in which the meaning of one's life is celebrated and life is appreciated for the gift that it is. Wendell Berry states: "Any definition of health that is not silly must include death. The world of efficiency is defeated by death; at death, all its instruments and procedures stop. The world of love continues, and of this grief, is the proof."[26]

Healing

Medical science has yet to generate a useful understanding of how healing occurs. Health statistics can offer calculated predictions of treatment outcomes, longevity probabilities, and health risk factors. The dynamics of healing largely remain a mystery. Our sophisticated and expensive enterprise of biomedical research cannot explain why spontaneous remission of serious illnesses occurs, how miracle or faith cures happen, or why persons who have excellent prognoses and expectations for cure unexpectedly do not survive. A growing body of knowledge about subtle energy, the placebo effect, and spiritual dimensions of experience offer promising clues toward understanding the healing process.

BOX 2–1
Parameters of the Holistic Health Model

Holism

The client is viewed as a totality. The person is treated, rather than the symptoms or the disease. The integration of the self-other environment is assumed.

The individual's uniqueness. The client is accepted as he or she is, rather than as a representative of a statistical aggregate. Two persons with the same disease might be treated very differently by a holistic practitioner.

Underlying unity. The person is regarded as a functional whole, in which there is a continuity among aspects of human–environment interaction. There is no artificial separation between body, mind, or spiritual experience, and disease is seen as a result of multiple contributing factors rather than a single cause. Treatment on one level impacts all levels.

Research on stress and resistance resources. Research investigates the relationship between the person-environment interaction and the individual experience of health and illness. Factors considered integral to health are social support; health practices; family illness patterns; personality traits; early social-structural, cultural, and child-rearing factors; and relatedness to nature and to the process of life.

Primacy of mind, attitudes, and belief systems. The effects of mental states and belief systems on health are a focus of client assessment and health teaching. The will to live, hope, and faith are considered important to recovery from illness and health maintenance.

Placebo effect. The placebo effect, or the client's expectation that the treatment will be effective, is considered part of the self-healing process and is actively enhanced.

Ecological view. A unified universe is postulated of which each person is a part and in which each person is interconnected to others, to nature, and to the world. Family, community, and global health or dis-ease are reflected in the individual. Support of healthy families, caring communities, and environmental health is seen as integral to individual well-being.

Focus on Health Promotion

Emphasis is on health promotion and disease prevention rather than on symptom relief. Lifestyle patterns and habits that maintain health are stressed. A preventative rather than crisis orientation to healthy living is important. Nutrition, stress management, rest, exercise, lifestyle choices, values, and belief systems are emphasized in optimizing wellness. Disease is seen as an opportunity for self-awareness and growth and as part of the life process.

Health as balance, integration, and harmony. Health is seen as a continuum with transitional states. The goal is high-level wellness, with emphasis on the quality rather than the length of life. The experiences of joyful aliveness, vigor, optimism, happiness, relational intimacy, and spiritual growth are considered as important as bodily health.

Preventive and promotional focus. Health-care resources may be better used when directed to health promotion and disease prevention, when compared to the cost and efficacy of treating disease and disability. Health is seen as more than the absence of sickness.

Meaning of illness. Illness is considered an opportunity for positive growth. Illness is thought to have meaning within the context of the person's life experience.

Illness and imbalance/dis-ease. Illness is seen as a shift in the homeodynamic balance of the individual, rather than as an attack from the outside. Treatments facilitate the restoration of balance, through which the person recovers by virtue of his or her own natural healing capacity.

Individual Responsibility

The person is seen as an active participant in the healing process and is not treated as a passive recipient of knowledge or treatment. Self-awareness and self-understanding can facilitate growth and health-enhancing lifestyle changes. This perspective, however, can also invite the person to blame him- or herself for illness, which is counterproductive.

Practitioners as Educators, Consultants, Facilitators

Emphasis on a collaborative working relationship recognizes the client's self-responsibility for health and decision making; the practitioner is part of the healing environment of the client.

continued

BOX 2–1 continued
Parameters of the Holistic Health Model

Warmth, caring highly valued. The relationship facilitated by the practitioner can be healing in itself, as well as establishing an environment conducive to the client's healing. Demonstrations of warmth, caring, and empathy are essential to a facilitative relationship. Compassionate touch is valued. Supportive involvement is considered more important than professional neutrality.

Egalitarian relationship. Status differentials and hierarchical structure are minimized between practitioner and client, providing respect for the client's equality within the relationship.

Mutuality in interaction. The practitioner and client participate in a healing encounter that actively involves them both and through which both change and grow. Both are seen as interconnected in the process of healing; what affects one, affects the other.

Practitioner as role model. Practitioners are expected to practice what they preach, thereby demonstrating credibility as health proponents and offering a demonstration of the efficacy and worth of holistic lifestyle behaviors.

Cultural Diversity in Healing Practices
A value is placed on multicultural pluralism. A wide array of approaches is acceptable, in contrast to a more standardized approach in the allopathic model.

Alternative Worldview/Consciousness
Humanistic concerns, along with a transcendental, antimaterialistic, spiritual worldview, are core values. Altered states are considered to be a means of emotional and spiritual growth, and natural means (e.g., meditation) are used to attain these states. The evolution of a here-and-now awareness, personal authenticity, self-knowledge, and responsibility to self and others within a web of interconnectedness is valued. Encouragement of a diversity of healing practices and lifestyles, emphasis on cooperation and community, and a desire to live in harmony with nature are among the contributions that the holistic paradigm offers.

Source: Lowenberg, JS: Caring and Responsibility: The Crossroads between Holistic Practice and Traditional Medicine. University of Pennsylvania Press, Philadelphia, 1989, with permission.

Subtle Energy

What differentiates a living system from a nonliving system? What animates the body during life but is absent after death? Western science does not purport to have the answers to these questions, which go to the core of life's mysteries. Rather, they have been left to philosophers, spiritual teachers, and poets. A theory of a life-stimulating energetic force, called vitalism, is one that explains life and health as more than a result of a mechanistic physical or chemical reaction. Many alternative/complementary therapies attribute their effects to the action of a vital force, called by various names: "chi" in China, "ki" in Japan and Thailand, "prana" in India, "mana" in Hawaii, "vital elan" in Europe.

The vital force is considered universal energy, the basic constituent and source of all life. This life force is thought to energize and flow through the energy field in health and to be decreased or become blocked in illness. Health is restored by altering the intensity or the flow of the ill person's life force. Although research exists on subtle energy healing modalities, their mechanism remains unknown because they defy conventional explanation and because valid, reliable measurement techniques have yet to be developed.

The idea of an all-pervasive energy is ancient. Around 500 BC, Pythagoras described a luminous body reflecting a vital force that he named "vital energy." Paracelsus, a 16th-century alchemist, described the aura and its effects on states of health and disease.

Late 18th- and early 19th-century Europe saw the concept of vitalism emerge as a reaction against the mechanistic reductionism of the new scientific revolution.[27]

In 1775, Mesmer proposed that a subtle healing force pervades the universe in a fluid form he named "animal magnetism."[28] Practitioners of naturopathy and herbalism attribute healing to the force of nature (*vis medicatrix naturae*), a term coined by a Scottish professor named Cullen.[29] Homeopathy, anthroposophy, osteopathy, chiropractic, acupuncture, acupressure, and Therapeutic Touch are among the healing practices that attribute healing to subtle energy and vital force. Research studies reveal some clinical efficacy in each of these modalities, although the healing dynamic is not yet clear.

Rubik[30] proposed a theory of energetic information transfer to explain possible mechanisms of subtle energy healing. She suggested that subtle energies could be exchanged, perhaps through the interaction of the electromagnetic fields emitted by the central nervous systems of the healer and the person healed. Bioelectromagnetic research shows that certain types of nonionizing electromagnetic fields can stimulate the healing response, specifically in healing bone fractures, insomnia, and mood disorders.[31]

Other bioelectromagnetic hypotheses point to a unifying concept of bioinformation that interacts with endogenous electromagnetic fields or at the level of membrane receptors in the organism. Although these theories are as yet hypothetical, they build on new discoveries in quantum physics and suggest a framework in which to consider the role of human participation as part of science.[32]

The Placebo Response

The placebo response is an impressive demonstration of the mind's power to affect the body. The word *placebo,* which means "I please" in Latin, refers to the healing influence that can be attributed to a treatment through a person's belief in its efficacy. The placebo response is responsible for approximately one-third of symptom relief in pharmacological studies.[33] An estimated 80 percent of the symptoms brought to primary care practitioners are self-limiting; self-healing can occur without, or irrespective of, treatment.[34]

The significance of the placebo, or a medically inert substance or intervention, is such that it is the standard by which treatment effectiveness is measured and has become a research requirement in the scientific method. When a drug or treatment fails to demonstrate better results than the research placebo, disappointment in the lack of demonstrated effectiveness can overshadow the good news that people are capable of self-healing, aided only by the expectation that their health will improve. This good news does not sell health products, but it does offer a powerful tool in the healing process that all practitioners can use to their clients' benefit.

Understanding the placebo response sheds light on how beliefs can either enhance or inhibit reactions to treatment. Placebo research indicates that establishing a positive expectancy and confidence in the desired health outcome definitely enhances treatment effects. Practitioner beliefs and the nature of the therapeutic relationship also have an impact on treatment effectiveness: proponents who believe in the efficacy of the treatment, and who establish empathic, supportive relationships with clients, observe better treatment outcomes.

Clients can be taught to use their own consciousness to influence the course of illness and recovery. Positive intention, visual imagery, and relaxation techniques can be integrated into ongoing client care. All healing is self-healing, and the placebo response is a demonstration of this natural phenomenon. Healing is experienced in the individual as the result of a shift in the flow of life energy between the person and the environment toward wholeness.

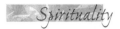 Spirituality

The experience of wellness or illness cannot be fully understood without the perspective of spirituality. Spirituality, which reflects the basic human need to experience connection to life and the life force, is the vital process of discovering meaning, purpose, fulfillment, and value in life. Spirituality is more than dogma or religion; rather, it is a source of power that supports active, intimate engagement in the process of living. One's spiritual health directly influences the healing process as well as how one copes with life's crises of illness, suffering, and loss. Spirituality is a way of being and experiencing that develops through awareness of a transcendent dimension characterized by certain identifiable values in regard to self, others, nature, life, and whatever one considers the "ultimate." A sense of disconnection from one's true source and from a meaningful orientation to one's life is a state of painful spiritual suffering.[35]

A great challenge facing the healing arts is to bring spirituality openly and consciously into clinical work. Peggy Burkhardt,[36] a major leader in the integration of spirituality in nursing, asserts that the first step to integrating spirituality in health care is acknowledging the presence of spirituality in all that we are and all that we do as human beings. Spirituality is addressed as much in our way of being with one another as in what we do for others. As we become more aware of and attend to the spiritual in all persons (including ourselves), we may find that we are integrating spirituality into health care as a way of seeing others and being in relationship with them.

The experience of illness may precipitate a state of spiritual distress in which the meaning one's life or one's relationship to God is challenged. Some clients may attribute their illness and suffering to their own lack of spiritual strength or to their perception of God, blaming themselves or a higher power for their painful experiences. Unfortunately, "pop" interpretations of the power of the mind and its connection to the body reinforce misplaced guilt and blame, which increases suffering and interferes with healing. Stephen Levine, who facilitates conscious healing during the dying process, addresses self-blame: "You are not responsible for your illness, you are responsible to your illness, to care for yourself and to understand what meaning this illness has in your life."[37]

A spiritual context of care allows us to answer crucial questions: Is it possible for a person with a chronic disease or a disability to be creative, happy, and healthy? Is there such a thing as a "good death"? Yes, if one's perspective goes beyond the view that health is a state of symptom-free comfort. A holistic view allows for the realities of the human condition—disease, disability, misfortune, aging, pain, and death—to be incorporated into the process of growth and transformation.

Larry Dossey, a pioneer in the field of holistic medicine, reminds us that Spirit cannot deteriorate like material health. "It does not need booster shots or annual exams. It simply is."[38] Both Levine and Dossey understand that disease is as much a part of health as wellness, and they value disease as grist for growth, an opportunity to deepen one's connection to self, others, and life, even unto death.

Pop holism, which equates health with unattainable bodily perfection, is not very different from the conventional paradigm that treats health as a commodity, numbs consciousness, denies death, and ignores the interconnectedness of all things. Joel Goldsmith, healer and spiritual teacher, said: "To seek healing means to desire to be rid of some ill, some pain, some discord, some malformation, or some disharmony. A reason for lack of healing is that very often we are seeking healing instead of wholeness.[39]

Holism is not just one more set of ideas and skills for self-improvement. A truly holistic perspective is the context in which a person can mature and thrive through illness, disability, deformity, or closeness to death, while maintaining a vital, creative connection to who one is and what one values. Holism goes beyond the pop culture questions "How should I look, feel, and think?" Instead, it helps to answer a more vital inquiry: "Who am I, and how do I choose to I live?"

Health requires self-transcendence, a state of being that encompasses the duality of wellness-illness, pleasure-pain, and fluctuating body and feeling states. Thomas Hora, founder of the spiritual school of metapsychiatry, described self-transcendence as the spiritual dimension. When conscious of the spiritual dimension as the ground of being, we find truth, love, joy, harmony, supreme intelligence, creativity, peace, assurance, healing, and freedom.[40] These are not feelings but rather capacities from which we express our integration as individuals within the larger web of creation. Gerber observed that our personal decisions and patterns of spiritual expression have impact on the global community in which we live:

> When individuals change, the whole planetary consciousness also changes. As above, so below. The evolving patterns of individual awareness can eventually produce larger changes in the global macrocosm. As increasing numbers of human beings begin to grow spiritually through the inner understanding of their illnesses and energy blockages, and as they begin to realize their true divine nature, they will also start to recognize that all people are subtly connected to each other and to the world around them.
>
> As the enlightened consciousness of this small segment of humanity grows, it will have a ripple effect upon the minds of the greater planetary whole. The rising tide of increased spiritual awareness will begin to affect larger numbers of people through a kind of cosmic resonance effect. When enough minds have changed to reach the critical threshold necessary to move the entire global consciousness to a new level of healing and awareness, we will have arrived at the New Age.[41]

Holistic Nursing

The emergence of the specialty of holistic nursing, along with the founding of the American Holistic Nurses Association in 1980, heralded the New Age of the profession of nursing. Based on the principles of holism, holistic nursing is a paradigm shift away from the biomedical model of individual care and cure toward an understanding of life as a unified, continuous, interrelated event as the context of human health. (See Box 2–2.)

BOX 2–2
Holistic Healing in Health Care and Nursing

Holistic nursing embraces all nursing that has enhancement of healing the whole person from birth to death as its goal. Holistic nursing recognizes that there are two views regarding holism: (1) that holism involves identifying the interrelationships of the biopsychosocial-spiritual dimensions of the person, recognizing that the whole is greater than the sum of its parts; and (2) that holism involves understanding the individual as a unitary whole in mutual process with the environment. Holistic nursing responds to both views, believing that the goals of nursing can be achieved within either framework.

The holistic nurse is an instrument of healing and a facilitator in the healing process. Holistic nurses honor the individual's subjective experience about health, health beliefs, and values. To become therapeutic partners with individuals, families, and communities, holistic nursing practice draws on nursing knowledge, theories, research, expertise, intuition, and creativity. Holistic nursing practice encourages peer review of professional practice in various clinical settings and integrates knowledge of current professional standards, laws, and regulations governing nursing practice.

Practicing holistic nursing requires nurses to integrate self-care, self-responsibility, spirituality, and reflection in their lives. This may lead nurses to greater awareness of the interconnectedness with self, others, nature, and God/life force/the absolute/the transcendent. This awareness may further enhance nurses' understanding of all individuals and their relationships to the human and global community and permit them to use this awareness to facilitate the healing process.

The philosophy of nursing is articulated by Lynn Keegan, a pioneer in holistic nursing practice and education:

Nursing is an art and science; its primary purpose is to assist others in finding the wholeness inherent within them. Wholeness can be present during high levels of wellness, during times of illness and disability, and during the process of dying. The concepts of holistic nursing are based on a broad eclectic academic background, a sensitive balance between art and science, analytical and intuitive skills, and the opportunity to choose from a wide variety of modalities to promote the harmonious balance of human energy systems.

Nurses have the unique ability to provide services that facilitate wholeness. The teaching/learning process enables nurses to help people assume personal responsibility for wellness. Within the purview of holistic nursing, disease and distress can be viewed as opportunities for increased awareness of the interconnectedness of body, mind and spirit."[42]

Theories of Holistic Nursing

The roots of holistic nursing emerged from the vision of Florence Nightingale. In her book *Notes on Nursing*, first published in 1860, Nightingale described the work of nursing as putting patients in the best condition for nature to act upon them, emphasizing touch and kindness along with the healing properties of the physical environment, including fresh air, sunlight, warmth, quiet, and cleanliness. Nightingale viewed people as multidimensional beings inseparable from their environment.[43] A more recent idea, based on the tenets of holism, is that the healing presence of the nurse is an integral part of the patient's environment[44,45] and that the mutual energetic process present in every caring act enhances the health outcome.

Three prominent nursing theorists have contributed to the evolution of holistic nursing: Martha Rogers, Margaret Newman, and Jean Watson. Rogers's theory, entitled the "Science of Unitary Human Beings," was first introduced in 1970 in her first publication, *An Introduction to the Theoretical Basis of Nursing*. Rogers was influenced by the philosophy and science of von Bertalanffy, Burr and Northrup, and Einstein. She viewed nursing as an evolving study of pandimensional human and environmental energy fields. Human beings are irreducible, unified energy fields and evolve irreversibly and unilaterally across space and time. The environmental energy field is in constant and meaningful interaction with the human energy field.

Newman, a student of Rogers, first published her theory in her book *Health as Expanding Consciousness* in 1994. She continues to develop her understanding of the "mutuality of interaction between nurse and client; uniqueness and wholeness of pattern in each client situation; and movement of the life process toward higher consciousness."[46]

Watson originated the theory called "Human Science and Human Care."[47] She proposes assumptions about the science of caring and identifies primary factors of caring that comprise the framework of her theory. Watson values what she calls "authentic presencing," which facilitates the caring moment between the nurse and the client. Watson includes the human spirit or soul in the formulation of her nursing theory. These three theorists propose core values of holism: nurse–client–environment interconnectedness, consciousness as a force, and the primacy of the healing relationship. At its best, holistic nursing offers heart-centered care, which provides an opportunity for the nurse, the health-care team, the client, and significant others to participate in the caring moment. The holistic nurse values client input and experience, acknowledging that each individual knows him- or herself best.

The nurse is also encouraged to value and use intuition as part of assessment, intervention, and evaluation of client care. Holistic nursing care is seen as a dynamic process that allows for individuality, creativity, and respect for the rhythms of life.

BOX 2–3
Case Study

Bonnie, certified as a holistic nurse, was caring for Carlos, who was admitted to the hospital with acute peritonitis and was in a semiconscious state. Prior to entering his room, she paused, took a deep breath, and held the intention of being fully present. Closing the curtains behind her to ensure privacy, she consciously greeted him in a respectful manner. She touched his arm lightly to make her presence known and told him the purpose of her visit. As with any of her clients, she was alert, calm, and caring. She reassured him of being safe and well cared for, knowing the nature of an innately whole and loving universe. His breathing eased. She noticed her own had done the same. Although her total time in the room was only a few minutes, she had made a profound connection with her patient.

Bonnie's ability to care for Carlos in this manner is not based on a particular dogma or religion. In a respectful, artful way, Bonnie simply acknowledges the science that substantiates spiritual wholeness. She facilitates a sacred healing environment in this manner.

In addition to giving nursing care to her clients, Bonnie is actively learning about her community's bioregion—the quality of its food supply, air, and water. She recognizes that the spiritual longing humans feel seems to be deeply rooted in knowledge that the natural world's beauty, pathos, and sustainability are integral to our total health. Her political presence as a holistic nurse is being felt as she advocates for awareness of the importance of this to her community's health.

Bonnie extends her holistic nursing knowledge by using her position in the community to teach, guide, and advocate for this vital relationship among self, community, and nature through offering a course on Ecospirituality and Human Health at the local community college. Bonnie's awareness of the limitations of viewing human health as separate from the health of the planet provides an important voice in the evolution of her community's consciousness. She knowingly participates in the opportunity to evolve to a higher state of order and harmony.

Bonnie and Lorraine, another holistic nurse, support each other's practices. Lorraine has extended her therapeutic use of massage to pediatric patients. She has worked with administrators at her community hospital to implement the use of complementary and integrative strategies. Both nurses feel strongly that the nursing profession needs to honor the individual strengths and preferred methods of each nurse. They serve as consultants to their state board of registration in nursing, developing policies to allow nurses the freedom to offer expanded services.

Ensuring that the public has access to a wealth of quality healing arts is an important focus for nurses during this transitional period in health care. Bonnie and Lorraine's involvement illustrates that nurses are in a powerful position to influence the direction of health care. Integrating ancient wisdom and state-of-the-art scientific discoveries is an ongoing responsibility of the profession to which holistic nurses are committed.

Symptoms are respected as body messages, and new patterns of etiology invite discovery. The crisis of disease is honored and perceived as an opportunity for healing and growth. (See Box 2–3.)

Related Research

Articles on the nature and the efficacy of holistic nursing are most frequently narrative in nature, whereas studies that quantify knowledge of this specialty are few.[48] Nurses tell poignant stories of the effects of conscious attendance to presence and the human spirit. Burkhardt[49] recognized the need for spiritual care in nursing practice. Hines[50] identified attributes associated with healing presence. McKivergin and Daubenmire[51] discussed presence as integral to healing. Andrews[52] described the relationship between feelings of connection and both personal and global health promotion. Ercums, Curtis, and DeMilley[53] relate how nurses bring their "ibeingness" into healing actions and how client receptivity is enhanced.

TABLE 2–2   **Interventions Most Frequently Used in Holistic Nursing Practice***

Acupressure	Healing presence	Play therapy
Aromatherapy	Healing touch modalities	Prayer
Art therapy	Holistic self-assessments	Reflexology
Biofeedback	Humor and laughter	Relaxation modalities
Cognitive therapy	Journaling	Self-care
Intervention counseling†	Masssage	Self-reflection
Exercise and movement	Music and sound therapy	Therapeutic Touch
Guided imagery	Nutrition counseling	Weight management

*See Dossey, B, et al: Evolving a blueprint for certification: Inventory of professional activities and knowlege of a holistic nurse. J Hol Nur 16:33–66, 1998.

†Used in circumstances of addictions, grief, relationship issues, unhealthy environments, abuse and violence, spiritual issues, support groups, wellness promotion, and lifestyle needs.

Holistic nursing is a specific philosophical orientation to the scientific art of caring. In addition to a curriculum focused on the principles of holism, holistic nurses learn about the role of complementary/alternative therapies in health and healing, and many extend their learning beyond their basic nursing education to become certified as holistic nurses. Some achieve additional training in various complementary/alternative modalities to use within their clinical practice.[54–62] Dossey and colleagues[63] identified the most frequently used modalities in holistic nursing practice. (See Table 2–2.) Many nurses also refer clients to other professionals for integrative care if they themselves do not practice a healing modality that a client needs or requests.

The scientific artistry of holistic nursing involves respectfully meeting a person in the moment and understanding which roles and skills are required while consciously basing care in a universal, unitary worldview. Holistic nurses may serve as guides, helpers, advocates, interpreters, managers, monitors, and therapists. In all cases, the holistic nurse is aware of a universe of transforming energy where the web of life holds a conscious potential for healing, growth, and evolution.

Nursing has a rich tradition of compassion and care, with its relational, spiritual, and environmental orientation, and has earned the public's trust like no other profession. Nursing has entered a new era with the evolution of holistic nursing practice, with its incorporation of the holistic paradigm within this specialty focus. Holistic practitioners hold the vision of health that will continue to transform client care, the means with which to restore wholeness to our beleaguered ecosystem, and the faith that healing possibilities are infinite.

RESOURCES

American Holistic Nurses Association
2773 E. Lakin Ave., Suite # 2
Flagstaff, AZ 86003-2130
Phone: (800) 278-2462
http://www.ahna.org

Institute of Rogerian Scholars
437 Twin Bay Dr.
Pensacola, FL 32534
Phone: (800) 985-9793

Seeds and Bridges, Incorporated
The Center for Holistic Nursing Education
P.O. Box 1243
Amherst, MA 01004-1243
Phone: (877) 917-3337
http://www.seedsandbridges.com

References

1. Monte, T: World Medicine. JP Tarcher, Los Angeles, 1993, p 318.
2. Quote appeared in New York Times, Letter to Editor, March 29, 1972.
3. Initiates, T: The Kybalion: A Study of Hermetic Philosophy of Ancient Egypt and Greece. Yogi Publication Society, Chicago, 1912, p 137.
4. Sheldrake, R: Rebirth of Nature: The Greening of Science and God. Park Street Press, Rochester, Vt., 1991, p 89.
5. Quoted in Gerber, R: Vibrational Medicine: New Choices for Healing Ourselves. Bear & Company, Santa Fe, 1988, p 435.
6. Keck, RL: Sacred Eyes. Synergy Associates, Boulder, 1992, p 164.
7. Bohm, D: Wholeness and the Implicate Order. Routledge, New York, 1980, p 2.
8. Initiates: The Kybalion, p 113.
9. Wilber, K (ed): The Holographic Paradigm and Other Paradoxes. Shambhala, Boston, 1985, p 5.
10. Initiates: The Kybalion, p 65.
11. Interview with David Bohm. New Age Journal, September/October 1989, p 110.
12. Quoted in Keck: Sacred Eyes, p 153.
13. Swimme, B: The Universe is a Green Dragon. Bear & Company, Santa Fe, 1984, p 45.
14. Keck: Sacred Eyes, p 153.
15. Brennan, BA: Hands of Light: A Guide to Healing through the Human Energy Field. Bantam, New York, 1987.
16. Bendit, L J, and Bendit, PD: The Etheric Body of Man: The Bridge of Consciousness. Quest. Wheaton, Ill., 1989.
17. Kunz, D (ed): Spiritual Healing: Doctors Examine Therapeutic Touch and Other Holistic Treatments. Quest, Wheaton, Ill., 1995.
18. Vithoulkas, G: The Science of Homeopathy. Grove Weidenfield, New York, 1980, p 40.
19. Wilber, K, Engler, J, and Brown, DP: Transformations of Consciousness: Conventional and Contemplative Perspectives on Development. Shambhala, Boston, 1986, p 7.
20. Gerber: Vibrational Medicine, p 470.
21. Bendit, LJ: The Spirit in Health and Disease. In Kunz: Spiritual Healing, p 93.
22. Newman, MA: Health as Expanding Consciousness. Mosby, St. Louis, 1994, p 4.
23. Newman, MA: The rhythm of relating in a paradigm of wholeness. Image: Journal of Nursing Scholarship 31:227, 1999.
24. Rubin, BD, and Kim, JY (eds): General Systems Theory and Huma Communication. Haydon Book Company, Rochelle Park, Ill., 1975, p 8.
25. Dossey, B: Keynote address at: Holistic Nursing Conference; New York University; New York; March 18, 1998.
26. Berry, W: Another Turn of the Crank. Counterpoint, Washington, D.C., 1995.
27. Lain Entralgo, P: Sensualism and vitalism in Bichat's *Anatomie Generale*. Jl Hist Med 3:29, 1948.
28. Ellenberger, HF: The Discovery of the Unconscious. Basic Books, New York,1970, p 55.
29. Kaptchuk, TJ: Historical context of the concept of vitalism in complementary and alternative medicines. In Micozzi, MS (ed): Foundations of Complementary and Alternative Medicine. Churchill Livingstone, New York, 1996, p 35.
30. Rubik, B: Energy medicine and the unifying concept of information. Altern Ther Health Med 1:34, 1995.
31. Rubik, B, et al: In J Swyers et al: Expanding Medical Horizons: Report to NIH on the Status of Alternative Medicine. U.S. Government Printing Office, Washington D.C., 1996.
32. Bendit: The Spirit in Health and Disease, p 93.

33. Ingelfinger, F: Medicine: Meritorious or meritricious? Science 200:942, 1978.
34. Benser, H, and McCallio, DJ, Jr: Angina pectoris and the placebo effect. N Eng J Med 300:424, 1979.
35. Gillman, J, et al: Pastoral care in a critical care setting. Critical Care Nursing Quarterly 19:10, 1996.
36. Burkhardt, MA: Reintegrating spirituality into health care. Altern Ther Health Med 4:56, 1998.
37. Levine, S: Healing into Life and Death. Doubleday, New York, 1984, p 78.
38. Dossey, L: Beyond Illness: Discovering the Experience of Health. Doubleday, New York, 1985, p 87.
39. Goldsmith, J: Living between Two Worlds. Harper & Row, New York, p 8.
40. Hora, T: Beyond the Dream: Awakening to Reality. Crossroads, New York, 1996, p 37.
41. Gerber: Vibrational Medicine, p 468.
42. Keegan, L: Holistic nursing: A revolutionary approach to improved patient care. Holistic Nursing Update 1:4, 2000.
43. Nightingale, F: Notes on Nursing. Dover, New York, 1989. (Original work published 1860)
44. Osterman, P, and Schwartz-Barcott, D: Presence: Four ways of being there. Nursing Forum 13:28, 1996.
45. Bright, MA: Centering: The healing path to healing presence. Alt Health Pract 1:191, 1995.
46. Newman, M: Experiencing the whole. Advances in Nursing Science 20:35, 1997.
47. Watson, J: Nursing: Human Science and Human Care. National League for Nursing, New York, 1988.
48. Montgomery, CL: The care-giving relationship: Paradoxical and transcendent aspects. Alternative Therapies 2:52, 1996.
49. Burkhardt, M: Spirituality: An analysis of the concept. Holistic Nursing Practice 3:69, 1989.
50. Hines, DR: Presence: Discovering the artistry in relating. Journal of Holistic Nursing 10:294, 1992.
51. McKivergin, M, and Daubenmire, MJ: The healing process of presence. Journal of Holistic Nursing 12:65, 1994.
52. Andrews, S: Promoting a sense of connectedness among individuals by scientifically demonstrating the existence of planetary consciousness? Alternative Therapies 2:39, 1996.
53. Ercums, J, Curtis, FR, and DeMilley, M: Nursing's caring paradigm: A story of mutuality and transcendent healing. Alternative and Complementary Therapies 4:68, 1998.
54. Berg, JA, et al: Integrative therapies in primary care practice. Journal of the American Academy of Nurse Practitioners 10:541, 1998.
55. Ching, M: Complementary therapies: Research, education, and practice in nursing. Contemporary Nurse 7:173, 1998.
56. Cole, A, and Shanley, E: Complementary therapies as a means of developing the scope of professional nursing practice. J Adv Nurs 27:1171, 1998.
57. Engebretson, J: Alternative and complementary healing: Implications for nursing. J Prof Nurs 15:314, 1999.
58. Eresser, S J: Complementary therapies and nursing research: Issues and practicalities. Complementary Therapies in Nurse Midwifery 1:44, 1995.
59. Raisler, J: Alternative healing in nurse-midwifery practice. J Nurse Midwifery 44:310, 1999.
60. Taylor, AG: A nurse-directed interdisciplinary center for the study of complementary therapies. Journal of Emergency Nursing 24:486, 1998.
61. Bauer, SM: Use of complementary therapies in cancer patients receiving chemotherapy. Developments in Supportive Cancer Care 1:11, 1996.
62. Hayes, KM, and Alexander, IM: Alternative therapies and nurse practitioners: Knowledge, professional experience, and personal use. Holistic Nursing Practice 14:49, 2000.
63. Dossey, B, et al: Evolving a blueprint for certification: Inventory of professional activities and knowledge of a holistic nurse. Journal of Holistic Nursing 16:33, 1998.

CHAPTER 3

The Bioenergetic Basis of Health

Philip M. Helfaer and Mary Anne Bright

Philip M. Helfaer, PhD, MA, has practiced bioenergetic analysis for 30 years and teaches in the United States, Norway, and Israel as a member of the faculty of the International Institute for Bioenergetic Analysis. After receiving degrees in philosophy and clinical psychology, Helfaer became a psychotherapist. He has written Sex and Self-Respect: The Quest for Personal Fulfillment.

Mary Anne Bright, RN, CS, EdD, the editor of this book, is an associate professor at the University of Massachusetts–Amherst School of Nursing. She teaches courses in holistic health and psychiatric-mental health nursing, conducts research on Therapeutic Touch, and is a member of the International Institute of Bioenergetic Analysis and of the American Holistic Nurses Association.

What Is Bioenergetic Analysis?

Many mainstream and alternative philosophies today consider the mind, body, and spirit of a person to be an integrated unity. In bioenergetic analysis, also called "bioenergetics," the integration of these three expressions of the person is understood to be based in the biological energies of the body. As a discipline, bioenergetic analysis offers both a theoretical understanding of this view and a clinical application. This chapter describes some of the energetic processes of the body and why they are important for understanding health.

As a first insight into bioenergetic analysis, consider its application in therapy. Conventional psychotherapy focuses on the psyche. This means, in essence, that the patient talks and the therapist listens and responds verbally. In bioenergetic analysis, the body is brought directly into the therapeutic activity. The bioenergetic therapist develops an understanding of the patient by looking at the patient's body as well as by listening to the patient. Moreover, the bioenergetic analyst works directly with the body by observing and drawing conclusions from its overall form and appearance, breathing patterns, movements, and deep muscular tensions. The therapist also supports emotional expression through bodily expression. For example, if a client reports feeling choked up with sadness, the bioenergetic therapist will guide him or her to express that sadness by crying.

Like traditional psychotherapy, bioenergetic analysis includes explorations of the client's past, dreams, associations, and current behavior, as well as the relationship between the client and the therapist. However, the somatic work in bioenergetics not only deepens and facilitates these explorations, it also explores the energetic, biological disturbance underlying them.

TABLE 3–1   What Is Health?

Understanding the biological basis of these capacities is the distinctive feature of bioenergetic analysis:
- The capacity for free and creative expression of emotion
- Freedom from crippling guilt, shame, and humiliation and the capacity for pleasure
- The ability to relate in a realistic and productive way with others
- The capacity for love and sexual fulfillment
- The capacity for productive work

Sigmund Freud, the founder of psychoanalysis, and his early students observed and identified specific capacities of a healthy person. Bioenergetic analysis takes the psychoanalytic process further. By examining the biological basis of those capacities, the therapist helps the client to experience and express feelings of which he or she is not aware. For example, the therapist may help mobilize a patient's suppressed anger by encouraging him or her to hit a pillow or kick a bed while verbally expressing angry feelings. Grief and other painful feelings are also controlled in the body by muscular tension and respiratory constriction. When the tensions are released through appropriate expressive movement, the client may be able to let go into deep crying, which is healing.

The question of how to understand, or even what constitutes, change, is an enduring one for therapists of all persuasions. We will not resolve the problem now, but, consider that the events of any therapy, verbal or bioenergetic, can be understood as falling in three large domains: the intrapsychic, the interpersonal, and the somatic. Changes occurring in the course of therapy can also be looked at as various kinds of events falling into these three domains. There are various ways to conceptualize the events of these domains, but these three domains will contain all events. Surely, we must include in our search for an understanding of the nature of change those changes, which actually occur in the aliveness of the tissues as we understand and can observe it from the energetic point of view. I believe the latter is a critical key to understanding the nature of change in therapy, since the energetic process underlies changes in the interpersonal domain and the intrapsychic domain.

To the bioenergetic analyst, an individual's expressive movements and many other bodily qualities reveal the person and the imprint of early development as deeply as do spoken words. Change through bioenergetic therapy is based on actual changes in bodily functioning. For example, improvement in health will be reflected in fuller breathing, less tension, more free energy, more graceful movement, and an increased capacity for pleasure. (See Table 3–1.)

Principles of Energetic Functioning

When a patient appears in the office of a bioenergetic practitioner, the practitioner looks, listens, and begins to gain an understanding of the underlying energetic problem or disturbance. Following is a discussion of a few of the basic principles of bioenergetic analysis.

Armor

Children commonly experience fear in their relations with adults, especially their parents, who are bigger, more developed, and frequently willing to use their superior strength to establish power and control. In addition, anger, threats, punishments, shaming, humiliation, rejection, sexual inappropriateness, and abandonment—to mention only a few things to which they may be subjected—are all frightening to children.

When children are frightened by their parents, they have a tendency to hold their breath, suck in their gut, tighten the musculature of their pelvic floor, and pull up in their shoulders. This autonomically organized pattern of activation and tension affects virtually the whole musculature and all the inner organs. If the child subsequently learns to express anger and cry freely, the tension will be discharged. Anger and crying are natural and normal release mechanisms for that kind of tension.

What happens when children are not free to release their tension by expressing anger and by crying? The tension is held and, through chronic activation of the sympathetic nervous system, remains as a pattern of muscular holding to which the body must adapt. This condition, bioenergetically termed a "contraction," is contrasted with a state of "expansion," which produces pleasurable feeling. Such contractions commonly persist into adulthood.

In childhood, a variety of symptoms can emerge from this form of chronic stress: nightmares, enuresis, school phobia, various somatic symptoms such as headaches and stomachaches, depression, and antisocial behaviors. In adulthood, the sexual component of the chronic contraction may be seen in a tightly constricted, held, or deadened pelvis. Associated with the pelvic holding may be limitations on sexual feeling and fulfillment, difficulties in establishing an enduring love relationship, shame, and guilt. All such patterns of muscular tension, apparent to the trained observer, are called "blocks," "muscular attitudes," or "armor."

These various types of muscular tensions form an integrated whole and can be quite complex. For example, deeply held turmoil, which is expressed as overactivation of a person's autonomic nervous system and armored defense patterns, often underlies depressive underactivation. The inner experience engendered by strong, long-lasting contractions is always some form of misery.

These complex muscular blocks consume enormous amounts of energy that the person might otherwise use for a more fulfilling life. The contractions causing blocked energy and the blocked energy itself (stasis) are agents harmful to the person and the body. Relative freedom from stasis and chronic contraction is a bioenergetic criterion of health. Bioenergetic analysis directly addresses the contractions with the goal of releasing the tension, freeing the trapped energy, and allowing the individual to find his or her own positive movement. The changes that take place are both bodily and psychological. (See Box 3–1.)

Sexuality

Bioenergetics has its origins in the study of sexuality. Freud established that a person's capacity for sexual love is one of the strongest indicators of his or her health. He also demonstrated that traumas, developmental conflicts, and violations of sexuality in childhood are primary underlying causes of emotional and relational difficulties in adult life (neurosis). Now, it is also known that whenever there is a disturbance in sexuality, there is a disturbance in self-respect. Developmentally, sexuality and self-respect are intertwined functions, each developing along with the other. Sexuality and self-respect[1] are thus two key avenues for exploration in bioenergetic analysis.

The "self" in bioenergetics is not a psychological entity, but a physical one. The body is the self. Self-respect, then, means to honor, accept, and live in accordance with one's own body, with its states and feelings—especially sexual feeling, needs, choices, and the individual's sense of him- or herself as a man or woman.

Wilhelm Reich advanced Freud's fundamental discoveries about sexuality. Long before modern sex research, Reich undertook serious experimental and theoretical investigations into the nature of orgasm, its various disturbances, and the meaning of orgasm for the life of the person and the health of the body. Reich showed that the core of neurosis is a specific kind of sexual dysfunction, which he called orgastic impotence.[2] Orgastic

BOX 3–1

The Roots

Bioenergetics has its origins in the pioneering work of Wilhelm Reich[1-3] (1897–1957), who advanced the psychoanalytic study of the self to a bioenergetic conception of health based on the functioning of the whole organism. A psychoanalyst and student of Freud, Reich was the first to work systematically with the body and respiration in the psychoanalytic process. He developed both a clinical technique for the treatment of neurosis involving the whole organism and a remarkable theory based on clinical observation of the energetic functioning of the person.

Alexander Lowen[4] (b. 1910) founded the International Institute for Bioenergetic Analysis in 1956. He had been Reich's student when Reich came to America shortly after the outbreak of World War II. Lowen developed Reich's therapy through numerous physical and analytic techniques. Breaking with the European psychoanalytic tradition, he got people up off the couch and onto their feet during the therapeutic process.

REFERENCES

1. Reich, W: Character Analysis. Farrar, Straus & Giroux, New York, 1972. (Original work published 1945)
2. Reich, W: The Function of the Orgasm. Farrar, Straus & Giroux, New York, 1973. (Original work published 1968)
3. Sharaf, M: Fury on Earth: A Biography of Wilhelm Reich. St. Martin's/Marek, New York, 1983.
4. Lowen, A: Bioenergetics. Penguin, New York, 1976.

impotence refers to many disturbances, dissatisfactions, and frustrations of sexual experience, not only male impotence. A man might be said to suffer orgastic impotence, for example, if he was able to have an erection and intercourse but was unable to establish a lasting love relationship with a partner, if he routinely suffered from diminished desire or incomplete orgasm, or if he treated his partner with a lack of respect. A woman might be considered orgastically impotent, for example, if reaching orgasm with her partner is a difficult struggle. Unfortunately, these and many other similar disturbances are common. It is important to recognize these sexual frustrations, to know that deeper fulfillment is possible, and to understand that they have a bioenergetic basis in the body.

Orgastic potency, on the other hand, is the capacity to experience a full and gratifying orgasm in the sexual embrace with a loved partner. Reich demonstrated that this capacity is an essential criterion of health. Orgastic potency reflects a free-flowing, unobstructed energetic state, the essence of a healthy body.

Sexual response can be broken down into a series of stages or capacities. (See Table 3–2.) A healthy person has the biological capacity for each stage of sexual response within the context of a loving relationship with another person. When sexual love is blocked, an

TABLE 3–2   Capacities for a Healthy Sexual Response

- The capacity for generating free energy (beyond that required for survival)
- The capacity for allowing that energy to become focused in sexual feelings, in yearnings for a loved partner, and in the buildup of tension
- The capacity to build the genital, sexual charge in love making with another
- The capacity for genital intercourse in which the genitals join and move together, further building the charge toward orgasm
- The capacity to surrender fully to the feelings, experience, and involuntary movements of orgasm, which includes:
  - the capacity to be overwhelmed by orgasm
  - the capacity for allowing the refreshment and relaxation that is the aftermath
- The capacity for maintaining the loving feeling and bond with the partner after sexual intercourse

energetic stasis results. Over the long term, sexual stasis throws the person back into the sexual conflicts of childhood, and symptoms appear that express the unfinished experiences of childhood. This is a bodily, bioenergetic process, not simply a psychological one. Stasis engenders misery and can lead to depression. It may also be the initiating factor in certain other illnesses.

Armoring is the underlying basis for orgastic impotence. Indeed, one major function of armor is to limit sexual feeling and expressiveness. As a therapy, bioenergetic analysis focuses on sexuality and helps the individual soften the armoring. Softening armor allows a freer movement of energy in the body, and this heightens the capacities for the several stages of sexual response. To understand more deeply the nature of armoring and the subtleties of its interference with sexuality, we need to consider the following sections on the rhythm of life and the bioenergetic nature of "character."

Health and the Rhythm of Life

The most distinctive observable feature of living tissue is that it is in constant motion. The heart beats, the breath goes in and out, and peristaltic waves move through the intestines. Under a microscope, single-celled organisms display a variety of fascinating movements: flowing, streaming, pulsating. These rhythmic movements, called pulsations or organismic movement in bioenergetics, are not only intrinsic to life, they are truly the rhythm of life. It could be said that living tissue moves because it is alive, but it would be equally true to say that the movements we observe are life itself. Dead tissue does not move.

There are two fundamental aspects to the biology of organismic movement that are the foundations of our experience of ourselves and of our health and that bioenergetics addresses. The first aspect is the expansion and contraction of tissue along with the cyclic wave between the expansion and contraction, called pulsation. The second aspect is the fact that living tissue produces excess energy, charging itself and then releasing the excess energy in discharge. The management of charge and discharge defines the energetic economy of the organism.

Pulsation is the fundamental beat of the rhythm of life. The basic emotions—anger, fear, grief, excitement, and pleasure—consist of patterns of expansion and contraction. Expansion, the basis of pleasure, is mediated by the parasympathetic branch of the autonomic nervous system. Contraction, the basis of anxiety, is mediated by the sympathetic branch, the branch pertaining to preparing the body for fight or flight. In a pleasurable state, we feel expansive and typically move out into the world. In an anxious state, we contract and pull into ourselves, away from the world.

The organism's energy economy is regulated through the ongoing creation and discharge of energy. In our adult lives, a fulfilling sexual love relationship offers the best and primary vehicle for that regulation through the regular, safe, and pleasurable expression of orgasm. The regulating function of charge and discharge can be looked at in broader terms, too. A healthy buildup and discharge of energy is possible through creative, pleasurable, and positive movement of many kinds found in work, the home, and virtually any area of life.

The bioenergetic basis of health is (1) the body's fundamental capacity for free pulsation and (2) the capacity for building a charge of excess energy and determining its discharge. Whatever limits pulsation, charge, and discharge limits health. When they are chronically limited, so is health.

Tissue that is pulsatory is said to have motility, the capacity to produce, hold, and allow the movement of energy. Armoring reduces motility. Softening armor increases motility and thus enhances the capacity for life itself. This is the goal of bioenergetics.

The bioenergetic process of heightening energy and motility requires working with an individual's character and grounding, discussed in the following two sections.

BOX 3–2
Bioenergetic Disturbances in Everyday Living

In daily life, without thinking twice about it, everyone actually makes bioenergetic observations of just the sort discussed in this chapter. It is easy to distinguish a tense person from a relaxed one, for example. Other characteristics of energetic functioning are also readily observable, and interested students might be surprised by what they learn when they start to practice making bioenergetic observations. We all know that a lively, healthy person has an energetic sparkle, a depressed one has little energy and a dull quality, and a withdrawn one has an unapproachable look associated with having little energy available for contact with the world. There are also patterns of over- and underactivation that can be distinguished on observation. Anxiety, turmoil, torment, obsessive-compulsive hesitancy, and overactivity are all patterns of overactivation that the individual has been unable to soothe or calm down.

Character

When we think of anyone we know well, we can visualize his or her particular way of moving, talking, or going about a task. In bioenergetics, this pattern of expression is called "character," short for "characteristic behavior." (See Box 3–2.) Character is the cumulative result of armoring that developed in childhood. It is a psychosomatic concept, because it includes psychological and somatic aspects. It is a concept that is obvious and yet also difficult to grasp.

In adults, pulsation and the healthy charge-discharge function of sex and life activity may be limited by character. Character is an actual modification of the person's biology and of the self at the level of pulsation. It develops in childhood as an adaptational necessity; it is a survival strategy. It is the outgrowth of the child's need to adapt to a maturational environment that is—in greater or lesser measure—negative, disrespectful, depriving, or traumatic in any of a number of possible ways. Character is difficult to change because it is embedded in the basic way the body becomes organized, and this organization is sustained by guilt, shame, humiliation, fear, and rage.

Bioenergetic analysis addresses the subtleties of character on the somatic and psychological levels. Individual character is, in fact, remarkably complex, and each individual is unique, making the exploration of character alternately fascinating and frustrating. The therapeutic issue, again, is softening the character to allow for greater expansion and charge and discharge.

Grounding

When we refer to "a grounded person," we usually mean someone who is "in touch with reality," an individual who has his or her "feet on the ground." This concept means that there is an energetic pulsation between the head and the feet such that there is a unified connection, vertically, throughout the whole body.

Character, with its chronic muscular holding patterns, distorts or breaks up the unification and disrupts one's connection with the ground and with reality. If you observe people as they walk and move, you can—even without special training—note differences having to do with grounding and character. Graceful movement will stand out, leaving an impression of beauty.

Movement is graceful when it is grounded. It requires a freely moving pelvis, and that is based on a sense of acceptance of and connection with the genitals. Gracefulness, in fact, is a criterion for health.[3] Grace is a function of free pulsation, healthy energy economy, freedom from character restrictions, and freedom from guilt and shame. This is the bioenergetic basis of health. It allows the person to have whatever joy, happiness, and fulfillment that life might bring among the stresses, hardships, and sorrows that are our common lot. Grounding, along with sexuality and self-respect, is another focus of

BOX 3–3
Bioenergetic Exercises

Bioenergetic exercises[1] are designed to relieve ourselves of the chronic stress of character armoring. They enhance respiration, foster the breakdown and release of tension, encourage the release of suppressed emotion, and enhance the capacity for the buildup of energy. When used regularly over a long period of time, they can produce changes on a deep bodily level, which are reflected in an individual's increased capacity to function in work, love, and interpersonal relationships.

Patients perform the exercises during each therapeutic session, in group exercise classes, and at home. All bioenergetic exercises involve respiration, the basic pulsation of the whole body. The production and utilization of energy depends on unrestricted and deep respiration. The expression of emotion also depends on unrestricted respiration. The primary way to inhibit feeling is to inhibit respiration. "Kicking" and "blanket roll" work directly with respiration.

Kicking

Lie on a bed and kick 20, 50, 100, up to 200 times. Each kick counts as one. Keep the leg straight and the ankle loose, allowing the foot to flop or snap, and bring the foot high up perpendicular to the bed. This exercise has healthy benefits on different levels. It gets the respiration going. It draws energy down into the feet, legs, and pelvis. In addition, and not to be dismissed lightly, it provides the opportunity to express whatever one has a "kick"—that is, a complaint—about or is angry about. It is a good tension reliever.

Blanket Roll

To make a blanket roll, an old wool blanket can be folded lengthwise into quarters and rolled up around anything firm and cylindrical, such as a roll of newspapers and magazines held firm by duct tape. Place the roll on the floor and lie on it so that the roll is right under the shoulder blades. Stretch the arms back. Notice the stretching and opening of the chest. Now allow an easy sound to emerge from the throat. Let the sound go all the way "to the bottom of the barrel." Then allow a crying sound to emerge from the throat, like a "hah-hah-hah" sound, so that the diaphragm pulsates. Experiment with this and its effects on breathing and, indeed, allowing crying to emerge. Crying is always healing.

Grounding

A third exercise is for grounding. Stand with feet about a foot apart. Make sure that your feet are parallel with each other, or perhaps have the toes pointed slightly pointed inward. Soften the knees, belly, shoulders, and jaw, and allow yourself to bend forward, rolling over one vertebra at a time, until your fingers touch the floor. Keep the knees soft and the legs not quite straight. Perhaps you will have to stretch a bit behind the knees. Breathe. Hold the position for a few minutes until you notice that there is a slight tremor, or "vibration," in the legs. Roll back up slowly. Feel your feet on the floor or ground throughout.

REFERENCES

1. Lowen, A, and Lowen, L: The Way to Vibrant Health: A Manual of Bioenergetic Exercises. Harper Colophon, New York, 1977.

bioenergetic therapy in which specific work is directed to fostering the energetic contact with the ground. Some of this work is done using the bioenergetic exercises discussed in Box 3–3.

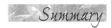 *Summary*

Bioenergetic analysis is a relatively new discipline that offers unique contributions to the understanding of healthy functioning and the maintenance and restoration of health. Through clinical practice and observation, bioenergetics has fostered the understanding of the basic energetic processes of the human organism. The bioenergetic basis of health is the body's fundamental capacity for free pulsation, the building up and discharging of

TABLE 3–3   Bioenergetic Criteria for Health

- Self-respect
- Grounding; energetic connection between feet and ground
- Graceful movement
- Orgastic potency
- Unrestricted respiration
- Freedom from chronic muscular tension, armoring, and character restriction to allow for full pulsatory capacity and a strong capacity for the charge-discharge function
- Energetic aliveness and the capacity for enjoying and expressing it

energy. Whatever limits pulsation limits health. From the understanding of the energetic processes of the body, bioenergetics has evolved these and other specific criteria establish a paradigm or definition of the nature of health. (See Table 3–3.)

In its clinical application, bioenergetics describes the developmental and post-traumatic disturbances of the body's energetic functioning. As a treatment, bioenergetics has the goal of relieving the body of the chronic stress of armoring and character disturbances. Through analytic and bodily techniques it heightens the energetic aliveness of the body by increasing the production of energy through fuller respiration. With the heightening of motility and the resolution of character issues, the individual may be freer to find his or her own positive, life-affirming movement in the world. Along with these developments, bioenergetics fosters the development of the capacity for joy, aliveness based in the fullness of feelings, and grace in living.

Every individual seeks fulfillment in love and a sense of freedom and dignity. Bioenergetic therapy focuses on the key related functions of sex and self-respect and the developmental relation between them. Out of a deep respect for the central life function of sex, the bioenergetic therapist takes seriously and respectfully the deep longings each person has for sexual fulfillment.

Even in a permissive society most people still struggle with shame, guilt, inhibition, and frustration; in addition, sexual abuse and emotional abuse affecting sexuality are still prevalent. For these common conditions, bioenergetics offers freeing work with the body guided by an understanding of energetic and developmental processes. At the same time, bioenergetics specifically addresses the development of self-respect at the deepest organismic level and supports the development of a healthy self-regulation that can extend into all areas of life.

RESOURCES

International Institute for Bioenergetic Analysis
1 Post Road
Fairfield, CT 06430
Phone: (203) 319-0521
Fax: (203) 319-0523
E-mail: iibanet@aol.com

REFERENCES

1. Helfaer, PM: Sex and Self-Respect: The Quest for Personal Fulfillment. Praeger, Westport, Conn., 1998.
2. Reich, W: The Function of the Orgasm. Farrar, Straus & Giroux, New York, 1973, ch 4. (Original work published 1968)
3. Lowen, A: The Spirituality of the Body: Bioenergetics for Grace and Harmony. Macmillan, New York, 1990.

CHAPTER 4

Psychophysiology of Mind-Body Healing

Elinor M. Levy

Elinor M. Levy, PhD, is an associate professor at the School of Medicine, Boston University. She has conducted extensive research on the effect of mood on immunity and is the coauthor of Ten Best Tools to Boost Your Immune System, *published by Houghton Mifflin.*

Can Emotions Influence Your Health?

Arguing with a friend can do more than make you angry—it could give you a migraine. Preparing for finals may cause stomach cramps. The death of a loved one can leave you with insomnia for months. As you probably know from experience, emotions generate significant changes throughout the body. A growing body of scientific evidence supports the mind-body connection, indicating that stress, anxiety, and depression may not only cause temporary discomfort but may also leave people vulnerable to illness.

To understand how moods and attitudes affect health, we must first understand the mechanisms that allow the mind to influence the body. This general area of research, variously called behavioral medicine, mind-body medicine, and psychosomatic medicine, remains somewhat controversial. Skeptics in the scientific and medical communities question whether the changes caused by nervous system mediators last long enough and are of sufficient magnitude to affect our overall health.

What Is the Immune System?

This chapter concentrates on one area of mind-body medicine: psychoneuroimmunology. This discipline, which has been studied extensively in recent years, considers the immune system to be an important mediator between psychological factors and health. Most researchers agree that as we react to our environment, the brain signals the rest of the body through the activation of neurons and the production of neurochemicals. This, in turn, activates or suppresses the immune system.

The immune system consists of a collection of cells and their products. The cells of the immune system circulate as white blood cells or are organized either into immune tissues that line the mucosal surfaces of the body (e.g., along the respiratory and gastrointestinal tracts) and the skin or into organs such as lymph nodes and the spleen.

The immune system can be separated into two major components: the innate, or nonspecific, immune system and the acquired, or specific, immune system. A law enforcement analogy can help our understanding. Try to think of the immune system as

FIGURE 4–1   Cells of the Innate Immune System: Functions of
Granulocytes and Macrophages

Cells of the Innate Immune System

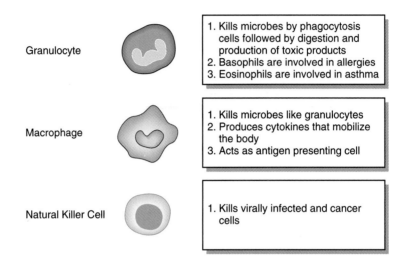

Granulocyte

1. Kills microbes by phagocytosis cells followed by digestion and production of toxic products
2. Basophils are involved in allergies
3. Eosinophils are involved in asthma

Macrophage

1. Kills microbes like granulocytes
2. Produces cytokines that mobilize the body
3. Acts as antigen presenting cell

Natural Killer Cell

1. Kills virally infected and cancer cells

the body's law enforcement agencies and the infectious agent or cancer as the disturber of the peace.

The Innate (Nonspecific) Immune System

The innate immune system acts as a first line of defense, analogous to the local police. The innate immune system rids the body of threatening organisms. For example, granulocytes and macrophages, which are major players in the innate immune system, are phagocytic white blood cells and are good at recognizing, gobbling up, and destroying bacteria. Natural killer (NK) cells, another innate component, are good at identifying and killing virally infected cells to stop the spread of virus. They also can kill cancer cells. Soluble (also called "humoral") components of the innate immune system include *complement* and *defensins*. These are serum proteins, largely produced by the liver and phagocytic cells, that can kill microorganisms. (See Fig. 4–1.)

The Acquired (Specific) Immune System

The specific part of the immune system is composed of certain white blood cells called lymphocytes and the antibodies they produce. This part of the immune system is more analogous to the FBI or CIA because it has more far-reaching and sophisticated methods and organization.

Lymphocytes are divided into two major subtypes: B cells, which are the source of antibodies, and T cells, which are essential for cell-mediated immunity. (See Fig. 4–2.) T cells provide the brains or muscle needed to deal with terrorists and criminal elements. They are further subdivided according to their function. Cytotoxic T cells kill infected or foreign cells or cells perceived as foreign, such as cancer cells. Helper T cells, as the name implies, assist B cells and cytotoxic T cells as well as cells of the innate immune system in doing their jobs. For instance, although B cells can make antibodies, they generally must have T cells assist them. Antibodies recognize and bind to antigens and directly or indirectly help decrease or neutralize them.

FIGURE 4–2   Functions of B and T Cells

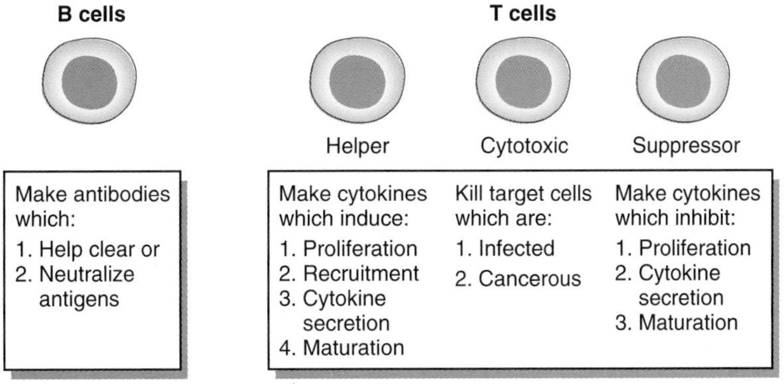

Some T cells are regulatory or suppressor cells, acting to rein in the response of other immune cells. Most T-cell suppression activity is provided by cytokines or interleukins.

Lymphocytes can circulate through the blood or lymphatic system. The lymphatic system flows through the body's tissues, carrying proteins to the lymph nodes. In this way, as well as through organization of lymphocytes in the lymph nodes, in the spleen, along mucosal surfaces and under the skin, the immune system patrols the body, searching for signs of danger.

All the cells of the immune system are produced in the bone marrow throughout life. The T lymphocyte, a nonphagocytic white blood cell, is unusual in that it leaves the bone marrow in an immature state and generally has to mature in the thymus before it becomes fully operational.

Cytokines act as messages or directives to other cells of the immune system and even affect nonimmune organs. (See Table 4–1.) For instance, the cytokine called interleukin-1 (IL-1) acts on the brain to induce fever and on a variety of other tissues to gear the body up to fight infections. Other cytokines, called chemokines, recruit immune cells from the blood and send them to the site of an infection. Still other cytokines call on the bone marrow to produce more white blood cells to join the effort.

The Role of the Lymphocyte

Lymphocytes differ from cells of the innate immune system in that their range of recognition is very limited. Think of the lymphocyte as a special agent assigned to track down a particular suspect, in comparison to a border guard trying more generally to turn back any foreigner lacking an entry permit.

Anything recognized by the immune system is called an antigen (the "suspect" in our analogy). These are usually foreign proteins. Any one lymphocyte has only one type of antigen receptor that can recognize just a small piece of one antigen or maybe a group of very closely related antigenic segments. The antigen receptor on B cells is a surface form of immunoglobulin (also called "antibody"). The strength of the immune system resides

TABLE 4–1   Pioneers of the Mind–Body Concept

PIONEER	APPROXIMATE DATE	PIONEERING CONCEPT
Walter Cannon	1910	Fight-or-flight response
Hans Seyle	1970s	General adaptation syndrome
George Solomon	1980s	Psychoneuroimmunology
Robert Ader	1980s	Conditioning of the immune response

in its billions of lymphocytes, each with a different receptor. This gives the specific immune system and the antibodies it produces the ability to recognize an incredible array of potential targets.

Generally, T lymphocytes do not recognize intact antigens. Instead they require an antigen-presenting cell, often a macrophage, to chew up the antigen into small pieces and display these pieces for the T cell. (See Fig. 4–3.) The individual T cells are interested only in the details. This is in some way similar to using fingerprints or DNA evidence to make an identification.

When a B or a T cell encounters an antigen in the proper form, the antigen interacts with the antigen receptor and a signal is passed across the membrane to the inside of the cell. Here the signal is propagated in a series of biochemical reactions from the outer membrane to inside the nucleus, where the transmitted signal turns on or off a variety of genes. (Our agents, the B and T cells, have spotted a suspicious suspect. With the approval from the field office, they shift from a surveillance mode to a pursuit mode.) The B and T cells are stimulated and produce additional cells or produce antibodies that recognize the same antigen. (The agents are given a backup team.) This process is termed *clonal expansion*. (See Fig. 4–4.)

The next time the body is challenged by the same antigen, many more cells will be ready to attack the organism that expresses that antigen. The initial contact also makes the cells better adapted for a quicker and more vigorous response. This provides the rationale for immunization. Immunization with a relatively harmless pathogen, such as the killed or weakened polio virus, primes the acquired immune system so that it can respond effectively when it next meets the more virulent form of the pathogen, thus keeping us

FIGURE 4–3   Antigen Presentation

Antigen-presenting cells (APCs) can take in large antigens and break them down into small pieces. These small fragments bind to the pocket of specialized molecules—major histocompatibility complex (MHC) proteins—and are displayed at the surface of the APC. T cells recognize the combination of the antigen fragment and the MHC carrier.

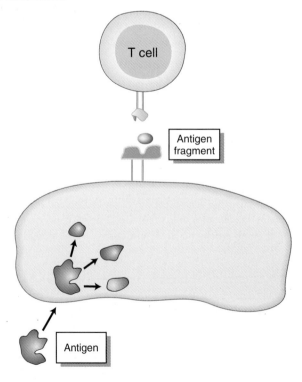

FIGURE 4–4   Clonal Expansion

When a lymphocyte receives a signal following interaction with an antigen-presenting cell bearing an antigen fragment it can recognize (for example, antigen 2), the lymphocyte divides to produce more cells that are able to recognize the same antigen.

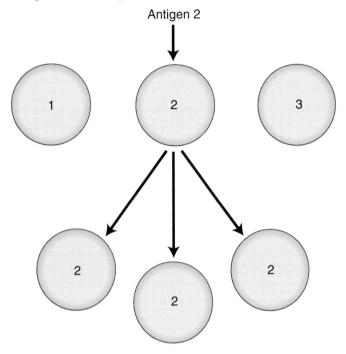

from getting sick. It serves the purpose of a realistic training exercise to prepare the agents for an actual attack. When the immune system is weakened, as dramatically illustrated in diseases such as acquired immune deficiency syndrome, people become more vulnerable to infections and the development of cancer.

The Immune System at Work: From Allergies to Toxic Shock

The receptors on newly developed lymphocytes recognize not only dangerous substances but also normal environmental antigens found in foods. Worse still, they can recognize components of our own body.

An ideally functioning immune system recognizes and destroys harmful substances while ignoring all harmless substances, especially self-tissues. When it fails to make this distinction, people develop hypersensitivity reactions (allergies) or autoimmune diseases. In allergies such as hay fever, a harmless antigen from ragweed pollen triggers the immune system to react, producing itchy eyes and a runny nose, as though responding to an infectious organism. An even worse situation results in autoimmune diseases, where the immune system reacts against the body's own tissues. For example, in certain forms of diabetes, disease develops after cells of the immune system attack and destroy the beta cells in the pancreas that normally make insulin. In extreme cases, hypersensitivity reactions and autoimmune diseases can be fatal.

The immune system can also be destructive when carrying out legitimate functions. For instance, certain pathogens induce a massive activation of the immune system with a tremendous outpouring of cytokines. These organisms contain what are called superantigens, which can activate large numbers of lymphocytes. Toxic shock syndrome is one example of a potentially fatal condition caused by the extreme reaction of the immune system to a superantigen in a *Staphylococcus aureus* infection.

These examples show the importance of regulating the immune system's tremendous power. Suppressor cells and regulatory factors provide one level of control from within the immune system, like an internal review board. The central nervous system provides another element of control, which is discussed below.

The Immune System and Nervous System Interact

The brain and peripheral nerves respond to threats and mood changes by producing messengers, referred to as neurochemicals, which direct other parts of the body to react. They influence everything from heart rate to sexual function to immunity. A list of neurochemicals that affect immunity is given in Table 4–2.

Neurochemicals influence immunity by binding to specific immune cell receptors that control activation. (See Fig. 4–5.) Depending on the mediator involved, this can either augment or block signals being delivered by antigens and cytokines.[1] More often than not, the neurochemicals suppress immune function. For instance, in response to stress, the central nervous system produces cortisol and norepinephrine. These stress hormones prevent T-lymphocyte activation and reduce cytokine production. (Cortisone is a synthetic form of cortisol and is a widely used medication to suppress inflammation.)

When stress or depression becomes prolonged or extreme, the body can adjust. Feedback mechanisms can turn down the production of neurochemicals such as cortisol and make target tissues less likely to respond, in part by causing a decrease in the number of receptors that bind neurochemicals. For instance, abnormal physiological responses to stress are seen in people with post-traumatic stress disorder (PTSD), in which stress has been so severe that the body's neurochemical response to stress in the future is forever changed, leaving the person more vulnerable to stressful stimuli.[2] Another example of long-term consequences of stress comes from research in which stressing a pregnant animal causes developmental alterations in the brain of her offspring, whose future neurochemical and immune patterns of response to stress remain abnormal even when it becomes an adult.[3]

A few neurochemicals, such as melatonin and prolactin, have an opposite effect and tend to stimulate cell-mediated immunity. Sometimes the interaction between neurochemicals—for instance, β-endorphin and cells of the immune system—can be very complex, with the outcome depending on how much of the neurochemical is present as well as the location and history of the responding immune cells.

Communications between the central nervous system and immune system are bidirec-

TABLE 4–2   Selected Cytokines and Their Functions

CYTOKINE	PRIMARY SOURCE	FUNCTION
IL-1	Macrophages	Lymphocyte activation, fever, metabolic changes
IL-2	T cells	T-cell proliferation, activation of killer cells
IFN gamma	T cells, NK cells	Activation of killer cells, mood changes
TNF–alpha	Macrophages	Activation of cytotoxic cells, fever
GM-CSF	T cells, Macrophages	Proliferation of granulocyte and macrophage precursors

[handwritten margin notes: "to much stress." "P.T.S.D -" "Post - traumatic - stress - disorder"]

FIGURE 4–5 Immunosuppression by Neurochemicals

Lymphocyte activation is regulated by nervous system signals. When a lymphocyte recognizes the antigen on an antigen-presenting cell, signals are transmitted from its membrane to its nucleus. Here genes are turned on to produce cytokines and proteins needed for cell division. Suppressive signals from neurochemicals weaken the signals coming from the antigen receptor so that fewer genes are turned on.

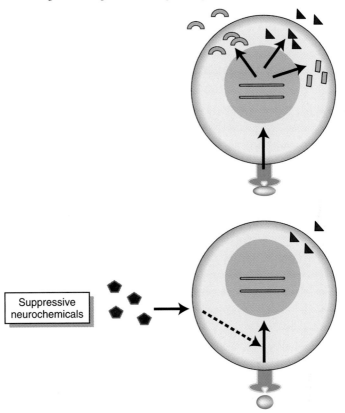

tional.[4,5] For instance, the immune system can alert the brain to an infection in the body by producing the cytokines interleukin-1 and interferon gamma. In response, the brain raises body temperature to produce a fever, inducing both moodiness and fatigue. Interleukin-1 can also increase cortisol production, which in turn suppresses a continuing immune reaction. (See Box 4–1.)

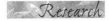 *Research*

Thoughts, Feelings, and the Immune System

Numerous studies have evaluated the effects of psychological events or mood states on immunity, and a variety of experiments have examined immune responses in people exposed to stressful situations. Some of the best controlled studies have assessed immune function of students during exam periods compared to the same students at nonexam times.[6] Immune functions studied included production of various cytokines, NK activity, and the ability of lymphocytes to divide when activated. Other populations studied include more chronically stressed populations such as recently divorced men and women, as well as caregivers for people with Alzheimer's disease.[7-9] These studies statistically exclude effects caused by a number of health behaviors likely to change with stress, for example, sleep patterns, smoking, and alcohol intake. Recently divorced men's and women's T lymphocytes were less responsive to stimulation and showed less ability to

BOX 4–1

Experimentation with the Role of the Central Nervous System on Immune Function

Several experimental approaches have been used to clarify the role of the central nervous system on immune function. In the simplest studies, neurochemicals are added to immune cells in the laboratory, or animals (usually mice) are injected with a test substance whose effect on immunity is measured.

Other studies confirm the role of neurochemicals in influencing immunity by adding or injecting an antagonist or blocker for the neurochemical of interest. For instance, naloxone blocks the binding of β-endorphin to its receptor. Naloxone can also block the effect of stress on natural killer (NK) cell activity in some models. NK cells are thought to be an important first line of defense against viral infections and certain cancers. They also seem to be the most stress-sensitive immune component. When naloxone blocks the effects of stress on NK activity, then it suggests that β-endorphin is a mediator between stress and NK activity under the conditions used in that experiment.

Another experimental approach has tried to show a connection between the central nervous system and the immune system by more directly looking at central nervous system components. Several researchers have destroyed specific areas of the brain and then measured changes in immunity.

The involvement of peripheral nerves is suggested by the work of Bulloch[1] and Bellinger and colleagues,[2] who have shown that nerves enter into areas where immune system cells such as lymphocytes and macrophages congregate, such as the lymph nodes, spleen, lymphoid areas of the gut, and other mucosal surfaces, where they exist in close proximity to lymphocytes. These nerves could be triggered by an ongoing immune response to release neurochemicals such as norepinephrine directly into the environment of responding lymphocytes.

Other experiments demonstrate that the immune system communicates with the brain in a feedback loop, from immune response (via the cytokines or messages produced by the brain) to the central nervous system and back again. The cytokines, particularly IL-1, can activate the hypothalamic-pituitary-adrenal (HPA) axis, inducing a release of corticotrophin-releasing hormone (CRH), which induces the release of adrenocorticotrophin hormone (ACTH), and finally cortisol. (See Fig. 4–6.) Increases in cortisol are seen in experimental animals not only in response to injected cytokines but also in response to various infections.[3]

The CRH also induces the sympathetic nervous system to release norepinephrine and other mediators responsible for suppression of T-cell and NK-cell activity.

References

1. Bulloch, K: Neuroanatomy of lymphoid tissue: A review. In Guillemin, R (ed): Neural Modulation of Immunity. Raven Press, New York, 1985.
2. Bellinger, D, et al: Innervation of lymphoid organs and implications in development, aging, and autoimmunity. Int J Immopharmac 14:329–344, 1992.
3. Riley, V: Psychoneuroendocrine influence on immunocompetence and neoplasia. Science 212:1100–1109, 1981.

suppress Epstein-Barr virus infections. Caregivers of those with Alzheimer's disease had less responsive NK cells than controls, which might help explain the greater number of days that they reported being ill.

To completely rule out the effect of behaviors on immunity, other studies have used experimentally induced stressors. For instance, in these studies the same subject's immunity is compared before and after an experimental stress in a controlled setting. Again, one sees immunological changes in response to stress in all these cases.

In one study, subjects were asked to recall and discuss in one session the most stressful or painful events they had experienced, and in another session their least stressful or most pleasurable experiences.[10] Subjects reported the degree to which they experienced emotions such as anxiety, excitement, or relaxation. Physiological measures (heart rate, blood pressure, and electrodermal activity) were measured before, during, and after the induced-emotion sessions. In addition, blood was drawn for immune analysis immediately after the emotion-recall session, and again 40 minutes later.

As anticipated, heart rate and systolic blood pressure increased while the subjects discussed negative emotions. The number of neutrophils in the blood, the predominant form of phagocytic white blood cell, also increased—a phenomenon commonly seen in circumstances of increased emotional arousal. At the same time, the ability of lymphocytes to divide when artificially stimulated decreased. The impaired ability to respond to a stimulus suggests the lymphocytes would be less protective against an infectious challenge.

Similar, although less dramatic, changes in blood pressure and immunity occurred during the discussion of positive emotions. These changes were interpreted as reflecting the excitement people reported feeling when recalling good times.

Fluctuations in feelings of anxiety strongly correlated with changes in heart rate, which increased; however, there was a negative correlation with changes in immunity (as anxiety increased, the ability of lymphocytes to divide in response to a challenge decreased).

Subjects who tended to react with the greatest emotion also reacted with the greatest physiological and immunological changes. These results are consistent with the hypothesis that the same neurochemicals, possibly catecholamines, are responsible for the changes in both systems.

Feeling Helpless Can Be Dangerous to Your Health

Another experiment demonstrated that individuals' reactions to stress depend on their interpretation of the stress. In a study by Sieber and colleagues,[11] subjects were divided into three groups, each of which was subjected to the same noise stress. Each group had

FIGURE 4–6   Hypothalamic-Pituitary-Adrenal Feedback Suppression of Immunity

(1) Activation of the immune system leads to the production of cytokines such as IL-1 and IL-6. (2) These cytokines bind to receptors in the brain and cause the release of corticotrophin-releasing hormone (CRH) from the hypothalamus. (3) CRH acts on the pituitary to cause the release of adrenocorticotropic hormone (ACTH) and also activates the sympathetic nervous system. (4) ACTH acts on the adrenals to cause the release of cortisol, which suppresses further production of cytokines and is generally anti-inflammatory.

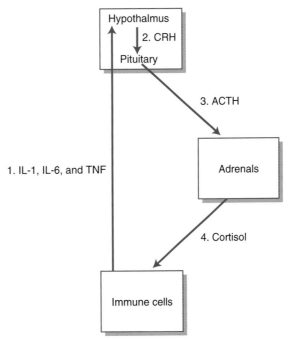

received very different instructions beforehand. Two groups were told that they could turn off the noise by tapping the correct pattern on a button in the cubicle. For one group this was true; but, for the other group, the noise would continue no matter what pattern they tried. The third group had no option but to sit and endure the noise.

Natural killer cell activity was measured before and after the session. The group given no option had lower NK activity after the noise exposure. The other two groups had unchanged NK activity. The authors interpret their data as showing that having some control or even having the perception of some control over a situation protects against the potentially harmful effects of stress. This work confirms the relevance to humans of earlier animal studies.[12]

A meta-analysis (which combines the results of many different studies) by Herbert and Cohen[13] in 1993 of human stress studies concluded that stress changes the number of immune cells circulating in the blood and, more importantly, causes a change in their ability to function. The analysis concluded that the total number of white blood cells increases with stress, whereas the number of lymphocytes decreases. T-cell functions, most notably the ability to multiply when challenged, are generally depressed by stress.

An indirect measure of T-cell function, based on their ability to keep herpesvirus under control, can also indicate when T cells are not working normally. For instance, all herpes viruses, including herpes simplex and Epstein-Barr virus, establish lifelong infections. Most of the time they remain latent, but when the immune system is less effective than usual, the virus can reactivate.

Natural killer cell activity is particularly sensitive to stress.[14] Individual studies also indicate a decrease in the ability to make cytokines, such as interleukin-2 and gamma-IFN. The ability to make antibodies is variably affected by stress; most studies show that immunoglobulin A (IgA) in the saliva decreases with stress, whereas immunoglobulin G (IgG) in the blood increases or is unchanged.

Is Stress Always Harmful?

Not all immune functions are suppressed by stress; some increase instead. In several animal models select macrophage activity increases, such as the production of the cytokines IL-1 and tumor necrosis factor (TNF). These cytokines help mobilize the cells of the immune system to fight infections.

Animal studies have compared the effects of a single exposure to a stressor with repeated exposure to stress. Most studies indicate that repeated exposure to the same stress, such as electric tail shock, has less of an effect on immunity than a single episode. It is reasonable to suppose that on repeated exposure the animals adapt to the stressor. This view is supported by a study in animals that no longer responded to a repeated stress but could still respond immunologically to a novel stressor. However, human immune function continues to be suppressed by chronic social stressors.

Stress, Infections, and Cancer

Psychoneuroimmunologists continue to research the effect of psychological stress on susceptibility to disease via an effect on the immune system. In a large majority of studies on animals, there is good evidence that stress affects their ability to resist infections and cancer. In studies of rodents exposed to foot shock or restraint stress, for instance, stressed animals showed impaired immunity to herpes simplex virus in in vitro tests and were subsequently more susceptible to such infections after in vivo challenge.[15]

Animals exposed to rotation stress, or to the stress of crowded housing, or to foot shocks were more susceptible to the growth of cancer cells. There are, however, a few contradictory studies in which stressed animals were more resistant to cancer and infection than controls.[16,17]

Although there have been only a few controlled human studies, these have generally indicated links between stress or mood states and health, such as two very carefully controlled studies indicating that psychological factors influence susceptibility to the common cold.

In each experiment, Sheldon Cohen and colleagues[18,19] exposed volunteers to a nasal spray of infectious virus. They were kept in isolation for a week after exposure to the virus.

The first experiment showed a linear relationship between the amount of stress the volunteers had reported experiencing within the previous year and their susceptibility to developing a cold. In the follow-up experiment, volunteers filled out questionnaires measuring social support before exposure to virus. Subjects with the greatest number of types of support networks—including family, work or religious groups, volunteer situations, and so forth—were most resistant to the development of colds. It is reasonable to hypothesize that the social support was able to buffer the effects of stress.

Other studies suggest a possible role for the mind on the progression of cancer. This effect should be distinguished from an effect on the incidence of cancer. Despite many studies, evidence for an influence of mood or personality on the initiation of cancer is at best very weak.[20]

However, an early prospective study conducted in England suggested that mental attitude can influence the progression of cancer. In 1985, Pettingale and colleagues[21] reported on a 10-year follow-up of a group of 57 women who initially had early-stage breast cancer. Among those who were judged at the start of the study to have a fighting spirit, 70 percent were still alive 12 years after diagnosis, compared to 20 percent of those having a hopeless attitude. Those who reacted with denial or with stoic acceptance had intermediate survival levels.

Social Support and Recovery from Illness

Studies have suggested that psychosocial interventions can decrease cancer progression and death. California psychiatrist David Spiegel and colleagues[22] studied a group of 86 women with metastatic breast cancer. The women met weekly for a period of a year. They participated in semistructured sessions in which they had the opportunity to share experiences, feelings, and advice. The women in the intervention group lived 36.6 months from the onset of intervention, significantly longer than the 18.9 months in the historical comparison group. This study is currently being replicated with immune measures to try to connect survival benefits with improved immune function in the women participating in the group sessions.

Encouraging results were also obtained in studies by California psychiatrist F. Fawzy and colleagues.[23] In these studies, half the patients diagnosed with malignant melanoma (a form of skin cancer) were assigned to a group that received a psychosocial intervention. The remaining participants served as a control group. Both groups had surgery to remove the melanoma, followed by standard medical care. The intervention consisted of a 6-week program that included health education about their cancer, instruction in stress-management techniques, instruction in coping skills, and psychological support from one another and the staff. The groups were evaluated after 6 months and again at 6 years. Those who received the intervention related less distress, depression, and fatigue at the 6-month evaluation than did the control group. They also exhibited a statistically significant increase in NK cell number and activity. NK cell activity is very sensitive to stress and is important in fighting tumor cells.

A number of authors have reported very strong data on the protective effect of social support, particularly for heart disease. In a study of people recovering from a heart attack conducted by Berkman,[24] the number of patients who died within 6 months of a heart attack was closely related to the number of types of sources they had for emotional support. In the most dramatic comparison, 69 percent of those over the age of 75 without any sources of social support died within 6 months, compared to 43 percent of those with one source of support and 26 percent of those with two or more sources of support. The effects were stronger in men than in women and in those over 75 compared to those aged 65 to 74.

Uchino and colleagues[25] reviewed the neuroendocrine mechanisms that could form the connection between social support and health, especially heart disease. The immune system, particularly macrophages, is important in the formation of atherosclerosis and also may be involved in inflammatory response to local infection, which some believe contributes substantially to heart disease. However, whether the immune system helps to mediate the clear psychological effects on heart disease in addition to the direct effects of neuroendocrine factors remains quite speculative at this time.

Summary

Abundant evidence supports the conclusion that the brain influences physiological and immunological reactions to stress, anxiety, and depression through the release of neuro-chemicals. The central nervous system signals the body to mobilize its resources in response to a perceived threat, be it physical or psychological. A long list of neurochemicals can influence virtually all aspects of immunity. The influence of neurochemicals depends on their concentration, type, and location, as well as the previous experience of the responding immune cell. The immune system can inform the central nervous system of infections in the body via interleukins, which can induce fever, fatigue, and mood changes.

The biological changes brought about by the central nervous system have an impact on health. A number of well-controlled prospective studies indicate that stress can leave us more vulnerable to infectious diseases. Evidence suggests that once cancer is established, psychological factors appear to influence its progression. Social support is associated with greater longevity, fewer infections, and less heart disease.

Skeptics point out that people who are depressed or stressed are less likely to eat and sleep well and more likely to engage in such self-damaging behaviors as smoking or drinking excessively. They may also be less likely to seek medical treatment. However, the experiments reviewed in this chapter have either been designed so that such behaviors are not relevant to the results, as in experimental exposure to virus in a controlled setting, or have considered those unhealthy behaviors in the data analysis. This body of evidence suggests that psychological factors can influence health over and above their effect on health-related behavioral factors.

Stress itself is not necessarily bad for us; rather it is our interpretation of stressors that makes them bad. If even a modest amount of control is experienced over the stressful situation, or if the situation is seen as challenging rather than threatening, then the stress becomes neutral or even positive for the immune system.

It is much easier to show an effect of stress or depression on specific components of the immune system than to show its effect on overall health. One explanation for this is that the immune system has so many potential pathways for protecting the body from infections that diminishing or even eliminating particular functions may not have a noticeable effect on health in most situations.

There is some concern that promotion of mind-body techniques leads some patients to feel guilty if they are unable to muster the right attitude to cure themselves. It should be realized that the mind has only a limited ability to change immunity and that the immune system itself is of only limited use against certain types of cancer and infections. We should appreciate the power of the mind to heal, but also be aware of its limitations. (See Box 4–2.)

BOX 4–2
Pioneers of the Mind-Body Connection

Walter B. Cannon

Cannon was an early proponent of the mind-body connection and is credited with the concept that an abrupt disruption of an organism's physiological equilibrium, or homeostasis, leads to consequences that can be characterized as a fight-or-flight response, meaning that the body mobilizes its resources for a response when threatened.[1] A disruption of our body's equilibrium can be caused by a physical or psychological challenge. In the early 1900s, Cannon suggested that the sympathetic nervous system (SNS) mediated this response via the catecholamines they produce.

Hans Selye

Selye expanded this concept with a description of the general adaptation syndrome as a response to a more prolonged anxiety.[2] Such adaptation is mediated by both the SNS and the hypothalamic-pituitary-adrenal axis. The hypothalamus is a region of the brain that controls temperature, sleep, and activities of the gut. The pituitary and adrenals are glands that respond to signals from the hypothalamus in response to stress. The cascade of neurochemicals produced includes cortisol and the catecholamine norepinephrine (also called "noradrenaline").

These and other mediators change our blood pressure, heart rate, skin temperature, and so forth, making our hearts start to race, our palms become sweaty, and so forth. In addition, less obvious changes affect metabolism, production of sex hormones, and much more. These changes prepare the body for flight or flight. Selye also suggested that the changes caused by prolonged periods of distress could lead to disease.

George Solomon

Solomon, a psychiatrist, is credited with coining the term *psychoneuroimmunology*.[3] He has championed the idea that individual personality and our psychological responses to stress can influence health via changes in the immune system, particularly for autoimmune diseases and AIDS. The immune system plays a central role in protecting us from infections of all kinds, including those caused by bacteria, viruses, and yeast. Extending the ideas of Cannon and Selye, George Solomon and Robert Ader viewed the immune system as an important stress-sensitive component of the body that could mediate some of the effects of stress on health.

Robert Ader

Ader conducted one of the most intriguing experiments in psychoneuroimmunology. In this early work, he demonstrated that mice could be conditioned by pairing a novel taste with a powerful immune suppressant.[4] Earlier, Pavlov had conditioned a dog to salivate by ringing a bell. This was achieved by a number of conditioning sessions in which the bell and food were paired, suggesting that the dog associated the two stimuli such that its brain responded to the bell as it would to food. Ader's experiment paired saccharine with an immunosuppressive drug during the conditioning sessions. Subsequent exposure to the saccharine alone caused moderate immune suppression, suggesting that the brain knew of immune changes caused by the drug, associated the changes with the novel taste of saccharine, and re-created those changes in the absence of an external immunosuppressive signal. (See Table 4–3.)

REFERENCES

1. Cannon, WB, and de La Paz, D: Emotional stimulation of adrenal secretion. Am J Psysiol 27:64–70, 1911.
2. Selye, H: The evolution of the stress concept. Am J Cardiol 46:81–87, 1970.
3. Solomon, GF, and Amkraut, A: Psychoneuroendocrinological effects on the immune response. Ann Rev Microbiol 35:155–184, 1981.
4. Ader, R, and Cohen, N: Behaviorally conditioned immunosuppression and murine systemic lupus erythematosus. Science 215:1534–1536, 1982.

TABLE 4–3   Neuroendocrine Factors That Directly Influence the Immune System

- *Neurotransmitters:* norepinephrine, serotonin, dopamine
- *Neurohormones:* corticotrophin-releasing hormone, cortisol, growth hormone, prolactin, insulin, vasopressin, oxytocin, somatostatin
- *Neuropeptides:* substance P, vasoactive intestinal peptide, endorphins, enkephalins
- *Others:* melatonin, estrogen, adrenaline

REFERENCES

American Psychosomatic Medicine Society
6728 Old McLean Village Dr.
McLean, VA 22101
Phone: (703) 556-9222
Fax: (703) 556-8729
E-mail: *info@psychosomatic.org*
Website: *www.psychosomatic.org*

International Society of Psychoneuroendocrinology
Dr. David Saphier, Secretary/Treasurer
511 Dudley St.
Shreveport, LA 71104
Phone: (308) 865-8175
Website: *www.ispn.org.*

Psychoneuroimmunology Research Society
Dr. Virginia Sanders, Secretary/Treasurer
Department of Cell Biology, Neurobiology, and Anatomy
Loyola University Medical Center
2160 S. First Ave.
Maywood, IL 60153
Phone: (708) 216-6728
Fax: (708) 216-6731
E-mail: *pnirs@pnirs.org*
Website: *www.pnirs.org*

Society of Behavioral Medicine
7600 Terrace Ave.
Middleton, WI 53562
Phone: (608) 827-7267
Fax: (608) 831-5485
E-mail: *sbm@tmahq.com*
Website: *www.sbmweb.org*

REFERENCES

1. Kiecolt-Glaser, J, et al: Marital discord and immunity in males. Psychosomat Med 50:213–229, 1988.
2. Yehuda, R., et al: Cortisol regulation in posttraumatic stress disorder and major depression. Biol Psych 40:79–98, 1996.
3. Sobrian, S., et al: Influence of prenatal maternal stress on the immunocompetence of the offspring. Pharm Biochem.Behav 43:537–547, 1992.
4. Kiecolt-Glaser et al: Marital discord and immunity in males.
5. Sieber, W, et al: Modulation of human natural killer (NK) cell activity by exposure to uncontrollable stress. Brain Behav Immun 6:141–156, 1992.

6. Glaser, R, et al: Stress depresses interferon production by leukocytes concomitant with a decrease in natural killer (NK) cell activity. Behaviora Neurosci 100: 675–678, 1986.

7. Kiecolt-Glaser, J, et al: Marital quality, marital disruption, and immune function. Psychosomat Med 49: 13–34, 1987.

8. Kiecolt-Glaser et al: Marital discord and immunity in males.

9. Esterling, B, et al: Chronic stress, social support, and persistent alterations in the natural killer (NK) cell response to cytokines in older adults. Health Psych 13:291–298, 1994.

10. Knapp, P, et al: Short-term immunological effects of induced emotion. Psychosomat Med 54:133–148, 1992.

11. Sieber et al: Modulation of human natural killer (NK) cell activity.

12. Laudenslager, M, et al: Coping and immunosuppression: Inescapable but not escapable shock suppresses lymphocyte proliferation. Science 221:568–570, 1983.

13. Herbert, TB, and Cohen, S: Stress and immunity in humans: A meta-analytic review. Psychosomat Med. 55:364–379, 1993.

14. Berkman, L: The role of social relations in health promotion. Psychosomat Med 57:245–254, 1995.

15. Sheridan, J, et al: Psychoneuroimmunology: Stress effects on pathogenesis and immunity during infection. Clin Micro Rev 7:200–212, 1992.

16. Aarstad, H, and Seljelid, R: Effects of stress on the growth of a fibrosarcoma in nu/nu and conventional mice. Scand J Immunol 35: 209–215, 1992.

17. Hermann, G, et al: Stress-induced changes attributable to the sympathetic nervous system during experimental influenza viral infection in DBA/2 inbred mouse strain. J Neuroimmunol 53:173–180, 1994.

18. Cohen, S, Tyrrell, D, and Smith, AP: Psychological stress and susceptibility to the common cold. New Eng J Med 325:606–612, 1991.

19. Cohen, S, et al: Social ties and susceptibility to the common cold. JAMA 277:1940–1944, 1977.

20. Fox, B: Depressive symptoms and risk of cancer. JAMA 262:1231, 1989.

21. Pettingale, K, et al: Mental attitudes to cancer: An additional prognostic factor. Lancet 1:750, 1985.

22. Spiegel, D, et al: Effect of psychosocial treatment on survival of patients with metastatic breast cancer. Lancet 2:888–891, 1989.

23. Fawzy, F, et al: Critical review of psychosocial interventions in cancer care. Arch Gen Psych 52:100–113, 1995.

24. Berkman: The role of social relations in health promotion.

25. Uchino, B, Cacioppo, J, and Kiecolt-Glaser, J: The relationship between social support and physiological processes: A review with emphasis on underlying mechanisms and implications for health. Psych Bull 119:488–531, 1996.

CHAPTER 5

Culture and Holistic Nursing

Dorothy Ann Gilbert

Dorothy Ann Gilbert, RN, PhD, is an associate professor at the University of Massachusetts–Amherst School of Nursing. In her current research she is investigating the influence of cultural differences on the communication in patient-nurse relationships.

The middle-class, European-American nurse was looking forward to working with Ms. G, a Spanish-speaking Puerto Rican woman whose chief complaint was described in her chart as "infertility." When the nurse asked her what had brought her to the clinic that day, Ms. G replied that she needed a fertility certificate. Ms. G explained that the man she had been living with for several years had kept asking, "Why don't you give me a baby? Why don't you give me a baby?" Eventually he broke up with her and took up with another woman, who gave him a baby right away. But now a new man had asked Ms. G to marry him, and she wanted to show him a fertility certificate; that is, a written guarantee prior to marriage that she could have children.

Although the nurse thought she understood Ms. G's concern, a fertility certificate was not an option. Fertility is not predictable, and it varies over the life span and between partners. For example, Napoleon and Josephine Bonaparte could not have children together, but each had a child with another partner. So no one could guarantee that Ms. G and her new partner would be able to have children together before they actually started trying to have them. Moreover, a workup for infertility routinely began with the man, because a sperm count is relatively inexpensive and less intrusive than most procedures for the woman. But the nurse was not sure a sperm count would be acceptable to Ms. G's new partner if he held traditional Puerto Rican values. Finally, the nurse did not know whether Ms. G and her new partner would meet the clinic's admission requirements for an infertility workup because they were not yet married.

This situation illustrates how patients and nurses from different cultures may have different health concerns and different ideas of how to address them. In this case the cultural differences centered on conception, but they might have included virtually any other aspect of health and healing. Holistic nurses need to understand the many characteristics of culture to appreciate how their care is influenced by their own culture, as well as to provide culturally competent care, especially to people of backgrounds different from their own. The situation involving Ms. G and the nurse will be considered again later in this chapter.

Culture: What It Is, What It Is Not

Sir Edward Burnett Tylor,[1] the founder of anthropology as a social science, developed one of the most frequently cited definitions of culture: "Culture . . . is that complex whole which includes knowledge, belief, art, morals, law, custom, and any other capabilities and habits acquired by [people] as [members] of society." More recently, the U.S. Office of Minority Health[2] described culture as "integrated patterns of human behavior that include the language, thoughts, communications, actions, customs, beliefs, values, and institutions" of various groups of people. Together, these two definitions provide essential characteristics of culture: social acquisition and the complexity and integration of beliefs, values, and behavior in human groups.

Social Acquisition   *became for generation*

The most widely accepted characteristic of culture is its social acquisition. As Tylor pointed out in his definition, culture is learned from other people as members of society. Scholars such as Margaret Mead[3] noted early in the 20th century that culture depends on education, broadly defined. A child born of Samoan parents will grow up to speak English and exhibit European-American beliefs, values, and behavior if raised by European-American parents in the United States. Conversely, a child born of European-American parents will grow up to speak Samoan and exhibit Samoan beliefs, values, and behavior if raised by Samoan parents in Samoa. At the time Mead first put forth these ideas, it was widely assumed that people's beliefs, values, and behavior could be attributed to such factors as race or human nature. Today the social acquisition of culture is considered to be a given.

Complexity and Integration

In addition to being characterized by social acquisition, culture is also characterized by complexity and integration. Culture is complex because, as indicated by Tylor and the U.S. Office of Minority Health, it consists of many elements considered simultaneously. Nevertheless, these elements tend to be integrated into patterned wholes. Barnett and Rabin[4] present a classic example of complexity and integration in a discussion of the refusal of some Navajo parents to use Frejka aprons to treat congenital hip dysplasia in their children. Health-care providers reasoned that, although congenital hip dysplasia ranges in severity, many children who are untreated are likely to walk with a limp and may develop painful arthritis of the hip joint in adulthood. From their viewpoint, a Frejka apron was essentially a harness to hold the head of long bone of an infant's leg against the hip socket so that a normal hip joint would gradually develop over a period of months. Thus it was a "low-tech," relatively inexpensive treatment that prevented deformity, adult arthritis, and much more difficult treatment later in life. Why, they wondered, would anyone refuse such a treatment?

In contrast, some Navajo parents wondered why anyone would accept such a treatment. Problems with bone formation were not obvious during infancy, and people who limped were not considered to be deformed. Instead, they were fully functioning members of society who married at the same age as everyone else. Further, Frejka aprons held infants' legs in a frog's leg position that was incompatible with use of the Navajo cradleboard that protected infants and enabled them to be easily carried on horseback or in a wagon. Risking their children's safety for some possible consequence that might not even develop in the distant future made the treatment seem much worse than the "problem." When all the relevant cultural elements of this situation were considered and understood to be integrated into a whole pattern, the rejection of Frejka aprons by some Navajo parents made sense.

The complexity and integration of culture have implications for the transferability of cultural elements. Although a particular treatment modality developed by one group of people might be isolated for investigation or used by those from another group, the modality may "heal" only within the cultural context in which it was developed. For example, the Amhara of highland Ethiopia experience an illness called *setir* (water on the knee or sprained knee). According to Young:[5] "From the Amhara's point of view, the ailment is produced when blood collects in the area of the knee, then becomes stagnant and thick, and distorts the alignment of the cords [that is, blood vessels and ligaments]. . . . *Setir* is usually treated by means of a therapeutic massage (to restore cords to their proper places) and bleeding (to draw off the intrusive blood that forced the cords out of place). During [bleeding], three hornfuls of blood are cupped and poured into a basin." Given the way the healer collects and stores the blood, it will inevitably coagulate and will appear stagnant and thick. For many Amhara, then, *setir* always heals in the sense that it produces the dark blood that the sick person, the person's kin, and the healer expect. In that same sense, *setir* could not heal anyone from another cultural context with different expectations. The practice can succeed only within Amhara culture as an integrated whole.

Three Clarifications about Culture as a Concept

The definitions of culture offered above emphasize characteristics of social acquisition, complexity, and integration. Nevertheless, three important clarifications are needed to further understand what culture is and what it is not: the point of view selected, the cultural variations within groups, and the way culture interacts with the environment.

The Point of View Selected

The description of culture may differ depending on whether the viewpoint is that of the people in the particular group or of the observer. The lists of cultural elements provided by Tylor and the Office of Minority Affairs offer observers' viewpoints that divide the world of a group of people into mutually exclusive and exhaustive categories for description and analysis. The people within the group, however, may have a different way of dividing their world, if they divide it at all.

Fadiman[6] describes the influence of the point of view selected when she explains her efforts to describe the experiences of a Hmong family, originally from Southeast Asia but now residing in the United States. Fadiman tried to create file folders for her extensive notes concerning the Hmong family, the family's American doctors, and the "collision" of the two cultures: "Should [some notes] go in the Medicine folder? . . . The Animism folder? . . . The Social Structure folder? [For the Hmong] medicine was religion. Religion was society. Society was medicine. . . . As my web of cross-references grew more and more thickly interlaced, I concluded that the Hmong preoccupation with medical issues was nothing less that a preoccupation with life. (And death. And life after death)." Fadiman's conclusion illustrates how the people's point of view can be very different from that of an observer. An understanding of culture may depend on which viewpoint is selected.

Intracultural Variation

Just as observers and people in the group are likely to have different points of view, there also may be varied perspectives among the people within the group. Unfortunately, some definitions may make culture seem codified and static, as if one blueprint were being followed by all members of a group, generation after generation. Some textbooks and articles try to describe in a few pages the culture of a particular group. This results in inaccurate overstatements, such as "Mexican-Americans believe in a traditional illness called *mal de ojo* (evil eye)," a traditional illness, which is caused by the stare or glance of a person with a powerful gaze.

It may be that some Mexican-Americans, especially those raised in Mexico who speak and read primarily in Spanish, have experienced *mal de ojo*, but even they may not necessarily agree on the exact nature of the illness or what to do about it. In a series of studies on intracultural variation in relation to four traditional illnesses reported in a Texas border community, Trotter[7] and others found variations in the diagnosis and treatment of *mal de ojo* and other illnesses. Further, experience with the illnesses was by no means universal because, in 20 percent of the 255 households surveyed, none of the four illnesses had ever been treated.

Similarly, Blumhagen[8] studied 103 European-Americans, most of them middle-class, who had a diagnosis of essential hypertension and were attending a clinic in Seattle. Although the clinic nurses explained that the cause of essential hypertension is unknown, more than 40 percent of the patients believed that the cause of essential hypertension was hyper-tension; that is, too much stress in their lives. If Trotter or Blumhagen had selected different communities at different times, their results would show variation. Thus information about phenomena such as traditional illnesses offers holistic nurses an idea of the range of knowledge, values, and behavior concerning cultural aspects of health and illness, but it does not offer a blueprint.

Lack of recognition of intracultural variation leads to stereotyping, which can be defined as generalizing from a few characteristics of some members of a group to all members. Thus stereotyping destroys the sense of diversity that an understanding of culture is able to provide. For example, Foster[9] tells of Buffalo Bill Chan, an Asian patient at a California hospital in which specialized treatment programs for Hispanics, African-Americans, and Asian-Pacific Islanders were available. Mr. Chan had never seen another Asian prior to his departure from Wyoming, nor did he like Chinese food, yet he was placed in the Asian treatment program and an Asian diet was ordered for him. Thus, in an effort to be responsive to cultural differences, the hospital stereotyped Mr. Chan by assuming he preferred to be treated with Asian treatment modalities and to consume an Asian cuisine.

Interaction of Culture with the Environment

Finally, culture is not insular. For purposes of presentation and discussion it is sometimes useful to consider examples—such as the rejection of Frejka aprons by some Navajo, treatment of *setir* by some Amhara, and variability in *mal de ojo* within one Mexican-American community—in which cultural elements operate apart from other influences. In reality, however, culture interacts with the wider physical, biological, and economic/social/political environments. The last of these environments is of particular importance today given the world-transforming effects of a global market, global labor processes, and the resulting unequal power relations among groups of people.

As Singer and colleagues[10] point out, phenomena such as drinking patterns among Puerto Rican men in Hartford, Connecticut have as much to do with the history of the economic and political relations of the island as with internal, cultural traditions. Under Spanish rule, alcohol was a medium of payment for indigenous Puerto Ricans, and it became widely consumed. After U. S. acquisition of the island and with the loss of individually owned land to large sugar plantations, many men became paid laborers for whom alcohol was an integral part of social life, a symbol of being a good provider, and a symbol of manliness in general. In addition, alcohol consumption was encouraged by extensive advertising by the rum industry, few restrictions on sales, ready availability, and low cost.[11] The Great Depression, continued loss of jobs in Puerto Rico, and postwar migration to places such as Hartford led many men to unskilled jobs or unemployment.

BOX 5–1

An Incompatible Meaning of "Culture"

The viewpoint presented in this chapter is that culture is socially acquired and comprises many integrated elements. This viewpoint is incompatible with the viewpoint which suggests that having only one element in common is a sufficient basis for culture, such as the "culture of poverty." For instance, Meleis and colleagues[1] suggest that a single common characteristic can differentiate members of a population from the mainstream, marginalize them, and leave them voiceless such that they share a common culture. Although it is true that marginalized people are likely to be in particular need of health care that takes their marginalization into account, their ways of life tend to vary based on such factors as class, gender, age, and geographic location. There is little evidence, for example, that impoverished people have beliefs, values, or behavior in common. Valentine[2] pointed out long ago that the culture of poverty, a notion introduced by Oscar Lewis,[3] is essentially a series of undemonstrated hypotheses. Schiller[4] argues that highlighting marginalized groups as culturally distinct serves to distance and subordinate them; it conceals more than it clarifies.

REFERENCES

1. Meleis, AI, et al: Diversity, Marginalization, and Culturally Competent HealthCare: Issues in Knowledge Development. American Academy of Nursing, Washington, D.C., 1995.
2. Valentine, CA: Culture and Poverty: Critique and Counterproposals. University of Chicago Press, Chicago, 1970.
3. Lewis, O: Children of Sanchez. Random House, New York, 1961.
4. Schiller, NG: What's wrong with this picture? The hegemonic construction of culture in AIDS research in the United States. Medical Anthropology Quarterly 6:237–254, 1992.

". . . drinking is culturally defined as a male thing to do, . . . [but] it is the combination of a cultural emphasis on drinking as proper, appropriate, and manly, with political and economic subordination in a system in which most alternative expressions of manliness are barred to Puerto Rican access, that is of real significance."[12] (See Box 5–1.)

Toward Cultural Competence

Culture, then, is the socially acquired, complex, integrated, ever-changing, and variable patterns of peoples' beliefs, values, and behavior that can be described from multiple points of view in the context of wider physical, biological, and economic/social/political environments. Understanding culture in this way enables holistic nurses to begin to move toward cultural competence. "Competence," according to the U. S. Office of Minority Health, "implies having the capacity to function effectively as an individual and an organization within the context of the cultural beliefs, behaviors, and needs presented by consumers and their communities."[13] Some basic steps toward cultural competence follow.

1. Identify the Influence of One's Own Culture on Care

First, to be culturally competent, holistic nurses need to identify ways in which their own culture shapes their knowledge, values, and behavior, thus influencing the care they provide. In the situation described at the opening of this chapter, for example, notice how the nurse made an analogy between the childlessness of Ms. G and the childlessness of Napoleon and Josephine. Although the nurse may have learned about these historical figures from her middle-class European-American background, it is not apparent that Ms. G would have any idea who Napoleon and Josephine were—nor that the analogy would be persuasive even if she did. Notice further that the nurse thought Ms G. might not have met the clinic's admission criteria, perhaps because she thought that sex was appropriate only after marriage. The nurse's beliefs and values are as evident in the situation as are those of Ms. G.

BOX 5–2
Ethnocentrism

Many people may not be aware of their own culture until they come into contact with another, perhaps because culture is so pervasive. We grow comfortable with what we are used to. ("I and my family and friends don't speak with an accent; other people speak with an accent.") Among people everywhere there is a tendency, known as ethnocentrism, to judge one's own way of life as the best or most appropriate. Ways that are different are deemed inferior, immoral, ignorant, or generally unacceptable.

Ethnocentrism has a long history: Herodotus, the father of history, wrote that ancient Egyptians were uncivilized because they urinated in private rather than on the street as proper ancient Greeks would do. Foster[1] pointed out the ethnocentric premises embedded in American-aided international health programs during the mid-20th century: that the American medical system as practiced in the United States was the appropriate model for the development of health services in all countries and that it would be readily accepted or, if it were not, that people in developing countries could be educated to understand the advantages of the American way.

When European-American, middle-class health-care providers conclude that some people from other groups are immoral or rude because they do not meet standards such as individualism, future orientation, or being on time, they are being ethnocentric. By the same token, when members of such other groups conclude that many health providers are immoral or rude because they do not meet standards such as familism, past orientation, or attending to important matters first, they, too, are being ethnocentric.

REFERENCES

1. Foster, GM: Medical anthropology and international health planning. In Logan, MH, and Hunt, EE (eds): Health and the Human Condition. Duxbury, North Scituate, Mass., 1978.

2. Respect Perspectives Other than One's Own

Cultural competence also requires holistic nurses to take the equally fundamental step of acknowledging and respecting perspectives other than their own. It is possible that nurses unfamiliar with cultural differences might ethnocentrically conclude that Ms. G was "uneducated" because she requested a fertility certificate. Similarly, such nurses might conclude that the Navajo parents who refused to use Frejka aprons were "noncompliant" or that Mexican-Americans who believed they had experienced *mal de ojo* were "delusional." An understanding of cultural differences, however, informs nurses that their way is not the only way. People learn their ideas and behavior as members of their societies over the course of their lifetimes, and their ideas and behavior must be respected. (See Box 5–2.)

3. Distinguish the Essential from the Nonessential

Third, Western medicine—and perhaps any system of beliefs, values, and behavior in which students are educated and in which graduates practice—can be conceptualized as a "culture." Thus, to be culturally competent, nurses must distinguish the essential aspects from the nonessential aspects of their practice. In the case of Ms. G, the routines of the infertility team, such as beginning a workup with a sperm count, might have been based on good and valid reasons as far as the team is concerned, but much of the routine could have been delayed, altered, or omitted without endangering Ms G.

Many techniques and products of Western medicine in current use are arguably effective, if "effective" is narrowly defined as prolongation of some lives, relief of many unpleasant symptoms such as pain or fever, or even facilitation of conception in some infertile couples. Veterinary medicine can also be effective in these ways. The problems arise when, along with the effective techniques and products, the customary behavior and views of Western medicine are prescribed because they are customary, not because they are essential. An awareness of a culture of Western medicine helps nurses tell which is which.

4. Learn about Traditional Ways of Life

Holistic nurses can improve their cultural competence by becoming familiar with traditional cultural patterns. By reading books and articles about different of ways of life or by learning about traditional life ways through other routes, nurses can broaden their horizons on values, beliefs, and behavior. For example, Ms. G's situation may have been influenced by traditional Puerto Rican ideas about gender roles. As described by Sanchez-Ayendez,[14] some Puerto Ricans conceptualize men as having authority over women, although the concept of maleness extends beyond a need to prove virility to being primary providers, protectors of the family, respectful to others, and worthy of respect themselves. And it is through motherhood, traditionally, that women realize themselves and achieve their greatest satisfactions in life. The world of women is said to revolve around the household and their children, even when they work outside the home.

5. Anticipate Variation

By anticipating variation, rather than uniformity, within cultures, holistic nurses can move toward cultural competence by looking at each client as unique rather than as a stereotype. Although it was useful to know some traditional Puerto Rican cultural patterns, it remained necessary to explore Ms. G's actual perspective rather than to assume she was following a traditional blueprint. Furthermore, her ideas about a fertility certificate were not likely to be found in a textbook about Puerto Rican culture. Ms. G had a perspective that may have been culturally patterned but was also unique to her.

6. Seek Other Relevant Perspectives

Variation can also be expected in the perspectives of other people relevant to the situation. In the case of Ms. G, her new partner was an obvious example, but her family and friends might also have played a critical role even though they were not immediately present. They may have offered her emotional support, or she may have deferred to them as the ultimate decision makers. The awareness of who these others might be and the roles they might play in a health-related situation is yet another aspect of cultural competence.

7. Negotiate Plans of Care

It is possible that once the first six steps have been accomplished, holistic nurses will discover conflicts among the various perspectives, or what Kleinman calls explanatory models of health and healing. When general, open-ended questions are insufficient to gain a full understanding of patients' experiences, Kleinman[15] recommends eliciting their explanatory models by asking a series of questions that will vary depending on the circumstances. The questions are approximately as follows:

1. What do you call your problem? What name does it have?
2. What do you think has caused your problem?
3. Why do you think it started when it did?
4. What does your sickness do to you? How does it work?
5. How severe is it? Will it have a short or long course?
6. What do your fear most about your sickness?
7. What are the chief problems your sickness has caused for you?
8. What kind of treatment do you think you should receive? What are the most important results you hope to receive from this treatment?

Kleinman's questions may be more applicable in episodes of acute illness, but the strategy could have been used in the case of Ms. G to identify some important themes. The nurse needed to explore what Ms. G called her problem, the nature of its cause (for example, jealous witchcraft by the other woman with whom her former partner subsequently became involved), and perhaps the time of onset if that seemed relevant. But for the purpose of this discussion, let us assume that Ms. G believed she had a problem that she called potential "barrenness." Ms. G seemed to think that women alone were responsible for barrenness, because she reported that the other woman had given her former partner a baby whereas Ms. G had not. She may have believed her barrenness would be lifelong unless she did something about it. If she subscribed to traditional Puerto Rican ideas of gender roles, she may have feared she would never be able to be a complete woman, a mother, or a wife, and these possible inabilities may have been a major problem in her life. As a person who might have understood the traditional role of Puerto Rican men, Ms. G apparently wanted to be able to assure her new partner, who did not just want to live with her but wanted to marry her, that she could "give him a baby."

After ascertaining the client's explanatory model, Kleinman recommends that health providers present their own explanatory model, consisting essentially of their answers to the same eight questions, in terms the client can understand. Before talking with Ms. G, the nurse called her problem "infertility." She did not know the cause or onset. Except for obvious explanations—such as that Ms. G's former partner had a sperm count of zero or that Ms. G. had had a hysterectomy— the "cause" of the infertility might only have become known when a particular treatment procedure, followed by intercourse with her new partner, resulted in Ms. G's becoming pregnant. Pregnancy, according to the nurse, requires an adequate fertility ratio that varies depending on the combination of partners. Based on the information provided, the nurse seemed most concerned about the general lack of fit between what Ms. G wanted (a fertility certificate) and the treatment the fertility team could offer (a workup).

After the two models have been presented, according to Kleinman, they can be openly compared in order to identify conflicts and to mutually negotiate a plan of care that is acceptable to both parties and to the client's family. From the nurse's viewpoint, for instance, a fertility certificate was not an option. She might have been able to offer Ms. G a report on her status, from a Western medical point of view, that might rule out obvious reasons why Ms. G could not have a baby. This would assume that the findings from a history, physical exam, and other relevant procedures were "normal." This plan also would have provided an opportunity for the nurse to learn more about Ms. G, her family, and so on, and for Ms. G to learn about the nurse and the infertility team. There is not enough information in the vignette to determine conflicts in the two models from Ms. G's point of view, her response to the nurse's suggestions, or alternative plans Ms. G might have suggested. Nevertheless, Kleinman's strategy could have been effective in the narrow, Western medical sense, and it could have promoted Ms. G's health and healing if it had reflected her perspective.

8. Recognize the Influence of the Environment

Strategies are not confined to the individual level, however. Recognition of the influence of wider environments extends holistic nurses' focus beyond the immediate encounter to the population level. For example, as noted earlier, Ms. G might have been influenced by her cultural perception of gender roles and by her positive valuation of children, but she might also have been influenced by unequal power relationships based on gender, and perhaps class, in her society. Promoting health and healing requires work at the social policy level and what is becoming known as refocusing upstream:[16] rather than spending all our time pulling drowning victims out of the river, let us look upstream to see what is pushing them in.

In this chapter, however, it is being recommended that the individual and population levels not be confused. Although it would be appropriate to "flag" for future understanding the fact that Ms. G may be at risk for violence because men seem to exercise a great deal of control of her life, it would not be appropriate for the nurse to explain to Ms. G that she is being oppressed by her male partners and that she needs to be emancipated. Similarly, although the nurse should be sure that she is not trying to retain Ms G. as a client for the financial gain of the infertility team, she should not be vilified for being a tool of the medical establishment that supports, and is supported by, a capitalist system.

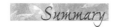
Summary

The encounter between Ms. G and the nurse illustrates basic steps toward cultural competence based on the understanding of culture that has been presented in this chapter. Given the increasing cultural diversity of people in the United States today, holistic nurses can anticipate the development strategies that are increasingly culturally competent. As this chapter was being written, the Office of Minority Health was soliciting feedback on proposed standards for cultural and linguistic competence. Readers may wish to consult that Website and the other sites provided in the Resources for further information.

RESOURCES

American Anthropological Association, Society for Medical Anthropology
Council on Nursing and Anthropology (CONAA)
4350 North Fairfax Dr., Suite 640
Arlington, VA 22203-1620
Phone: (703) 528-1902
www.people.memphis.edu/~sma/conaa.html

American Nurses Association
International Nursing Center
600 Maryland Ave. SW, Suite 100W
Washington, DC 20024
Phone: (800) 274-4262
www.ana.org/anf/inc/index.htm

Montana Area Health Education Center
333 Culbertson Hall
P.O. Box 170520
Montana State University
Bozeman, MT 59717-0520
Phone: (406) 994-6001

National Association of Hispanic Nurses
1501 16th St. NW
Washington, DC 20036
Phone: (202) 387-2477
www.NAHNHG.org

National Black Nurses Association
8630 Fenton St., Suite 330
Silver Springs, MD 20910-3803
Phone: (301) 589-3200
www.nba.org

National Council for International Health
1701 K St. NW, Suite 60
Washington, DC 20006
Phone: (202) 833-5900
www.ncih.org

Office of Minority Health Research Center
U.S. Department of Health and Human Services
P.O. Box 37337
Washington, DC 20013-7337
Phone: (800) 444-6472
www.omhrc.gov

REFERENCES

1. Tylor, EB: Primitive Culture. John Murray, London, 1871, p1.
2. Meadows, M: Moving toward consensus on contemporary competency in health care. Closing the Gap [newsletter of the Office of Minority Health, U.S. Department of Health and Human Services], May 2000, pp 1–2.
3. Mead, M: Coming of Age in Samoa. New American Library, New York, 1949. (Original work published 1929)
4. Barnett, CR, and Rabin, DI: Collaborative study by physicians and anthropologists: Congenital hip disease. In Adair, J, and Deuschle, KW (eds): The People's Health. Appleton-Century-Croft, New York, 1970.
5. Young, A: Some implications of medical beliefs and practices for social anthropology. American Anthropologist 78:5–24, 1976.
6. Fadiman, A: The Spirit Catches You and You Fall Down. Duxbury, North Scituate, Mass., 1997, pp 61-68.
7. Trotter, RT: A survey of four illnesses and their relationship to intracultural variation in a Mexican-American community. American Anthropologist 93:115–125, 1991.
8. Blumhagen, D: Hyper-tension: A folk illness with a medical name. Culture, Medicine, and Psychiatry 4:197–227, 1980.
9. Foster, SW: The pragmatics of culture: The rhetoric of difference in psychiatric nursing. Arch Psychiatr Nurs 4:292–297, 1990.
10. Singer, M, et al: Why does Juan Garcia have a drinking problem? The perspective of critical medical anthropology. Med Anthropol 14:77–108, 1992.
11. Ibid.
12. Ibid, p 93.
13. Meadows: Moving toward consensus, p 1.
14. Sanchez-Ayendez, M: The Puerto Rican American family. In Mindel, CH, Habenstein, RW, and Wright, R (eds): Ethnic Families in America. Elsevier, New York, 1988.
15. Kleinman, A: Patients and Healers in the Context of Culture. University of California Press, Berkeley, 1980.
16. McKinlay, J: A case for refocusing upstream: The political economy of illness. In Conrad, P, and Kern, R (eds): The Sociology of Health and Illness. St. Martin's Press, New York, 1986.

CHAPTER 6

Global Health Issues

R. Brooke Thomas and Mary Anne Bright

R. Brooke Thomas, PhD, is professor of anthropology at the University of Massachusetts–Amherst. He teaches courses on human ecology, biosocial aspects of poverty, and human adaptability. Thomas is a fellow of the American Academy of Sciences and has served on the Executive Committees of the American Association of Physical Anthropology, the U.S. Man in the Biosphere Arctic and Alpine Directorate, and the Institute of Ecology. He has worked for three decades in the Peruvian high Andes on problems of biocultural adaptation, health, and political ecology.

Mary Anne Bright, RN, CS, EdD, the editor of this book, is an associate professor at the University of Massachusetts–Amherst School of Nursing. She teaches courses in holistic health and psychiatric-mental health nursing, conducts research on Therapeutic Touch, and is a member of the International Institute of Bioenergetic Analysis and of the American Holistic Nurses Association.

Michael Perlman, the author who was to write this chapter, died on Earth Day, April 22, 1998. As a writer, educator, and environmental activist, Michael dedicated his life to expressing his concern about the ongoing abuse of the planet. This chapter is a tribute to Michael's vision of restoring global health.

For Michael, human health, in its broadest sense, is constructed from a balance of well-being between ourselves and that which surrounds us: our homes and families, communities and local places, nature and the planet. His ultimate pessimism lay in the continuing and systematic severance of these linkages taking place around him and the futility of his best efforts to communicate these concerns. In writing this chapter we attempt to honor these efforts and carry forward the connections he saw so clearly, exploring solutions to changing our consciousness about human and planetary health, and in the end providing hope.

We knew Michael too briefly. Our last contact with him, before he passed away, was at an Earth Action Conference held at Greenfield Community College (Greenfield, Massachusetts) and organized by Larry Buell, a professor, environmental activist, and founder of the Earthlands intentional community. The conference brought together more than 40 practitioners—healers, herbalists, outdoor educators, solar technology specialists, organic farmers, and environmental activists—who were seeking alternative ways of interacting with the earth, life, and one another. They gathered so that students and members of the regional community could meet and share ideas with like-minded people who, in various ways, saw these interconnections and were committed to making a difference in their own lives, if not the lives of others. Among the array of conference display tables, there was a lone young man with nothing obvious to distribute save a few books. This man was Michael Perlman, a soft-spoken, humble person, more intent on talking about ideas than selling the books he had written.

As the conversation progressed, he pointed to his book *Hiroshima Forever: The Ecology of Mourning*[1] (other works are listed in the References section). In Michael's opinion, the ecological movement began when the atomic bomb was dropped. At that point, he explained, we realized the human potential to destroy life across the planet—if not the planet itself. This notion challenged the artificial separation we had created between environment and humanness, and forced consideration of a dialectical relationship between the two: humans shaping nature and it, in turn, shaping humanity. New interconnections and a new consciousness about how to join things long kept separate were born out of the bomb as we gasped at the immediate and total devastation of two cities in Japan. We pondered the consequences of radiation, mutation rates, the distortion of life forms, and what the ubiquitous perception of vulnerability—no, annihilation—was to mean to all of us for the foreseeable future. Bomb drills and fallout shelters became but hollow gestures in response to intercontinental ballistic missile attacks, and visions of a nuclear winter fostered widespread pessimism and protest.

Michael Perlman's insights were impressive, as was the ease with which he glided from subject to subject, weaving them into a tapestry of interrelations. He revered trees, especially old-growth forests, because of their history. And in his book *The Power of Trees: The Reforesting of the Soul*,[2] he traced how their connections entwined with other aspects of the environment, and with an array of humans who relied on them, while finding them beautiful.

Michael's environmental concerns echoed those of the evening's main speaker, Michael Colby of Food and Water, an activist group in Vermont. Colby asked what capitalism and hyperconsumption were doing to us, to our environment, and to the less fortunate in the world. He pointed out how politics affects the foods we eat and how the campaign by the meat-packing industry to irradiate its product was being justified as a way to sanitize the unhygienic slaughtering conditions that large packing houses had created. Colby also explained how politics, industry, banking, and the media were merging for competitive advantage, and in the process compromising the quality of the food and water we consume, as if quality were a secondary consideration to profit.

These political and economic issues are not topics we normally associate with health in any immediate physical sense as laid out for us by biomedicine. Yet all have a direct bearing on how our physical, mental, and spiritual health is constructed. The social, political, and environmental aspects of daily living, as they impact health, are often invisible yet very real. Consider the context from which our food emerges. Much of what we buy at the grocery stores comes from overfarmed, pesticide-laden land. These products are grown and harvested by poorly paid farmworkers or imported from parts of the world where poverty—and hence an inability to obtain adequate diet and health care—is the norm.

There is an invisible but direct link between the food we eat and what is happening in the world. As nutritionist Dorothy Blair[3] has written: "A food system built on social injustice and ecological imprudence undermines social health, because the system is productive at the expense of the underclass both here and abroad, and at the expense of the environmental resources we owe our offspring." Rachael Carson,[4] in her book *Silent Spring,* which first alerted us to the present ecological crisis and drew connections among radioactive fallout, pesticides, and health risk, remarked, "There is an ecology of the world in our bodies."

Health Practitioners: Reconstructing a Sense of Health

As we entered the 21st century, many of us sensed a momentary euphoria. It was as though we had left behind a society capable of ignoring sordid histories, abusive socioeconomic structures, and outdated ways of thinking that had increasingly encumbered our actions. Entering the new millennium created the illusion that we had emerged into an era filled with new possibilities, one capable of better meeting people's needs and aspirations. The euphoria, of course, was not built on reality, for the date was but an artifact, and history does not easily yield its grip on the trajectory of global processes already in motion.

Nonetheless, there is a gathering momentum, a fresh wind, felt in disparate arenas of life (classrooms, conferences, public discourse, alternative lifestyles, and the occasional demonstration) signaling that significant change—even transformation—is imminent in how we will interact with family, community, workplace, consumption, health, and environment. It has arisen from recognition of and discontent with the fact that economic progress, materialism, individualism, technological solutions, and the authority of experts have guided our modernist ways of understanding and acting. In its wake, we have been left with high levels of dependence on a global system designed to serve profits first and to divert our imaginations with the rewards of lifelong hyperconsumption.

The result has left even those of us who benefit from the global system isolated and somewhat frantic: floating individuals devoid of meaningful connections to history, place, community, spirituality, nature, and even the future of our children. The seductions of our lifestyle place us in conflict with the possibilities that we sense are within our grasp— possibilities for a healthy, viable future for all people and for the earth itself. Such a contest is the dynamic and great debate of our time—both within ourselves and in society at large.

This chapter therefore seeks to explore how we might envision such a transformation as it pertains to linkages between global and individual health. In doing so, it is designed not so much to instruct or inform the reader, but to initiate a reconsideration of how *you* might affect health care and *your* participation in it. As you have undoubtedly realized in choosing a health-care vocation, health-care practitioners place themselves in the center of a most complex and powerful set of relationships. People arrive to you vulnerable, disconnected, and out of balance. How you perceive their state and engage a set of healing skills to bring about their well-being and what relationships you choose to emphasize—or ignore—will make all the difference to those you serve.

Health care is one of the arenas in which the aforementioned contradictions (seemingly irresolvable alternatives) abound for both professionals and users alike. In response, many have sought health and cures for illness beyond the biomedical tradition, embracing a range of alternative practices and therapies. Diagnoses, likewise, have reached beyond physical symptoms to those of the mind and spirit, and curing has incorporated social relations,[5] spirituality,[6,7] and interconnections with the environment.[8,9] ·

Beyond Biomedicine

Biomedicine, which achieved prominence only 100 years ago, is a relatively new phenomenon that emerged from a materialist worldview. As such, it treats what can be seen and measured as the only reality, it considers the body as a mechanistic entity, and it views humans as separate from the rest of nature. This view of reality is a radical departure from past medical traditions, both Western and Eastern. In the West, the 15th-century Swiss physician Paracelsus proposed "a correspondence, if not a unity, between the microcosm [the human body] and the macrocosm [all of nature, including relationships among natural forces on earth, plant and animal life, and the cosmic influences of planets and stars]."

Eastern medicine rests on similar assumptions. For example, from a Chinese perspective the human being is viewed as a microcosm of the universe: the human body is an ecosystem, and associations are based on metaphors from nature. As depicted in Figure 6–1, "Chinese medical thinking is holographic: each aspect of bodily life reflects the whole of which it is a part, all parts are in constant interaction with each other, and universal patterns are replicated at every level of human existence."[10]

The ascendancy of biomedicine as the dominant Western system of knowledge that effectively suppressed other medical truths has been well documented in other chapters.

FIGURE 6–1   Views of the Human Body, West and East

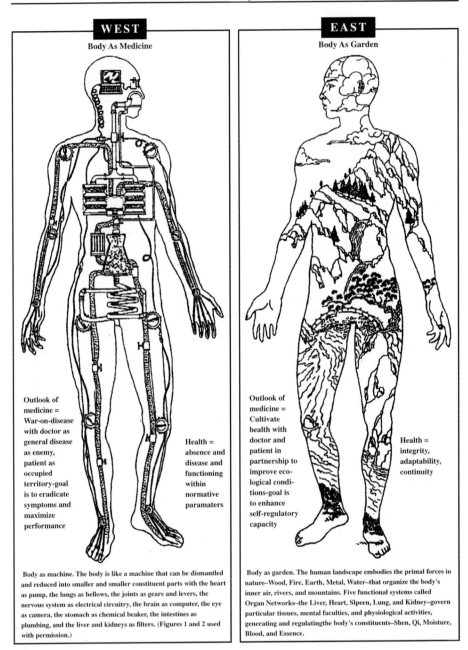

WEST
Body As Medicine

Outlook of medicine = War-on-disease with doctor as general disease as enemy, patient as occupied territory-goal is to eradicate symptoms and maximize performance

Health = absence and disease and functioning within normative paramaters

Body as machine. The body is like a machine that can be dismantled and reduced into smaller and smaller constituent parts with the heart as pump, the lungs as bellows, the joints as gears and levers, the nervous system as electrical circuitry, the brain as computer, the eye as camera, the stomach as chemical beaker, the intestines as plumbing, and the liver and kidneys as filters. (Figures 1 and 2 used with permission.)

EAST
Body As Garden

Outlook of medicine = Cultivate health with doctor and patient in partnership to improve eco-logical condi-tions-goal is to enhance self-regulatory capacity

Health = integrity, adaptability, continuity

Body as garden. The human landscape embodies the primal forces in nature–Wood, Fire, Earth, Metal, Water–that organize the body's inner air, rivers, and mountains. Five functional systems called Organ Networks–the Liver, Heart, Slpeen, Lung, and Kidney–govern particular tissues, mental faculties, and physiological activities, generating and regulatingthe body's constituents–Shen, Qi, Moisture, Blood, and Essence.

From: Alternative Therapies in Health and Medicine 1(1):46 March, 1995, with permission.

However, in the past decade popular response to alternative health care has been overwhelming. This is significant not only because the public has effectively gone beyond the authority of conventional medicine but also because such a trend shows how orthodoxy in general might be challenged, and therefore changed, to better serve humanity.

Recent trends toward increased use of complementary and alternative modalities are only now influencing the practices of conventional Western health-care practitioners. Wallace Sampson, of Stanford's Medical School and editor of *The Scientific Review of Alternative Medicine,* states that nearly all the alternative medicine courses and centers he examined in a recent survey were "developed and driven by advocates." The movement is "really a secular religion" and poses a threat to scientific medicine that is more serious than anyone realizes.[11] Nevertheless, more than 70 U.S. universities now offer some sort of alternative medicine program. Even the prestigious National Institutes of Health has recently (1998) created—albeit because of political pressure—the National Center for Complementary and Alternative Medicine to assess the efficacy of "unconventional" curing techniques.[12]

With such questioning and controversy going on in the field of health, these are, indeed, exciting times that avail themselves to new ways of combining forms of medicine. Biomedicine, therefore, stands uneasily at a crossroads, firmly convinced of its own efficacy but increasingly aware that it must go further—much further. Naively, it is convinced that it can evaluate alternative techniques through the rigor of its own scientific method (things that can be measured), overlooking the subtle and complex phenomena that elude empirical cause-and-effect verification.

Critical of such an effort, Hufford and Chilton,[13] in a chapter entitled "Politics, Spirituality and Environmental Healing," warn: "Alternative healing techniques are a great opportunity for social change. Such change must be careful not to be assimilated into the powerful institutions of biomedicine for they will be disempowered from radical possibilities."

Holistic Health: A Balance with Nature

Does the health of the environments we construct around us or, in a larger perspective, the health of the planet have anything to do with human health in the narrow biomedical sense? And what are the interconnections that might make this plausible?

While the intention here is to challenge the hegemony of biomedicine as a cosmology that subjugates other truths of healing, we do not seek to discredit its outstanding successes—after all, biomedicine stands as one of the most impressive accomplishments of human reductionist science. Nevertheless, at a time when human activities are severely threatening the environmental relations on which we all depend, and short-term secular goals divert our attention from the broader impact we are having on ecological, social, and spiritual health, we feel it is important to emphasize the need for a more complementary and expansive perspective.

A holistic perspective of health asks us to move beyond ego, symptomatology, suppression, and the quick fix. This serves as but a starting point on a pathway to explore the interconnections of life and how life forms—human and nonhuman—try to maintain a balance in an ever-changing world where it is easy to lose one's "footing."

In its emphasis on understanding linkages (to society, nature, the planet, and ultimately our place in the universe), holistic health asks us to inquire broadly—and at multiple levels—into the life systems that surround us in order to comprehend health and healing. This, then, requires a definition of well-being that incorporates an assessment not only of the biological but also of the mental, social, material, and spiritual. Such a holistic perspective (in embracing health, food, agriculture, and nature as interactive entities) consequently finds commonalties in "mad cow disease", bovine growth hormone, pesticide toxicity in the food chain, and red tide from waste runoff. In a similar sense, it is capable of linking cancer and cardiovascular disease with lifestyle and psychosocial stress, and attributing these factors to broader societal and environmental processes.[14]

Indigenous Perspectives

It is important to recall that biomedicine is a reflection of a system of knowledge of a particular society at a particular moment in history. It is a way of curing that is consistent with a constructed reality, emphasizing certain relationships of importance to that society and neglecting others. Identifying what biomedicine excludes is central to the concept of health it reproduces. Biomedicine's success in its own right has propelled the spread of this particular way of healing. Nevertheless, public health officials working in conjunction with missionaries, military missions, and development agencies, in an attempt to control minds and resource flows, have actively promoted its acceptance over large sections of the world. As such, Western medicine has become part of the standard development package accepted by/imposed on the third world that has actively traditionalized, trivialized, and labeled as "backward" indigenous systems of knowledge regarding their attachments to nature, obligations to community, and broad-based healing practices.

Indigenous perspectives—which integrate spirit with body, individual with community, community with environment, and past with present and future—have received considerable attention because they contrast so starkly with more Western notions of human domination over the world. These are other systems of knowledge that respect and are committed to the maintenance of human-nature linkages and are based on obligation to ancestors, those presently living, and generations yet unborn. As such, in offering alternative ways of perceiving, organizing, and acting upon the world, they hold out renewed understandings of human health.

Unfortunately, when these systems of knowledge become eroded or lost, a process of separation occurs. Local resources are extracted by outsiders, human labor is recruited away from social support and community projects, and information on health and nature built up over generations is discarded as irrelevant. Lost are a sense of identity, place, purpose, and an ability to control human interaction with both nature and the spiritual domain. *And when indigenous cosmologies are eliminated and systems of knowledge undercut obligations that bind people with one another, nature and their future are undermined.*

Andrea Carman, an Alaskan Yaqui from Chicaloon, addresses this dilemma in discussing her group's cosmology in terms of the corporatization of the natural world:

> This [water] right here—the blood of our mother earth—this ba'am, every rock, every stone, every blade of grass, every animal is part of that life in which we are all a part. The corporate worldview, on the other hand, sees the world as something dead, as only to be used, and used for profit. The indigenous worldview is based on respect . . . and the recognition of the interrelationships of all aspects of this sacred creation. The corporate world divides, divides, divides.
>
> [The earth] is a woman. She feels pain, she feels suffering. Our elders have said, and every nation's prophesy has told us, that she will not let this go on forever. . . . In order to protect her life which is the life of every one of us—every bug to the eagle to the fish to the moose—she will take a step from her own power, her life-giving and life taking power, to end this exploitation. This will happen unless we make a decision right here and now to end our participation and look at what that means in terms of every aspect of our life, which is interrelated.[15]

Bill Tallbull, of the Northern Cheyenne Tribe in Lame Deer, Montana, describes this unity of life in terms of the Medicine Wheel Alliance, a group of regional tribes that use a circular pattern of boulders formed on a 10,000-foot mountain in the Bighorns of Wyoming as a vision quest site:

> The Medicine Wheel Site itself is a lodge, which houses the spirit that helps us. The spirits to represent the environment—the natural forces—are there. Many of our mountains have these. . . . Mountain ranges, prairies, great rivers have these.
>
> It may sound strange that we live in a spiritual world—every one of you has a spirit. How well do you know your spirit? What does it do? We are familiar with those who live in the mountains, the spirits

that live there. And it has special meaning for us when we go there because through the generations people have been selected by those spirits to come to be workers. My grandfather always told us that his spirit would not go where the rest of us would go, that he was summoned to a mountain to be a worker on the mountain. All these mountains [the spirits that are there] were once people.

Our survival depends upon our spiritual relationship with all spirit life on this earth. . . . The things I say may sound strange to you, but they are a fact, they are real. We have lived this way and survived for thousands of years, and survival has been going back to nature. Understand it. Listen to it. Feel it. Take your shoes off. Your survival lies there.[16]

How strange Western people must seem to others in the manner in which we have constructed ourselves as unique and separate. We often perceive ourselves as individual flagships quite apart from, and mostly unconcerned with, the processes that created and sustain us, separated from the flow of evolution or the flow of energy that passes from the sun to allow earth-bound life forms to grow, move, and replace themselves. We have distanced ourselves from biological communities (the flora and fauna) of which we are a part, and only recently do we seem to have discovered the biosphere—that thin layer of life coating the earth. Without an understanding of our linkages to nature, the planet, and the universe, it is difficult to understand who we are and whence we came. And it is difficult to have obligations, as a conscious species, to the relationships that sustain both health and life. Holistic health, therefore, reaches out to comprehend our place in these extrahuman relationships, and, in the words of David Abram,[17] inquires "how had western civilization come to be so exempt from this sensory reciprocity?"

Outlandish Premises

This said, we propose six rather "outlandish" premises that link the origins of the universe to our contemporary sense of dislocation. In their remoteness, the premises whisper for a more holistic health. As previously mentioned, the absence of such perspectives from conventional Western thought regarding human health stands in lonely contrast to the cosmologies and curing practices of non-Western groups that have tied their origins and existence to these processes.

1. Created approximately 14 billion years ago, out of a supercharged, subatomic particle, in what our origin theory calls the "big bang," we are one with the universe, having been ultimately formed by its forces and materials (energy and matter). We share this experience with the makeup of the earth, the sun, other stars in our Milky Way galaxy, and ultimately the billions of other galaxies of the expanding cosmos.[18] As Vanderbilt University theologian Sally McFae observes, "We are brothers and sisters to the sun and moon, cousins to the distant stars."[19]

2. Life (self-replicating forms) appeared on earth about 4 billion years ago, an event that, from our present vantage point, seems extraordinarily rare—possibly unique—in an otherwise lifeless universe. Earth's living forms, therefore, share a similar origin and an ongoing interconnectivity as life itself has evolved over eons along diverse routes. These are lifelines relying on energy, materials, and genetic information from their predecessors. They constitute life strings along which life itself jumps from body to body before senescence sets in, hoping to avoid extinction.[20]

3. At a given time a dynamic ecological balance exists among facets of the contemporary web of life: this affects the sustenance, health, and reproductive potential of all these diverse life forms. Just as interconnections bind us to our evolutionary past, present living forms are linked to one another in a set of interdependency relationships that affect collective well-being. Although we distinguish between the

nonliving and living, and among different species within the latter group, James Lovelock's Gaia hypothesis proposes that the planet, in its entirety, is one huge, living creature that self-regulates the conditions necessary to sustain life.[21]

4. Human activities, driven by a growing anthropocentric and egocentric consciousness that prioritizes consumption and the economy over other considerations, are severely destabilizing this balance. This has especially been the case for the last 50 years, as connections among life forms are being severed at an extraordinary rate. "Like the dinosaurs 65 million years ago, human society now finds itself in the midst of a mass extinction: a global evolutionary convulsion with few parallels in the entire history of life. Unlike the dinosaurs, however, we are not simply the contemporaries of a mass extinction, we are the reason for it."[22]

5. Human health, either directly or indirectly, is also being impaired by these destabilizing processes. Not only are health risks increased through greater exposure to long-recognized environmental stressors, but newly emerging conditions and diseases combine with perceptions of greater vulnerability,[23,24] adding a psychological assault to our overall well-being.[25] Mike Davis, writing about Los Angeles, with its earthquakes, fires, and riots, entitles his book *The Ecology of Fear: Los Angeles and the Imagination of Disaster.*[26]

6. Solutions lie in changing our mode of interaction with the planet: with our natural environment and the social, political, and economic realities we construct around us. Although appropriate technology and social redistribution of resources will be important to the collective well-being of humanity, ultimately we must transform our consciousness about what it means to live sustainably—both locally and globally—in a manner that equates with environmental and social justice. New behaviors and actions will be derived from this change in consciousness.[27,28]

These premises rest on a growing awe of, and attachment to, the world around and beyond us. After NASA's first photos of our bluish planet, most of us began to confront what a small speck we are in such a vast, inert universe. And when subsequent photos of the earth's surface showed us eroded soils turning the seas off Madagascar red (as if the island were hemorrhaging), or the spreading sands of the Sahara Desert with accompanying drought across the Sahel, or the vast burning of forests in the Amazon and Indonesia, or dead forests and lakes along acid rain corridors, or the holes in the ozone layer, or the disappearing ice fields on high mountains and at high latitudes, we began to sense the danger we were heading into and the tragedy it could signal.

The vision of a pearl-like planet circling an insignificant star is fascinating because it shakes us out of our anthropocentric complacency and asks us to contemplate the fragility and preciousness of all life forms. It also reminds us that we as humans may be unique in our ability to comprehend the condition we—and the rest of life—are in. And so we wonder—and worry—about mass extinction, rampant extraction, gluttonous human consumption, life-harming waste and pollution, and the outright environmental destruction that we have presided over in the seas, across the land, and into the thin veil of atmosphere that surrounds us.

Some Recent Changes on Earth

Humans have significantly altered their environments since the advent of fire, and this has clearly accelerated with agriculture and industrialization. However, in the past 50 years—with heavy extractive equipment, bulk transporters, and political and economic incorporation of most nation states into a world trading system—resources almost anywhere in the world have become available for exploitation. A brief summary of these recent changes is provided in Table 6–1.

TABLE 6–1 Recent Changes on the Planet

"We live today as if there were no tomorrow—as if we had no children." (L. Brown)

- Population explosion
- Economic debt
- Military expenses
- Growing inequities
- Sustained impoverishment for one-fifth of the human population
- Increasing violence, rebellion, and warfare
- Newly emergent diseases
- Ecological debt
  - deforestation, desertification, mountain degradation
  - habitat and species extinction
  - soil erosion and pollution
  - water scarcity, diversion, pollution
  - overfishing
  - radiation contamination
  - toxic wastes and acid rain
  - air pollution, global warming, ozone depletion

"Addressing the global environment requires nothing less than a radical change in the conduct of the world economy and policy." (UNEP)

Taken as isolated events, these changes constitute uncomfortable background noise in the daily media. Considered together, however, and with the realization that so much of the destruction has occurred within our lifetime, the noise turns to a deafening roar. The cause for dire concern is not just destruction on so many fronts, but its magnitude and ongoing inertia that may be irreversible for the foreseeable future. This level of destruction should cause widespread alarm, yet, as Lester Brown[29] of the WorldWatch Institute states in discussing the future of growth, "in effect, we are behaving as though we have no children, as though there will not be a next generation."

Here are some of the trends. The present world population of 6 billion will probably not level off until we reach 10 billion people around 2050: pressures created on the land and in human societies will be especially serious in the third world. People already living on the margins will have pushed these margins still further, causing further degradation of the forests, soils, mountain slopes, river ways, and coastal resources. Growing economic debt, in part fueled by the need to support standing armies (a new phenomenon), will mandate that more natural resources be sold abroad in order to produce revenue to pay off loans. To achieve this, resources (timber, minerals, fisheries) from national lands will be put up for bid and small-scale farming will be restructured to produce commercialized, export-oriented crops (e.g., ornamental flowers bound for U.S. markets replace corn and other edibles compromising local food security in Latin America).

The human consequences of this have been to push self-sufficient forest peoples and small-scale farmers into low-paying, high-risk wage labor positions. And when these lifestyles are no longer sustainable locally, people leave the homes of their ancestors and migrate to urban slums. Currently, immense streams of migrants—some seasonal, some permanent—flow within and between national boundaries, especially from poorer to richer regions. Such conditions frequently force families to live apart from one another, with women and children being left at home bearing the increased pressures of household maintenance, agricultural production, and financial insecurity.

We will soon be a world where most people live in cities and, therefore, the justifiable demands of urban residents for better living conditions will override policy addressing rural and environmental concerns. Growing material inequities everywhere in the world already mean that one-fifth of the world population cannot meet their basic needs of adequate food and shelter. This could grow to one-quarter of the world population by the middle of the 21st century should the trend continue. It is not coincidental that violence, rebellion, and warfare, which in recent times have caused so much human misery and environmental destruction, exist in regions of economic insecurity, undernutrition, and high rates of illness. Nor is it surprising that conditions are being created for newly emerging and recurrent diseases of epidemic proportions, as people move into unfamiliar environments and into crowded, unsanitary slums and refugee camps, and as modern transportation allows for rapid migration to locations throughout the world.

These are the human dimensions of a world that has come to rely on models of consumer capitalism, economic development, and globalized free trade that challenge the legitimacy of national laws designed to protect people and the environment. For many, modernization has vastly improved their quality of life; however, the same processes have thrust 20 to 40 percent of humanity into an intolerable or barely tolerable existence.

The price does not end here, because the ecological debt we have incurred is immense. We have borrowed from biotic and geologic reserves built up for millennia, with no means or intention to pay them back. The great temperate and tropical forests are disappearing, as are the great fisheries. Coral reefs around the world, which protect the shorelines and host a diversity of marine life, are being degraded, as are forests protecting mountain slopes from erosion. Reservoirs and rivers silt up, and desertification spreads as aquifers, springs, and rivers dry up. The battle for water rights is bound to be a basic human struggle in the future. Species, too, are struggling for their existence, ending their evolutionary paths at such a rate (1000 per year) that Leakey and Lewin[30] have called our times "the sixth extinction."

Finally, the waste products of human consumption have polluted our air, soil, and water, while toxic wastes and pesticides work their way into the food chains of people and animals. Acid rain kills forests and lakes, radiation contamination refuses to go away, pollutants eat away the ozone layer and expose us to greater levels of ultraviolet radiation, and the greenhouse effect fuels global warming. Acknowledging this unremitting attack of human activities on the planet, the United Nations Environmental Program stated: "Addressing the global environment requires nothing less than a radical change in the conduct of the world economy and policy." To this Lovelock responds: "We are amazingly unprepared for our journey into the future. We try to guard against local hazards, but tend to ignore threats global in scale."[31]

The process of reviewing our unique place in the universe and tracing out the last few decades of ravaging life on the earth provides a sobering reminder of the contradictions that modern society must solve. So, too, are the words of indigenous peoples who warn us of distorted values and ask us to entertain changes in a lifestyle that is engulfing everything. These words from our contemporaries reflect experiences and traditions that provide a coherent sense of how humans are integrated into the world of creation. This outlook acknowledges a world of obligation in which the past informs the present as to how to act into the future, and in which individual action is responsible to ancestors, the community of living things, and generations yet unborn.

The Problem with the Current Complementary and Alternative Medicine Movement

Today's alternative health-care movement, while a definite expansion beyond the bio-medical model, has been limited to the health of the individual. Yet individual health exists in the context of the environment. A singular focus on individual health, without concern for the environment, is like treating fish in an aquarium for illness created by the contaminated tank water but doing nothing about the water. The current emphasis on individual health maintains the illusion that we are improving or lengthening our lives in a sustainable fashion. But Antonovsky[32] states: "Looking within the skin prevents understanding the social burdens that pressure people to behave in pathogenic fashion— From a moral point of view, the focus on the 'health within' is at the very least a passive and unconscious approval of the status quo."

Given this epistemological nearsightedness, the challenge seems to be how to peer out of our respective body orifices and view the macroscape constructing human heath: the social relations, economy, politics, and nature that form the interactive environment on which our immediate and ultimate well-being is so dependent. In this regard holistic health holds out considerable hope not only for medicine but also for creating a concept of well-being that embraces biological as well as psychological, social, material, and spiritual dimensions.

Impediments to Change

Individual nearsightedness is only one impediment to the changes required to reverse trends toward the healing of the earth and to promote sustainable life on the global level. Why do individuals avoid involvement in environmental action? Robert Jay Lifton[33] identified a psychological process that he called "psychic numbing."

Psychic numbing is the diminished capacity to feel. Symbolization is impaired, often with a marked separation of thought from feeling; one is able to receive information cognitively but ceases to experience its impact. In extreme versions of psychic numbing, one can become anesthetized to the cognitive dimension as well—psychic numbing is thus invoked, usually unconsciously, to prevent the self from being overwhelmed and perhaps destroyed by the images and events around it. In being inactivated, the self undergoes a temporary death in the service of preventing a permanent one—the numbing itself becomes a permanent feature that can color all experience. With its feeling level increasingly diminished, the self becomes even more detached and disaffiliated from the outside world.

The Health Belief Model (HBM), discussed in Chapter 1, offers a framework in which psychic numbing and environmental inaction can be understood. The HBM postulates that persons are more likely to take action for health when they do one of the following:

• Perceive that they are susceptible to a threat to health
• Perceive the health threat to be severe enough to warrant action
• Perceive that there are worthwhile benefits to action
• Perceive the barriers to action as surmountable

Susceptibility

Global threats to health can seem unreal to the average American who has been insulated from direct experience of the effects of acute overpopulation, deforestation, economic crisis, and so forth. Health problems linked to poor water and air quality, such as asthma and digestive disorders, have biomedical solutions in this culture that reinforce the illusion that all health problems are treatable. Frequently the illnesses associated with nuclear radiation and toxic waste occur long after exposure. Industries' nonaccountability for health disruptions and communities' dependence on these industries for their livelihood are all influences that numb the individual's willingness and ability to feel vulnerable to the realities of environmental health threats.

Severity

People are engaged in mass denial of the seriousness of "business as usual," unconcern with environmental consequences. Environmentalists are often depicted as doomsayers or "Chicken Little" alarmists, seeing impending disaster where there is none. Status quo social, political, and economic forces benefit from current environmental policies that compromise global health. These forces keep environmentally conscious groups—even groups that enjoy high prestige and influence, such as the United Nations, the World Health Organization, the Union of Concerned Scientists, and the Physicians for Social Responsibility—under fire as being naive idealists and under siege by political opposition. People find comfort in messages that assuage the fear of environmental decline, because the idea of extinction is both unthinkable and horrifying.

The perception of severity can work against a person's perception that health action is worthwhile. In a study of nurses' attitudes toward preventing nuclear war, Winder and Stanitis (Bright) [34] discovered that the perception of a severe threat to health could be associated with a sense of hopelessness and helplessness, as well as a sense of the uselessness of preventive or proactive citizen involvement. If people feel that their actions cannot make a difference, they may "fiddle while Rome burns." In addition, they found that the perception that a threat to health was perceived as severe required a larger system solution, which minimized a sense of personal involvement in the solution to the health threat.

Benefits of Action

Can one person, or a small group of concerned citizens, make a difference? This is the question that must be answered affirmatively for an individual to decide to become involved in environmental health advocacy and action. The benefits of environmental action may not be visible or immediate, and cultural norms favoring instant gratification and the quick fix can work against the optimism that sustains environmental advocacy efforts. Those who believe in the efficacy of their efforts are inclined to agree with Margaret Mead, who challenged the idea that small citizen action groups cannot create change.

Barriers to Action

The demands and distractions of daily life can be perceived as impediments to environmental action. It is hard to make time to "save the environment" when there is work to do, not to mention people to take care of, bills to pay, personal goals to achieve, and so forth. The complexity of modern life sets up seemingly impossible, competing demands on time. "Living for today," without taking into consideration the impact of our decisions on future generations, creates a false sense of separation from the continuity of life. Crisis and stress—illness, poverty, family and social violence, racism and sexism, crime, relocation, and other threats to individual survival and security—consume attention and energy. A tendency to avoid thinking about upsetting issues that are considered "out of sight, out of mind" and attitudes that perpetuate "not in my backyard" decisions (e.g., locating toxic waste sites where poor and politically disenfranchised people live) are barriers to appropriate action. A sense of alienation from nature—that nature needs to be brought under control, or that we are superior to other species, or that our needs are separate from those of other forms of life—inhibits an empathic connection to the life around us, and thus action on its behalf.

What Are We to Do?

An effective response to global health issues is a monumental and formidable task. Yet we have enacted many seemingly impossible dreams and visions: mastering flight, controlling disease, desalinating water, cultivating deserts, developing organisms that can digest petroleum waste products, linking communication worldwide, exploring atomic and cosmic space, and walking on the moon. Why not save the earth next?

Former vice president Al Gore[35] is among those who envision the need for "bold and unequivocal action: We must make the rescue of the environment the central organizing principle for civilization." He identifies six strategic goals toward this end:

1. Stabilization of world population from a dynamic equilibrium of high birth and death rates to a stable equilibrium of low birth and death rates.
2. Rapid creation and development of environmentally appropriate technologies capable of accommodating sustainable economic progress without the concurrent degradation of the environment. These new technologies must be transferred quickly to all countries.
3. A comprehensive change of the "rules of the road" by which we measure the impact of human action on the environment and establishment of new standards of accountability from the individual to the macroeconomic level.
4. Creation of a new generation of international agreements that will embody the myriad processes necessary for an overall plan that will succeed. These agreements must be sensitive to the vast differences in capability and need among developed and less developed nations.
5. Establishment of a cooperative plan to educate the world's citizens about global environmental needs, including researching and monitoring current changes. People of all nations need to be involved in this process, especially students. Information dissemination will help foster new thinking patterns about the relationship between civilization and the environment.
6. Establishment of social and political conditions throughout the world that are most conducive to sustainable societies. These societies will demonstrate certain characteristics: social justice; equitable arrangements of land ownership; a commitment to human rights; adequate nutrition, health care and shelter; high literacy rates; and greater political freedom, participation, and accountability.

These goals should be pursued simultaneously within the larger framework of a global Marshall Plan, with all policies integrated into the central organizing principle of saving the global environment.

New Visions: Deep Ecology and Ecofeminism

Individual action that entails new ways of thinking about relationships and connections lies at the core a transformation of how we interact with the environment. Two holistic frames of reference that engender new ways of perceiving this interconnectedness are those of deep ecology and ecofeminism.

Deep Ecology   Interaction with the universe.

The concept of deep ecology was developed by the Norwegian philosopher Ame Naess in the early 1970s. This approach was a departure from "human-centrism," which emphasizes human domination and primacy over nature, to a broader "biocentrism," which sees all life forms as sharing the rights that have been co-opted by humans. Principles of deep ecology locate the place of humanity in part of the organic whole of life. Devall and Sessions[36] assert that the work of becoming a whole person includes the attainment of spiritual maturation and the unfolding of the self in relation to the environment:

> *This process of the full unfolding of the self can be summarized by the phrase, "No one is saved until we are all saved," where the phrase "one" includes not only me, an individual human, but all humans,*

TABLE 6–2   Dominant Worldview vs. Deep Ecology

DOMINANT WORLDVIEW	DEEP ECOLOGY
Dominance over nature	Harmony with nature
Natural environment as resource for humans	All nature has intrinsic worth/biospecies equality
Material/economic growth for growing human population	Elegantly simple material needs (material goals serving the larger goal of self-realization)
Belief in ample resource reserves	Earth "supplies" limited
High technological progress and solutions	Appropriate technology; nondominating science
Consumerism	Doing with enough/recycling
National/centralized community	Minority tradition/bioregion

Source: Devall, B, and Sessions, G: Deep ecology. In Smith, MJ: Thinking Through the Environment. Routledge, London and New York, 1999, with permission.

whales, grizzly bears, whole rainforest ecosystems, mountains and rivers, the tiniest microbes in the soil, and so on.

The worldview of deep ecology contrasts sharply with the current dominant worldview. Basic principles of deep ecology foster a vision of the interconnectedness of life that offers an alternative to the consumptive, destructive, exploitative path we are currently following. (See Table 6–2.)

Ecofeminism

Ynestra King[37] asserts that ecology is incomplete without a feminist perspective. The ecofeminist perspective envisions a connection between eradicating the hatred and domination of nature and eradicating the hatred and domination of women. Ecofeminists equate the idea of dominating nature with a patriarchal view that is inconsistent with the continuity of life on the planet. King observes: "Paradoxically, the human species is utterly dependent on nonhuman nature. We could not live without the rest of nature; it could live without us."

Ecofeminism reflects the value of staying in touch with our bodily nature, an awareness that is intrinsic to women's experience. Identification with the body facilitates a more intimate experience of nature, heals barriers to our sense of connectedness to other forms of life, and supports an awareness of nonhierarchical relationships in nature.

Joni Seager[38] observes that women in all countries constitute the most vulnerable segment of society and that a disproportionate share of the impact of environmental problems falls them. It is most often women who initiate grassroots movements to improve the safety of food, water, and sanitary conditions when the health of their children is threatened. Women are subject to reproductive disorders, which are a serious indicator of environmental deterioration, and carry the burden of caring for children made ill or disabled by microbial and toxic waste contamination, without the benefit of sufficient protection and support from larger systems. Ecofeminism recognizes relationships between women and nature, between women and the patriarchal system that oppresses and divides them, and between women and the solutions to ecological survival.

Seager describes how an ecofemminist culture and politics can merge to create a healing culture:

> *Ecofeminists are taking direct action to affect changes that are immediate and personal as well as long-term and structural. Direct actions include learning holistic health and alternate ecological technologies, living in communities that explore old and new forms of spirituality which celebrate life as diverse expressions of nature, considering the ecological consequences of our lifestyles and personal habits, and participating in creative public forms of resistance, including nonviolent forms of civil disobedience.[39]*

The ecological movement cannot ethically proceed without the active inclusion and participation of women in environmental issues. For example, attempts at population control will not only fail, but will engender deeper resistance, if imposed in ways that disregard women's needs, rights, and centrality in childbearing and child rearing or that do not respect cultural values and norms. Emancipation and mobilization of women's vision, unification of women across boundaries of race, class, role and age, and active engagement of women's leadership and strength are critical to the ultimate success of the ecological movement.

A New Consciousness

As we become increasingly aware of the contradictions between how we act in our daily lives and what we must do to stop becoming "thieves of life,"[40] proposed solutions abound. According to Guha,[41] these fall into three general categories: (1) appropriate technology and environmental management/policy, (2) more equitable distribution of resources, and (3) a transformation of consciousness as to how we must interact with nature and our fellow human beings. The first solution operates largely within the confines of the existing status quo, attempting to find more efficient ways of doing the same thing while preventing, through management and laws, the more disruptive aspects of the capitalist economic system.

The second solution acknowledges the growing and grossly inequitable distribution of resources by region, class, and race, and seeks to reorder social relations, or at least to redistribute/reallocate resources. This is especially needed for the 20 to 40 percent of humanity who are barely getting by when third world elites and average people in the first world are consuming so much.

The third solution, a transformation of consciousness, underlies the first two in that we need to acknowledge that the health of all life—in both the short and long term—depends on renegotiating our interactions with nature and people. It builds on the fact that we cannot go on living this way, at least not for long. As such, it advocates a new systems of knowledge—a new consciousness—that might better achieve environmental and social justice.

The Old Consciousness: A Mechanistic Worldview and Its Consequences

As Stephen Marglin[42] observes, the mechanistic or modernist worldview, which is made up of countless specific domains of knowledge (e.g., medicine, engineering, agriculture), is in itself "a theory of knowledge with its own rules of acquiring and sharing knowledge, its own distinctive ways of changing the content of what counts as knowledge, and finally its own rules of governance, both among insiders and between insiders and outsiders." As such, it has its own priority categories and relationships between these categories, which encourage us to perceive, experience, and take for granted the world in certain ways while ignoring other possibilities.

Thus "health" is a category that has come to mean "symptom free" in the context of biomedicine, and nature is distorted into "natural" resources. These terms, in turn, are incorporated in priority relationships that we unconsciously accept. Thus "biomedicine" constitutes legitimate curing and "profitability" in an overarching assessment system that directs the use of medicine and natural resources to people who can pay more: this is how the system works.

Marglin refers to our current level of consciousness as a way of knowing that most of us have been socialized into and that dominant nations have successfully imposed on most of the world, especially in the last 50 years, with devastating effectiveness. Marglin asserts:

> *The ideological dominance of a single knowledge system justifies particular forms of acting in and on the world that threaten the sustainability of both material and social processes. . . . The problem comes when such knowledge refuses subordination to a cosmology, but pretends itself to be a cosmology, a theory of reality. As a cosmology it leaves no room, at least on the ideological level, for any other, equally necessary system of knowledge.*
>
> *As a cosmology, such knowledge gives us scientific management, which turns the worker into an appendage of the rule book and the machine for whom work has no meaning other than the paycheck at the end of the week. It gives us scientific forestry and scientific agriculture, which threaten to degrade the environment and exhaust the world's resources. It gives us scientific medicine, which transforms the person into a set of laboratory readings and poisons our bodies with chemicals as it prolongs life empty of meaning. It gives us scientific politics and administration, which transfers disembedded forms of instrumental and rational politics of the Third World, aiding and abetting the creation and maintenance of authoritarian and repressive regimes. In short, we see a dominance of a particular knowledge system as the thread that connects apparently disparate practices and beliefs about self, work, the environment and the body politic's practices and beliefs that threaten the sustainability of the present course of world development.*
>
> *How we come to think about the world depends in large part on the processes of socialization and education to which we are exposed. These processes surround us physically and mentally, molding and reinforcing daily routines, expecting certain types of social and economic interaction, and justifying political structures. As such, most of us live out our lives largely within the rules and constraints of a sociocultural cocoon. Nevertheless, there are times in history when the internal contradictions of life tear away at the social web of the cocoon and its system of knowledge. This occurs when the reality a knowledge system pretends to represent is challenged by other ways of organizing information and knowing—when people sense they are living a lie.*

As Marglin suggests in his rather grim portrayal of modern life, and as proponents of deep ecology and ecofeminism have observed, the contradictions in our lives challenge the complacency of our consciousness about the world we live in. The quality of our food, state of our health, our social responsibilities, sense of belonging, and obligation to something beyond ourselves prompt us to question this complacency.

These concerns have surfaced in the past and are still here today. The civil rights and women's rights movements in the United States, the fall of the Berlin Wall, the dissolution of the Soviet Union, the end of apartheid in South Africa, the Zapatista rebellion in Mexico (which started the day the North American Free Trade Agreement went into effect), the movement for universal health care, and the environmental movement are all such events. As disparate as these transformational movements may seem, they are connected as attempts to achieve a fairer world in a political-economic system reluctant to yield its privileges. A decade before each took place, they were but talk and protest from the margins; change seemed almost inconceivable. Yet as the contradictions—which had existed for so long—were debated, people of all sorts had to decide which reality was right and just. And so the world has changed in a dramatic manner—many would say for the better—in recent times. Our concern for the well-being of life and the health that fosters it is a challenge—undoubtedly the greatest challenge of our times—that still lies ahead. In the next section, a way of acting that serves as a pathway to hope is described.

Radical Ecology: Hope, Interconnectivity, and Balance

Carolyn Merchant,[43] in her book *Radical Ecology*, proposes a framework for understanding and participating in an ecological transformation. It is based on how growing contradictions can lead to a change in our consciousness, which, in turn, propels us to create more just environmental and social relations. In essence, Merchant's ecological transformation addresses the grand contradiction; that is, how to sustain the essential ecological processes that maintain all life when we are extracting, consuming, and despoiling at rates that vastly exceed replacement capacity. This situation seems especially dire because the human population is expected to increase by at least 50 percent by the middle of this century, consumption norms and expectations are increasing throughout the world, and inequities are expanding everywhere. The challenge, therefore, becomes how to change the present world system, made up of subsystems that reify economic development, free trade, and profitability, into one that emphasizes environmental sustainability and the environmental and social justice this implies.

Figure 6–2 presents three mutually reinforcing spheres—production, reproduction, and consciousness—representing both human and nonhuman life. Within and between these spheres lie the contradictions affecting all contemporary life. Starting in the center, the "ecological core," the sustenance of life, is dependent on a myriad of biogeochemical (nutrient) cycles and energy flows. How these are intertwined in food webs among plant and animal populations affects the web of life: its ability to thrive, grow, and hence produce and reproduce. Humans risk reducing both the diversity and abundance of production when we attach ourselves to these flows; simplify ecological systems by eliminating competitors or nonuseful species; export "products" from local areas so that they cannot be recycled; and impair the life-giving potential of air, soil, and water with our wastes ("postconsumption products"). And as this rate of extraction and exportation increases beyond the capacity of nonhuman populations to replace biomass productivity, the web of life starts withering. The strands start to unravel, and interdependencies are severed.

Birds are seen less frequently, the croaking of frogs becomes silent, polar bears laden with PCBs and dioxin far across the sea produce fewer offspring, types of trees disappear from yet more epidemics, chemical rain trickles down upon the land, bays turn red from animal waste, overfished spawning grounds never do recover, and, as the climate heats up, more powerful hurricanes and typhoons roar across the land and sea as glaciers melt into rising oceans. If "in God we trust," then "God help us, please!"

Declining biotic production, of course, affects the ability of populations to replace themselves, and as human populations both grow and increase their consumptive norms, nonhuman populations must give way by losing habitat and sometimes going extinct. A similar process takes place in terms of human social reproduction when whole ways of living, languages, and knowledge about nature and the supernatural are eliminated. And within societies of the "developed" world, when family values, ethics, and means of socialization become distorted by the profit motive, accumulation, and hyperconsumption (which comes to define individual aspiration and status), a hollowness of being settles over groups of people. Apathy, depression, and suicide cast a gloom over the young and old alike as community participation and volunteerism decline, reciprocity dries up, and antisocial behaviors become the fodder of the evening news.

Merchant's diagram (Figure 6–2) is effective in that it places in front of *us* the various processes that make our present way of living on this planet unsustainable. She then

FIGURE 6–2   Ecological Revolutions

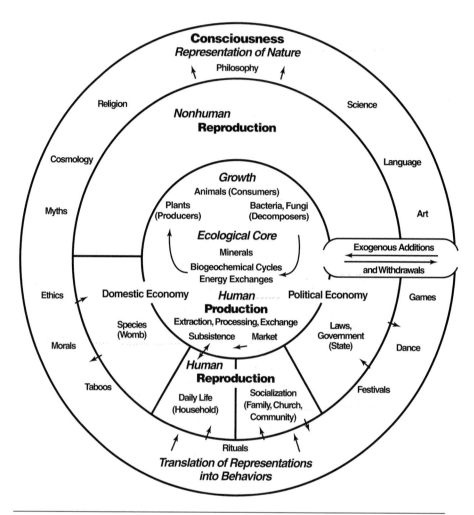

RADICAL ECOLOGY

From: Merchant, C: Ecological Revolutions: Nature, Gender, and Science in New England. University of North Carolina Press, N.C., 1989, with permission.

confronts us (our consciousness) with a series of steps (enumerated after this paragraph) designed to address and act on the aforementioned contradictions. In doing so she invites *us* to participate in the transformation. This is done with the confidence that as individuals challenge the existing dilemma in ways they feel appropriate, to the capacity they can, a momentum will be generated. And as this becomes more pervasive—making it easier for others to act—a transformation begins. Merchant[44] makes the following recommendations:

1. *Confront the illusion that we can commodify the world and live a life of accumulation. This is either blissful denial or just plain greed.*

2. *Be aware of deep-seated contradictions as to the sustainability of our behaviors.*

3. Reflect on ways we have absorbed roles and norms of the larger society: individualism, competition, materialism, hyperconsumption.

4. Ask what could be: new patterns of production, reproduction (both biological and social), and consciousness. Also how the present political and economic order is preventing fulfillment.

5. Search for alternative ways to resolve the present contradictions: a) between the sustainability of the ecological core and the effect human productive activities have upon it; b) between the non-human reproductive potential as influenced by human biological and social reproduction (material, legal, moral); and c) how these actions on nature perpetuate conscious representations of nature, our role in society, and our own identity.

6. Support social action that fosters new forms of consciousness toward environmental and social justice, and informs the public of how these representations can influence more fulfilling and sustainable human behaviors. In essence, by challenging the construction of our present consciousness toward nature and social interaction we open up new possibilities of thinking and acting. The outer ring of Figure 6–2 suggests domains in which some of these possibilities could take place.

While space does not permit elaboration, *you*, the reader, are encouraged to explore these possibilities, particularly in the context of expanded constructions of health and well-being. What, for instance, might be new modes of scientific inquiry that would diminish its cosmological stance and address, in a less hierarchical manner, a range of perspectives and practices related to health? And what about changes in the language of health (germ warfare, invasions) that set up barriers and obfuscate that which we are trying to accomplish? How might new forms of art, games, dance, festivals, and rituals bring people and their aspirations together rather than turning them into competitors? And how might they be brought into well-being maintenance and curing?

Can taboos, ethics, and morals be expanded in ways that provide meaningful commitment and obligation to environmental and social justice? And can myth, cosmology, and religion return a spiritual dimension to counter or complement our obsession with physical and material well-being? Within each of these domains of consciousness lie multiple possibilities with direct application to an expanded well-being.

The hope is that, as individuals confront the conditions that structure their lives and begin to address the contradictions that surround them, changes in consciousness will promote altered representations of nature, interdependency, and health. And these altered representations, in turn, will be translated into behaviors that affect others: humans, animals, plants, and nonliving materials that have been and will become life once more.

In this manner, challenges to the status quo gather momentum and the debate achieves greater legitimacy. Is this hope real? Does an ecological transformation have a chance of succeeding in a world where the global economy is encompassing all and consumption aspirations show no end? The outcome remains unclear, yet the grand debate continues with increased intensity—and this in itself seems to be considerable reason for optimism. Look around and notice flashes of light across the global landscape as people step forward, as groups are being formed, and as tired, tried ways are being challenged.

A life based on material accumulation, relatively void of social and spiritual attachments, and with people chronically out of time has generated sets of well-recognized stressors and pathologies. Today, more then ever, people are becoming concerned about their personal health, the food they eat, the conditions under which it is produced, and what this form of food production—filled with growth supplements, antibiotics, herbicides, and pesticides—is doing to the environment and our bodies.

Areas of life once segmented are now seen as a set of interdependencies. Environmental management, policies, and laws have become the business of communities, nations, and international bodies. And when governments have been unable or unwilling to address problems, concerned individuals, citizen groups, and nongovernmental organizations have proliferated. Frequently, these groups and organizations combine both environmental and social concerns (environmental racism, World Trade Organization protests), seeing linkages between the two agendas and not being constrained by the specific goals of government bureaucracy. Even foresighted corporations, practicing the concepts advocated by Paul Hawken, Amory Lovins, and L. Hunter Lovins in *Natural Capitalism*,[45] are seeing profitable advantages from an understanding of how the economic system can function in conjunction with the way nature works. In short, increasing numbers of citizen action groups and organizations are articulating the concerns and contradictions discussed here. And this is cause for an immense amount of hope that things will change—for the better.

Summary: New Vision, New Action

This chapter ends, as it started, with a tribute to Michael Perlman and his commitment to the beauty he sensed in the natural world around him. He saw, more clearly than most, the delicate connections that sustain our physical and spiritual balance, and lamented the callousness that blinds so many of us to the acts we are committing—plundering life and causing disease in order to achieve or sustain a middle-class existence. Indeed, Michael's seemingly intentional passing on Earth Day appears to have been a poignant last plea—the very most he could offer—to gain our attention and point to the seriousness of the struggle for our lives, for life, and for our precious little blue planet.

Michael Perlman's[46] vision included images of connection, celebration, and dreams:

> Most of us [who] want the ecological connection recognize that if community is to realize its promise it must include the hospitality to strangers, human and other. Most of us imagine far more than we realize. Most of us desire a different, friendlier world. Our capacities to dream of the Earth are crucial to the health of the future. If we think more boldly, we can sense the Earth [is] itself an expression of a kind of dream—or is itself dreaming, creatively generating forms, images, possibilities.

Hope for a transformation and the dreams that carry this theme were important elements in Michael Perlman's thinking. And thus he ended his essay with hope of what we might become:

> Ecological and social healing could go together and provide a framework for international peace that would encourage sharply-diminished reliance on other weapons, military spending, and violence. Taking better care of the health of Earth could provide renewable energy for the hope of international peace that the end of the Cold War too fleetingly occasioned. Facing the specter of all out climatic mayhem—and our participation in that dream of Earth—could disrupt disparity while nourishing cooperation among and within groups; counter consumerism while enhancing true material well-being; temper technological disconnection from Nature while encouraging reconciliation between the design of machines and the living world: and reveal to us the needlessness of our animosity toward difficult but hope-enhancing change. If we listen to our distant dreams, they will speak to where we presently are.[47]

Drawing from Michael's words—which live on and are passed onward—the question becomes how we will put these ideas to use. As health practitioners, you are situated in the center of these contradictions and a set of relationships that attempt to bring interconnectivity, balance, and hope to those you serve. Your dreams can shape the future of what health could be. These issues lie at the threshold of your primary health center, the refugee camp, the clinic, the hospital, your home, and your life. The times are right. Will you challenge your imagination to explore these linkages and come to a more comprehensive vision of health and care? And can you find ways to take these dreams to initiate a transformed ecology of health?

If not you, then who?

REFERENCES

1. Perlman, M: Hiroshima Forever: The Ecology of Mourning. Station Hall Arts, Barrytown, N.Y., 1995.
2. Perlman, M: The Power of Trees: The Reforesting of the Soul. Spring, Dallas, 1994.
3. Blair, D: Eating for wellness: Beyond the self. Unpublished manuscript.
4. Carson, R: Silent Spring. Houghton Mifflin, Boston, 1994. (Original work published 1962), p 12.
5. Antonovsky, A: Sociological critique of the "well-being" movement. ADVANCES: The Journal of Mind-Body Health 10:6, 1994.
6. Dossey, L: Recovering the Soul. Bantam, New York, 1989.
7. Taylor, E: A Psychology of Spiritual Healing. Chrysalis, West Chester, Pa., 1997.
8. Roszac, T: Ecopsychology: Restoring the Earth, Healing and the Mind. Sierra Club, San Francisco, 1995.
9. Winter, DD: Ecological Psychology: Healing the Split between Planet and Self. HarperCollins, San Francisco, 1996.
10. Beinfield, H, and Kornold, E: Chinese traditional medicine: An introductory overview. Alternative Therapies in Health and Medicine 1:44. 1995.
11. Quoted in Storkstad, E: Stephen Straus's impossible job. Science 288:1568, 2000.
12. Marshall, E: Bastions of tradition adapt to alternative medicine. Science 288:1571, 2000.
13. Hufford, D, and Chilton, M: Politics, spiritualitiy and environmental healing. In Chesworth, J (ed): The Ecology of Health. Sage, Thousand Oaks, Calif., 1996.
14. Steinberg, EM: The Balance Within: The Science of Connecting Health and Emotions. Freeman, New York, 2000.
15. Quoted in Gaul, KK, and Thomas, RB: Indigenous perspectives: Ecology, economy and ethics. Journal of Human Ecology (Special Issue No. 1), 1991, p 17.
16. Quoted in ibid, p 18.
17. Abram, D: The Spell of the Sensuous: Perception, Language, in a More-Than-Human World. Pantheon, New York, 1996, p 241.
18. Hawking, SW: A Brief History of Time: From the Big Bang to Black Holes. Bantam, New York, 1990.
19. Moyers, B (interviewer), and Pellet, P (producer): Spirit and Nature [video]. Mystic Fire Video, New York, 1991.
20. Dawkins, R: The Selfish Gene. Oxford University Press, Oxford, England, 1976.
21. Lovelock, JE: Gaia: A New Look at Life on Earth. Oxford University Press, Oxford, England, 1979.
22. Tuxill, J: Losing Strands in the Web of Life: Vertebrate Declines and the Conservation of Biological Diversity (WorldWatch Paper No 141). WorldWatch Institute, Washington, D.C., 1998, p 2.
23. Platt, A: Infecting Ourselves: How Environmental and Social Disruptions Trigger Disease (WorldWatch Paper No. 129). WorldWatch Institute, Washington, D.C., 1996.
24. Epstein, PR: Climate and health. Science 285:347, 1999.
25. Gallagher, W: The Power of Place: How Our Surroundings Shape Our Thoughts. Poseidon Press, 1993.
26. Davis M: The Ecology of Fear: Los Angeles and the Imagination of Disaster. Holt, New York, 1998, p 68.
27. Noble, V: Getting consciousness in the nineties: Turning the tide, healing the earth. Revision 17:30, 1995.
28. Macy, J, and Young, MY: Coming Back to Life: Practices to Reconnect Ourselves, Our World. New Society, Stony Creek, Conn., 1998.
29. Brown, L: The future of growth. In State of the World 1998: A WorldWatch Institute Report on Progress Toward a Sustainable Society. WW Norton, New York, 1998, p 2.
30. Leakey, R, and Lewin, R: The Sixth Extinction: Patterns of Life and the Future of Humankind. Doubleday, New York, 1995.
31. Lovelock, JE: A book for all seasons. Science 280:830, 1998.
32. Antonovsky, A: Sociological critique of the "well-being" movement. ADVANCES: The Journal of Mind–Body Health 10:6, 1994.

33. Lifton, RJ: The Protean Self. Basic Books, New York, 1993.
34. Winder, AE, and Stanitis (Bright), MA: Nuclear education in public health and nursing. American Journal of Public Health 78:967, 1988.
35. Gore, A: Earth in the Balance: Ecology and the Human Spirit. Plume, New York, 1993, pp 305–307.
36. Devall, B, and Sessions, G: Deep ecology. In Smith, MJ (ed): Thinking Through the Environment. Routledge, London and New York, 1999, p 200.
37. King, Y: Ecology and feminism. In Smith, MJ (Ed): Thinking Through the Environment.
38. Seager, J: Deep ecology and feminism. In Smith, MJ (Ed): Thinking Through the Environment, p 337.
39. Ibid, p 339.
40. Quinn, D: Ismael. Bantam, New York, 1995.
41. Guha, R: Eco-development debate: A critical review. South Asian Anthropologist 6:15, 1985.
42. Marglin, S: Sustainable development: A systems of knowledge approach. The Other Economic Summit/ North America 6:5, 1990.
43. Merchant, C: Radical Ecology: The Search for a Liveable World. Routledge, New York, 1992.
44. Ibid, pp 1, 2, 9, 13–14.
45. Hawken, P, Lovins, A, and Lovins, LH: Natural Capitalism: Creating the Next Industrial Revolution. Little, Brown, Boston, 1999.
46. Perlman, M: Imaginal Memory and the Place of Hiroshima. State University of New York Press, Albany, N.Y., 1988.
47. Perlman, M: The health of the earth. Unpublished manuscript.

Holistic Healing Modalities

CHAPTER 7

Meditation

Melissa Blacker

Melissa Blacker, MA, is an instructor in the Stress Reduction Program at the University of Massachusetts Medical School in Worcester, Massachusetts. She is also the coordinator of the Teacher Development Intensive Program, which is a part of the Professional Education Program at the Center for Mindfulness in Medicine, Health Care and Society at the University of Massachusetts. She has been a meditator since 1981 and guides meditation groups in Worcester and surrounding areas.

Imagine a life in which what is actually happening in the moment is what really counts. Whatever is present, whether painful or joyful, is experienced fully, without distractions. Worries about the future and regrets about the past have no power over you. Entering into the moment in this way, everything falls into perspective, and problems become manageable, no longer overwhelming. Calmness and alertness exist together. You are truly alive and awake. This state of mind can result from the practice of meditation, a healing modality that people have used ever since they first discovered the joy of sitting quietly and contemplating their inner and outer worlds.

The word *meditation* can be used to describe many different methods of quiet contemplation or observation. According to one definition, meditation means "to dwell on anything in thought; to contemplate deeply and continuously; to ponder; to ruminate; to reflect."[1] In this chapter, however, we will use the word to mean a certain kind of paying attention to something either real or imagined.

Just as the words *healing, holy,* and *whole* share a common root and meaning from the Old English word *hal,* meaning "healthy, whole, hale,"[2] the word *meditate* shares a root in Latin with the word *medical.* Both words derive from the word *mederi,* meaning "to cure." But *mederi* itself comes from an older Indo-European root, *med,* which means "to measure."[3] As Jon Kabat-Zinn, PhD, founder of the Stress Reduction Clinic at the University of Massachusetts Medical School in Worcester, Massachusetts, points out, both medicine and meditation are concerned with measuring. In meditation, we measure, or observe, our own internal state of mind and body, with an attitude of attentiveness and curiosity, checking to see if we are in balance. Kabat-Zinn calls this taking our "right inward measure." Medicine, he writes, is "the means by which right inward measure is restored when it is disturbed by disease or illness or injury." Meditation is "the process of perceiving directly the right inward measure of one's own being through careful, nonjudgmental self-observation."[4] We might say that the ideal practice of medicine as well as of meditation allows us to perceive things as they actually are, by taking a careful and accurate measure.

Categories of Meditation

All forms of meditation can be said to fall into two major categories: concentration meditation and mindfulness meditation. The two types are distinguished by their relationship to the object of meditation. Meditation can be practiced alone or with the assistance of an experienced practitioner who guides the process.

Concentration Meditation

In concentration meditation, the meditator focuses on something specific in the external environment or on something internal. Any object or stimulus in the external environment—a candle flame, a picture, music, or other sounds—can be used to focus the mind in meditation. Alternatively, the meditator can focus on an internal physical sensation, such as the breath, pulse, or heartbeat, or any other sensations present in the body. Emotions and thoughts can also be used as a focus.

In another form of concentration meditation, sometimes called "visualization," the person is guided to focus on something imaginary, such as a peaceful landscape inhabited by make-believe people. Sometimes a guide instructs the person to envision performing a difficult task, encouraging the meditator to feel a sense of ease in the performance that can then later be experienced in reality. For example, a student could imagine the successful completion of a difficult course of study. By seeing oneself in an enjoyable nursing practice, a student could better manage the anxiety of a rigorous nursing program.

Meditators can also focus on single words, phrases, or prayers, which are repeated internally. A word or phrase is often linked with a physical sensation, such as the breath. In some meditation traditions, the individual counts while inhaling and exhaling as a method of focusing awareness.

Mindfulness Meditation

When the object of attention is broad and/or continually changing, we speak of "mindfulness meditation."[5] In this form, the meditator directs awareness to whatever presents itself, whether an external object or sound, or an internal sensation, emotion, or thought. The meditator is instructed to notice the passing object of awareness but not to follow it or to attach to it. This form of meditation evokes a sense of resting in the present moment; one is awake and aware of whatever may come.

Awakening to Reality

Meditators can learn to see everything in their world as a means of awakening to the true nature of reality. Concentration meditation facilitates the development of a keenly focused awareness, whereas mindfulness meditation develops one that is broad and flexible, sometimes called a choiceless awareness. These meditation methods allow the meditator to experience the world directly, without judgment or ideas intervening between the observer and what is observed. The two forms of meditation complement and reinforce each other, leading to a condition of awareness that is not the everyday mental state of human beings. This state of alertness can lead to a feeling of being alive, healthy, and vibrant, no matter what the mental or physical condition of the body. (See Boxes 7–1 and 7–2.)

Research

In 1979, at the University of Massachusetts Medical Center in Worcester, Massachusetts, Jon Kabat-Zinn, a professor of medicine, started a research- and education-focused

BOX 7–1
Mind-Body Medicine

In Eastern thought, and especially in the teachings of Buddhism, the mind and body are not considered as separate entities, with the mind influencing the body or the body influencing the mind. The influence of meditation on the body-mind, as it is often called, is assumed to be naturally beneficial. A new branch of Western medicine, sometimes called mind-body medicine, is related to this concept. Both Herbert Benson's and Jon Kabat-Zinn's work have influenced the development of this new field.

The theoretical split between mind and body first described by René Descartes in the 18th century has led to certain practices in Western medicine that overlook the mind's influence on the body and the body's influence on the mind. Mind-body medicine suggests a more integrated approach, in which the physiological component of an emotional illness is presupposed, and vice versa. Anything that influences the mind "or" body can have an impact on disease, regardless of the category, physical or mental, into which the disease falls.

One effect of using meditation to heal an illness is the recognition that the split between physical and mental illnesses is an illusion and that the condition of the body-mind involves a complex interaction of so-called physical and mental processes. Even the idea of healing an illness may be "seen through" as an illusion.

The concept of "healing" is not easily defined. In medicine, there is often an expectation of curing a disease, which usually means eradicating it, and returning to "normal" healthy functioning. "Healing," however, may not necessarily involve curing the disease, but rather returning the entire organism to wholeness, rebalancing the body-mind. This can mean that the disease process itself has not been stopped or destroyed, but that certain attitudes toward the disease, and ways of relating to it, have shifted. This process gives the ill person new resources upon which to draw, thus making his or her life fulfilling and satisfying. An end to the illness is also possible as a result of the rebalancing and new sense of wholeness, but it is not necessarily the goal.

program. Kabat-Zinn, founding executive director of the Center for Mindfulness in Medicine, Health Care and Society, and his associates teach a combination of concentration and mindfulness meditation derived from Buddhist meditation methods, which they call "Mindfulness-Based Stress Reduction." Currently, the Stress Reduction Program operates as a part of the Center for Mindfulness at the University of Massachusetts Medical School.

In 1980 Herbert Benson, a Massachusetts physician, founded the Mind-Body Medical Institute in Boston, affiliated with Deaconess Hospital and Harvard Medical School. Benson and his associates teach and do research on his adaptation of Transcendental Meditation, which he calls the "Relaxation Response."[6] This is primarily a concentration practice. Kabat-Zinn's and Benson's pioneering research have generated widespread interest in the study of meditation and its effect on health and healing.

Research studies on meditation and healing have two general focuses: the physiological and mental effects and the impact on the disease process. The earliest studies of the effects of meditation, conducted in the 1930s, focused on the physiological changes in Indian practitioners of yoga and yoga meditation, primarily a concentration practice. Replications of these early studies continued until the 1970s and documented measurable changes in heart and pulse rates, brain waves, blood pressure, skin temperature, and respiration.[7] Beginning in 1957 and continuing into the 1960s, Kasamatsu and Hirai published a series of studies on Zen Buddhist practitioners. A significant finding of this research was that accomplished Zen meditators were able to maintain a spontaneity and freshness of perception in daily life.[8,9] Deikman, in a 1966 study, described the results of this kind of meditation as "a manipulation of attention that produces

BOX 7–2
Meditation as a Religious Practice

Meditation is a central or peripheral part of most religions, often used to enter into states of mind that facilitate spiritual awakening. The contemplative components of Judaism (Cabalistic meditation), Islam (Sufism), and Christianity (Eastern Orthodoxy's Philokalia and Roman Catholicism's Centering Prayer) often take the form of a concentration practice such as the inward recitation of words and prayers.

Meditation also plays a major role in Hinduism. The Sanskrit term for meditation, *dhyana,* describes "any absorbed state of mind brought about through concentration,"[1] and many traditional Hindu meditation practices emphasize focusing on an internal or external object.

Buddhist meditation, which arose in India 2500 years ago, was initially derived from Hindu practices. As this meditation practice spread from India to China, Tibet, and Southeast Asia, it mixed with indigenous practices and adopted some of the character of the cultures it encountered. There are therefore many forms of Buddhist meditation, some of which can be characterized as concentration meditation and some of which as mindfulness meditation. Chinese Taoism and Indian Buddhism blended to create the sect known as *Ch'an* in China and *Zen* in Japan, Korea, and Vietnam. Ch'an or Zen practices include both concentration and mindfulness.

Southeast Asian Buddhist meditation, which developed in Burma (Myanmar), Thailand, and Ceylon (Sri Lanka), produced many refinements of both concentration and mindfulness meditation, as did the mixture of Tibetan *Bon* and Indian Buddhism.

Both Western and Eastern forms of religious meditation have recently become popular in the West. One of the most well-known Hindu-based practices is Transcendental Meditation (TM), but there are also many other schools of meditation derived from the Hindu yogic tradition. Various Buddhist meditation traditions have taken root as well, especially Central Asian forms such as Ch'an and Zen practices, Southeast Asian *Vipassana* or insight meditation, and Tibetan Buddhist practices.

These Eastern forms of meditation have captured the interest of medical researchers, who have studied the effects of these practices on both mind and body. A number of studies (see the References and Bibliography) have shown that meditation has a significant and measurable impact on both mental and physical health. In addition, some Western practitioners of meditation have explored the effects of teaching meditation to people with illnesses, with the intent of relieving mental and physical woes. The relief of mental and physical symptoms has often been noted as a "side effect" of meditation. Such qualities as compassion for others, peacefulness and equanimity, and a deep wisdom are also thought to arise out of the practice of meditation.

REFERENCE

1. Fischer-Schreiber, I, et al: The Shambhala Dictionary of Buddhism and Zen. Shambhala, Boston, 1991.

---

deautomatization—an increased flexibility of perceptual and emotional responses to the environment."[10]

In addition to these perceptual and attitudinal findings, a great number of studies, some building on the early yoga studies, have linked meditation to improvements in physiological conditions. More than a thousand studies sponsored by the Transcendental Meditation Society, including some by Herbert Benson and his associate Keith Wallace in the 1970s, showed cardiovascular, cortical, hormonal and metabolic changes, as well as behavioral effects and alterations of consciousness.[11] Later studies duplicated these results, demonstrating changes in the cardiovascular system, lowered blood pressure, and changes in brain-wave patterns.[12]

Other physiological studies have linked meditation with positive effects on various states of disease: diabetes, asthma, fibromyalgia, premenstrual syndrome, Crohn's disease, psoriasis, and cancer.[13] Jon Kabat-Zinn and associates, in a number of studies in the 1980s, indicated that when patients with chronic pain practice meditation, their pain diminishes.[14–16]

A small number of studies have linked meditation to a lowering of stress-induced adrenal hormone levels, and others have shown a similar reduction in blood lactate, which is associated with anxiety and high blood pressure.[17] In a 1992 study, Kabat-Zinn and associates[18–20] showed reductions in anxiety and depression, and other research[21] has pointed to reductions in addictive behaviors and sleep disorders. Studies have shown that meditation, in addition to alleviating disease, has also been effective in promoting health, well-being, and enhanced states of sports performance.[22]

A recent study by Richard Davidson, Jon Kabat-Zinn, and associates[23] compared people taking an 8-week Mindfulness-Based Stress Reduction training course with a control group. In comparison with the control group, the experimental group showed significant increases in activation of a region of the brain associated with effective processing of "negative" emotions under stress, as well as significant increases in antibody titers to an in vivo immune system challenge. These results provide strong evidence that training in meditation and its application to daily living have profound and measurable effects on biological factors influencing both emotional and physical health. (See Box 7–3.)

Summary

As Rose's story in Box 7–3 demonstrates, meditation seems to affect the entire mind-body. Rose reported changes in physical symptoms as well as positive changes in attitudes and behaviors. Her new ability to observe herself and her own life with greater awareness influenced her thoughts and feelings—and even her medical symptoms.

The ability to choose different attitudes and behaviors often accompanies increased mindfulness. Certain personality traits that researchers have traditionally believed to be unchangeable—such as self-esteem, feelings of competence, and the ability to withstand stress—can shift in positive directions through the practice of meditation.

The healing that occurs through meditation exists on all levels, although not everyone experiences Rose's dramatic reduction in symptoms. Patients with potentially fatal diseases often find that their health continues to deteriorate. However, these patients report that the quality of their life changes as a result of meditating. The life that remains, with all its pain and suffering, becomes more accessible, richer, and more appreciated. Chronic pain can diminish, but even if it does not, patients sometimes report that their relationship to the pain changes: it is no longer the enemy. Using the practice of mindful awareness, one can choose to engage with pain—or with anything else, for that matter—with a sense of curiosity and attentiveness. Paradoxically, when this mindful attending is engaged, pain may diminish.

Graduates of the Stress Reduction Clinic often report that their lives have changed in ways they had not initially expected. Mostly, they find that the new self they may have wanted—healthy and whole—and the new life—filled with joy and peace—were always available to them. All they had to do was learn to stay still and pay attention. Through these simple but powerful means, lives become healed.

BOX 7–3
Stress Reduction in Action

The Stress Reduction Program at the Center for Mindfulness at the University of Massachusetts Medical School offers an 8-week program designed to help people manage stress and lead more productive and fulfilling lives.

The story of one participant in the program, who will go by the name of Rose, illustrates the process of change one experiences when taking the program. Rose's problems were initially related to work and had begun 6 months prior to her interview for the program. A responsible and self-motivated worker in a large retail outlet, she was highly regarded by her employer. When the company began experiencing financial difficulties, Rose's workload increased as fellow workers were laid off. She began to show symptoms of the overload, sleeping poorly and feeling exhausted during the day.

Rose's blood pressure increased, and she became anxious in any situation away from home, afraid that people would harm her. She had frequent, severe headaches and recurrent indigestion. Her doctor prescribed medication for her anxiety and for her high blood pressure, but she felt no relief. Finally, unable to work or even to leave the house, she notified her company that she had to take a medical leave. She was advised to see a psychiatrist, who referred her to the Stress Reduction Program.

The program consists of eight weekly classes, each lasting about 2½ hours. During the sixth week, there is an additional all-day class. During interviews conducted before and after the program, data are collected on each participant's medical and psychological symptoms and behaviors. Goals are set in the intake interview and evaluated during the final interview. During the 8-week period, participants are expected to practice the skills of concentration and mindfulness meditation each day.

During the intake interview, Rose reported being unable to concentrate, feeling depressed, worrying a lot, and having frightening dreams. She described headaches and digestive problems, as well as extreme anxiety about being with other people. She was concerned about attending a class with 20 to 40 other participants.

By taking the class, Rose hoped to gain more control over her emotions and body sensations, eliminate her fear afraid of going out in public, and feel good about herself. Her biggest concern was that she would feel better and go back to work at her company, only to find that "everything would go back the way it was."

In the first class, Rose explained she was taking the class to deal with her anxiety. She mentioned nothing about her work life, her physical problems, or her fears of public places and strangers. She did add that she had always been a good, dutiful person, helpful to other people when she could be. This last statement became the source of her own personal revelation in class.

In the weeks that followed, Rose—like all the class participants—learned the skills of concentration and mindfulness meditation through various exercises designed to increase awareness of the body and the mind. In an exercise called the "body scan," participants were trained to notice feelings in their bodies without trying to change them in any way. Students were then instructed to perform this exercise at home each day, using a 45-minute tape for guidance.

Eventually, mindful yoga exercises were added to the daily routine, as well as quiet sitting with attention to the process of breathing. After the fourth week, participants practiced mindfulness meditation on a daily basis, using the body scan, breath meditation, and yoga as supplementary practices. Discussions in class focused on the experience of performing these mindful practices, the nature and mechanics of stress, and mindful communication and nutrition. Everything was presented and discussed within the frame of increased awareness.

Rose said very little during the first few weeks of class, except to report that she was having difficulty concentrating and that her anxiety seemed to be increasing. She also found herself falling asleep during meditation practice at home. These are typical experiences for many in the program, and other participants supported her by sharing their own similar difficulties.

continued

BOX 7–3 continued

Stress Reduction in Action

Rose began to participate more in class discussions and often mentioned noticing how little attention she paid to herself and her own needs. Her desire to be "good" was beginning to be toxic to her. During the fifth class Rose revealed that she had been able to stay awake during a body scan meditation at home and had experienced being awake and relaxed at the same time. This was a completely new experience for her. When she attended the all-day class—in which more than 80 people participated, including ones from other classes running concurrently with hers—she reported feeling relaxed and comfortable in the large crowd, at home with herself.

During the last class, participants were encouraged to talk about what they had learned from the course. Rose spoke movingly about how all her life she had placed others before herself, trying hard to be good. She had been a good mother, wife, daughter, sister, and worker, but she had ignored her own needs. Through the practice of meditation, Rose had come to know herself, her own body and mind. She now believed that by knowing herself in this new way, she could change her life.

As Rose revealed in her final interview, she was also surprised to notice an improvement in her physical health. Her headaches had disappeared, her digestion had improved, and her blood pressure had returned to normal. With her doctor's permission, Rose had stopped taking medication. She felt somewhat more at ease in public, although going out still challenged her. She had come a long way in meeting her goal of being able to control her emotions and physical sensations.

Rose's scores on medical symptom checklists had improved dramatically as well, in one case by 50 percent. In her own words, Rose had learned to "focus on calming my anxiety to the point where I could control it instead of it controlling me. . . . When I feel anxiety building, I immediately stop, breathe, respond. I look at situations differently and choose the best response for me. . . . In the past [before the stress reduction program] my reactions were almost automatic. Now I am more able to accept my thoughts and feelings without allowing them to trap me and frighten me."

RESOURCES

Stress Reduction Program
Shaw Building
University of Massachusetts Medical School
55 Lake Avenue North
Worcester, MA 01655
Phone: (508) 856–2656
www.umassmed.edu/cfm
The clinic, founded by Jon Kabat-Zinn, offers classes in Mindfulness-Based Stress Reduction as well as professional education programs

The Mind/Body Medical Institute
Division of Behavioral Medicine
New England Deaconess Hospital
185 Pilgrim Road
Boston, MA 02215
(617) 732–9530
Herbert Benson's clinic

REFERENCES

1. McKechnie, JL (ed): Webster's New Universal Unabridged Dictionary, ed. 2. Dorset & Baker, New York, 1983, p 1118.
2. Compton's Interactive Encyclopedia. Compton's New Media, San Francisco, 1995.
3. Kabat-Zinn, J: Full Catastrophe Living. Dell, New York, 1990, p 163.
4. Ibid.
5. Fischer-Schreiber, I, et al: The Shambhala Dictionary of Buddhism and Zen. Shambhala, Boston, 1991, p 56.

6. Benson, H: The Relaxation Response. William Morrow, New York, 1975.

7. Murphy, M, and Donovan, S: The Physical and Psychological Effects of Meditation. Institute of Noetic Sciences, Sausalito, Calif., 1997.

8. Kasamatsu, A, et al: The EEG of "Zen" and "yoga" practitioners. EEG Clinical Neurophysiology, 9(suppl):51, 1957.

9. Kasamatsu, A, and Hirai, T: An EEG study on the Zen meditation (Zazen). Folia Psychiatrica et Neurologia Japonica 20(4):315, 1966.

10. Deikman, AJ: De-automatization of the mystic experience. Psychiatry 29:324, 1966.

11. Murphy and Donovan: The Physical and Psychological Effects of Meditation, p 85.

12. Ibid, pp 45–80.

13. Ibid.

14. Kabat-Zinn, J: An out-patient program in behavioral medicine for chronic-pain patients based on the practice of mindfulness meditation: Theoretical considerations and preliminary results. Gen Hosp Psychiatry 4:33, 1982.

15. Kabat-Zinn, J, et al: The clinical use of mindfulness meditation for the self-regulation of chronic pain. J Behav Med 8:163, 1985.

16. Kabat-Zinn, J, et al: Four year follow-up of a meditation-based program for the self-regulation of chronic pain: treatment outcomes and compliance. Clin J Pain 2: 159, 1986.

17. Murphy and Donovan: The Physical and Psychological Effects of Meditation.

18. Kabat-Zinn, J, et al: Effectiveness of a meditation-based stress reduction program in the treatment of anxiety disorders. Am J Psychiatry 149:936, 1992.

19. Miller, J, et al: Three-year follow-up and clinical implications of a mindfulness-based stress reduction intervention in the treatment of anxiety disorders. Gen Hosp Psychiatry 17:192, 1995.

20. Kabat-Zinn, J, et al: The relationship of cognitive and somatic components of anxiety to patient preference for alternative relaxation techniques. Mind/Body Medicine 2:101, 1997.

21. Murphy and Donovan: The Physical and Psychological Effects of Meditation.

22. Kabat-Zinn, J, and Beall, B: A Systematic Mental Training Program Based on Mindfulness Meditation to Optimize Performance in Collegiate and Olympic Rowers. Paper presented at: Department of Athletics, Massachusetts Institute of Technology, Cambridge, Mass., 1987.

23. Davidson, RJ, et al: Alterations in brain and immune function produced by mindfulness meditation. Manuscript submitted for publication.

BIBLIOGRAPHY

Borysenko, J: Minding the Body, Mending the Mind. Bantam, New York, 1988.

Goldstein, J, and Kornfield, J: Seeking the Heart of Wisdom: The Path of Insight Meditation. Shambhala, Boston, 1987.

Goleman, D, and Gurin, J (eds): Mind/Body Medicine. Consumer Reports Books, Yonkers, N.Y., 1993.

Hanh, TN: The Miracle of Mindfulness: A Manual on Meditation. Beacon Press, Boston, 1988.

Kabat-Zinn, J: Wherever You Go, There You Are: Mindfulness Meditation in Everyday Life. Hyperion, New York, 1994.

Moyers, B: Healing and the Mind. Doubleday, New York, 1993.

Suzuki, S: Zen Mind, Beginner's Mind. Weatherhill, New York, 1970.

CHAPTER 8

Imagery

Rothlyn P. Zahourek

Rothlyn P. Zahourek, RN, CS, HNC, is a clinical nurse specialist with a private psychotherapy practice. She is also a PhD candidate in New York University's Division of Nursing. Her professional affiliations include the American Holistic Nurses' Association, American Nurses' Association, and American Psychiatric Nurses' Association. Among her publications is Relaxation and Imagery Tools of Therapeutic Communication, *published by WB Saunders in 1988.*

At an Olympic trial, an athlete stands quietly with her eyes closed, envisioning the achievement of her personal best. An actor contemplates the experiences of Hamlet, imagining he is the character, prior to the actual performance. A woman in labor visualizes the easy birth of a healthy baby.

Human beings use imagery to envision a desirable outcome, develop solutions, distract themselves during pain and anxiety, and enjoy fantasy. Imagery brings thoughts and perceptions to life.

What Is Imagery?

Imagery is a multidimensional mental representation of reality and fantasy that includes not only visual pictures in the mind but also remembrances of situations and experiences such as sound, smell, touch, movement, and taste. According to Epstein,[1] both imagery and intuition are aspects of nonlogical thinking, which connects us with our inner subjective reality. Imagery is also a powerful component in memory. According to Horowitz,[2] imagery exists as "memory fragments, reconstructions, and reinterpretations or symbols which stand for objects, feelings, or ideas which enable us to create, to dream and to know."

Historically, people have believed that imagery could magically influence present and future health and prosperity. The power of imagery in healing can be seen today where indigenous "primitive" medicine is practiced by shamans using ancient ritual healing rites.[3,4] In such cultures mind, body, and spirit are never divided but are viewed as a whole. The rituals, visions, and images used by shamans are believed to be the bridge between the physical world and the healing power existing in the spiritual universe.

Although our contemporary culture values practical science and technology, there is a growing move among caregivers and recipients, as well as among scientists, toward a holistic perspective that regards consciousness and imagery as integral aspects of personal health. Within this system, a person's imagery is tied to his or her physiology, sense of well-being, and experience of the world.

Therapeutic Uses of Imagery

Imagery is a versatile intervention often used in conjunction with relaxation, hypnosis, biofeedback, desensitization, and cognitive behavioral techniques. Health problems of all kinds respond to the use of imagery. For example, imagery is used to manage the pain of chronic illness, burns, surgery, and arthritis, as well as for the normal physiological processes of childbirth.

Imagery can be used at any stage of the therapeutic process—even in stressful diagnostic procedures. For example, physical assessment through magnetic resonance imaging (MRI) involves confinement in a tunnel-like metal tube that can trigger claustrophobia and panic in some clients. A clinician might help a client imagine the tube as a comforting, womblike apparatus that contains everything needed to sustain life. Anticipating surgery is a universal fear: a client can be guided to imagine waking up without any trace of illness.

Imagery techniques can also be integrated into psychotherapy for such problems as obsessions, habit disorders, overeating, phobias, anxiety, depression, chronic pain, substance abuse, problems associated with dying and/or grief, and post-traumatic stress disorder. Imagery interventions include visualizing one's self in a past situation that was pleasant or in the future when the problem is resolved. Such interventions enhance the therapy process by sidestepping resistance and by engaging the client in a novel, often enjoyable, approach.[5]

As adjunctive treatment in addictions, imagery helps people to imagine what life might be like for them sober. For patients recovering from phobias and anxiety, imagery helps by providing a chance for behavioral rehearsal (living the feared moment) in the imagination rather than in the real world. Imagery has been used in Therapeutic Touch, during which practitioners might imagine soothing scenes or colors.

Imagery also plays a role in the process of emotional attachment and subsequently the capacity to let go in grief. Clients experiencing unresolved grief can be guided to have imagined conversations with those who have died, which helps to resolve unfinished business. Images of resolving difficult times with a lost loved one can enhance grief resolution, and memories of pleasant times can offer comfort. (See Box 8–1.)

Types of Imagery

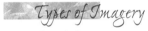

Experiential

Receptive imagery occurs spontaneously, often in early stages of sleep or just prior to awakening. These images are dreamlike and can yield creative ideas and/or solutions to problems.[6]

Active imagery is consciously created. According to Achterberg, Dossey, and Kolkmeier,[7] one can communicate directly with the body using this type of imagery.

Process imagery is the rehearsal of a procedure or event. For example, the Olympic athlete preparing for competition envisions success.

Therapeutic

Guided imagery and interactive guided imagery are used as therapeutic interventions. Guided imagery may be performed using a technique tailored to the individual or through a pre-existing scripted process. Interactive guided imagery is used to elicit a person's own imagery and then interact with it. Often the individual will envision what needs to be healed, dialogue with it, and learn the processes necessary to complete the healing.[8]

BOX 8–1

Theories of Imagery

There are numerous theoretical frameworks to help us understand the process of imagery. Recent advances in biological diagnostics corroborate the mind's effects on the body and increase the credibility of imagery's role in healing.

Early Psychoanalytic Theory

Many psychoanalytic theorists, including Freud and Jung, described the importance of imagery in understanding how people think and experience reality. Freud acknowledged the importance of his clients' imagery as early as 1890, when he conducted an imagery procedure. Freud pressed on the client's head; when he relaxed the pressure, he asked the client to relate the images experienced. According to Freud, clients reported seeing images, in rapid chronological succession, related to the central conflict.[1]

Jung[2] believed that the "psyche consists essentially of images. It is a series of images in the truest sense, not an accidental juxtaposition or sequence, but a structure that is throughout full of meaning and purpose." He employed the technique of "active imagination" to encourage exploration and expression of images from the unconscious, which he believed were always present but most accessible during dreams and when the individual focused on images that emerged spontaneously.

Brain Theories

In 1971 Pavio[3] described how the brain stores information as pictures and words. He demonstrated that words are more easily remembered than abstractions and images are recalled better than words.

In 1985 MacLean[4] described a trilevel organization to the brain. The inner, most primitive level generates reflexive and survival activities. The intermediate level is responsible for emotions and behavior as well as for imagery and other states of altered awareness. The highest level, the cortex, is responsible for verbal and rational levels of thought.

Achterberg[5] reviewed the research on brain laterality (right and left brain) in image formation. Imagery comes from the right hemisphere and logical thought from the left. The right hemisphere aids in processing emotions and in making judgments. During stress and worry, images are activated in the right hemisphere and then relayed to the autonomic nervous system. Achterberg contends that the healing nature of imagery is based on thought being translated into images. These images have a profound impact on the responses of the body.

Holographic Theories

The holographic model of imagery is fascinating to consider in relation to the healing potential of imagery. This model, developed by Pirbram[6] and explored by Epstein[7], describes the brain as a hologram in how it receives, transmits, and stores information. A hologram is a specially processed photograph that produces a three-dimensional image when a laser is shown through it. Any part of the hologram is capable of producing a complete whole image. This metaphor has been used to explain the powerful healing nature of imagery as well as phantom limb phenomena, kinesthetic body boundaries, and the way memory is retrieved even after significant brain damage.[8]

Because each nerve cell has the capacity to stimulate several other neurons at the synaptic cleft, many thousand synapses are possible. Subsequently, an infinite number of patterned associations are also likely. When any part is stimulated, the whole is reproduced—just as with a hologram. A specific smell, for example, may produce a cascade of memories. Regarding the storage of images in the brain, the image is everywhere at once and has no time/space dimension.

Holistic and Functional Theories

In 1979 Lang[9] proposed a holistic imagery theory whereby imagery produces both structural and functional coding systems in the brain. The type and degree of response is related not only to the specific content but also the meaning of the image. For example, imagining the proximity of a warm fire—a comforting scene—promotes relaxation, increases body temperature, and causes perspiration.

continued

BOX 8–1 continued
Theories of Imagery

Functional theories depend on the biochemistry in the brain and in the central and autonomic nervous systems. Messages and images are transmitted via neurotransmitters throughout the body—not only to nerves and muscles but also to organs and glands. For example, the mental image of a lemon stimulates the physiological response of salivation. Through biochemical networks of memories, which are located throughout the body, not only in the brain, responses related to past experiences can be evoked.

REFERENCES

1. Sheikh, AA, and Jordan, CS. Clinical uses of mental imagery. In Sheikh, AA (ed): Imagery: Current Theory, Application and Research. Wiley, New York, 1983.
2. Jung, CG: The Structure and Dynamics of the Psyche (RFFC Hull, trans; Collected Works, vol 8). Princeton University Press, Princeton, N.J., 1960. (Original work published 1926)
3. Pavio, A: Imagery and Verbal Processes. Holt, New York, 1971.
4. MacLean, P: A Triune Concept of the Brain and Behavior. Toronto Press, Toronto, 1985.
5. Achterberg, J: Imagery in Healing: Shamanism and Modern Medicine. New Science Library, Boston, 1985, p 122–126.
6. Pirbram, K: What the fuss is all about. In Wilbur, K (ed): The Holographic Paradigm and Other Paradoxes. Shambala Press, Boulder, 1982.
7. Epstein, G: The image in medicine. Advances (3):22–31, 1986.
8. Achterberg: Imagery in Healing, pp 122–126.
9. Lang, PJ: A bio-informational theory of emotional imagery. Psychophysiology 6:495, 1979

Classification Systems

Images can be categorized. According to Horowitz,[9] images are organized according to vividness, context, and interaction with perception and content. Imagery may also be understood on a continuum. On one end, a mental image appears as a vague, dreamlike perception with little form or content. On the other end, the image is extremely vivid. Many believe that the clearer the image, the more potent is its effect in changing physiological phenomena.[10] An example of the power of a clear mental image is perspiring and feeling nauseated when imagining a loved one in a car accident.

Ashen's ISM system establishes a relationship between the type of image used and the therapeutic outcome. Ashen[11] has classified images into an integrated system of three components:

- Imagination or imagery (I)
- Somatic response or feeling (S)
- Meaning (M)

For example, an image (I) can be described—a white house with red shutters. The image elicits a somatic response or feeling (S)—one's heart starts to beat more quickly. Finally, the image has meaning (M)—this is the house where one spent a tumultuous adolescence. Practitioners can use these three components as a guide in planning and implementing interventions with clients. Ashen's ISM system can be taught to clients to help them understand their own imagery and ultimately to direct physiological responses.

Research in Imagery

Imagery involves powerful physiological connections that are now considered a vital component to many forms of healing and holistic health interventions. Over the past 20 years, research on the effects of imagery on physiological and psychological responses in people in numerous conditions has increased dramatically.

Imagery and the Immune System in Cancer Patients

In the early 1970s, Achterberg and Lawlis[12] developed a system for investigating an individual's imagery experience of cancer (a projective test called "Image CA"). Their system became a prototype for later studies in arthritis, diabetes, and pain. The researchers asked patients to describe aspects of their experience by asking such questions as: "How do the cancer cells look in your mind, and how do your white blood cells fight the disease?" Patients were asked to draw what they "saw" in their imaginations.

The information was scored on several scales, including vividness, activity, strength of the cancer cell, and the relative comparison of strength and activity of the body's defenses. Researchers were able to predict those who would die or suffer deterioration with 100 percent certainty and those who would go into remission with 93 percent certainty.

Trestman[13] studied the effect of color and the symbolic nature of the images on cancer patients. Those individuals with a "good" prognosis described their cancer as black or red, while those with poorer prognosis visualized lighter colors. Symbols of powerful archetypal figures—such as God or King Arthur—representing their immune systems were nearly always associated with a good response. Vague, amorphous symbols—such as clouds or snowflakes—were associated with a poor response. The worst prognoses were associated with an inability to imagine or draw the immune system and a very powerful image of the cancer.

Similarly, the more symbolic the images, as opposed to being anatomically correct, the better the prediction of a positive outcome.[14] Achterberg cautions that healing or helpful images vary across cultures and emerge as patterns, rather than as cause-and-effect relationships, in determining prognosis. (See Box 8–2.)

In her summary of research findings, as of 1985, Achterberg[15] drew the following conclusions:

- Images are related to physiological states and may be either causative or reactive.
- Images can originate in the conscious and subconscious mind—such as in a dream—or be produced through a deliberate action such as an electrical stimulation.
- Images might be produced through the conscious processing of information, which in turn causes physiological responses.
- Images affect both the (voluntary) peripheral and the (involuntary) autonomic nervous systems.

In the late 1970s Simonton, Mathews-Simonton, and Sparks[16] conducted pioneering research on the mind-body connection with severely ill cancer patients. Their work and Seigel's[17] best-selling book about an exceptional cancer patient popularized the use of imagery to enhance the immune system in cancer and AIDS patients. Simonton and colleagues used individual and group psychotherapy, as well as relaxation and imagery, with 225 patients. Their initial work showed that the imagery intervention extended life beyond the median life expectancy.

Additional studies have investigated how imagery enhances immune function as well as longevity and quality of life. The now-famous study of metastatic breast cancer patients by Spiegel and colleagues[18] demonstrated that those in a support group where hypnosis and imagery was used doubled their length of survival compared to those in the control group.

In a small study of 13 patients, Gruber and colleagues[19] found that stage-1 breast cancer patients using a combination of relaxation, biofeedback, and guided imagery experienced a positive effect on their immune systems, including increased natural killer cells and lymphocytes. Richardson and colleagues[20] conducted a pilot study with breast cancer patients to identify the effects of imagery and support on coping, life attitudes, immune function, quality of life, and emotional well-being. A control group was used. As compared to patients receiving support, those receiving imagery tended to have more

BOX 8–2

Case Study

Celia had been diagnosed with a rare form of obstructive pancreatitis, which developed after a routine cholecystectomy. She was told that her pancreatic ducts were blocked and that her chronic pain resulted from the pancreatic juice's seeping out and essentially digesting her pancreas.

When not in terrible pain, she was nauseated and could not eat. Large doses of morphine sulfate maintained comfort, but, as a result, she was perpetually sleepy and constipated. She was a single mother of four children, all of whom had significant learning and behavioral disabilities.

In the first consultation with the clinician, Celia related strengths as well as problems. First, she loved the sun and warmth of summertime sunbathing. Describing herself as having a good sense of humor and being flexible, Celia acknowledged being successful in helping her children and prided herself on having exceptional patience. When asked to draw a picture of herself with her pain, she drew a simple body in black ink with angry-looking red areas in the midsection. The face grimaced. When asked her to clarify what she wanted from therapy; she said, "I just want to be able to cope a little bit better."

Two important points are illustrated in this encounter. First, it is important to be clear about the client's problems, strengths, and desired outcome for an intervention. Images can be metaphorically and directly built on that information. Second, clients may be fearful of or have misconceptions about imagery interventions. Emphasize that the process is interactive and that it is the client—not the clinician—who ultimately has control of his or her images and experience.

During the next few sessions Celia was taught relaxation techniques, using a basic progressive muscle relaxation exercise. She was also shown how to use a variety of imagery techniques, such as picturing and feeling the warmth of the sun on her face and body and allowing that sensation to spread throughout her body. This helped her to feel comfort and calm. The warmth of the sun was also a battery of energy for her to draw on as she continued to develop coping skills.

During the next session, the classic film *Fantastic Voyage*, which she had seen with her children several years earlier, was discussed. In the film, the main characters want to save a person who has suffered a blood clot to the brain. After being miniaturized, the film characters are injected into the person's body and begin their "fantastic voyage" through various systems of the body, including the circulatory, respiratory, and immune systems.

Celia was asked to relax, close her eyes, and visualize herself gently traveling through her body fixing things as she went. When she entered the pancreatic ducts, she was encouraged to begin gently cleaning and opening them up.

The following week Celia explained that she had been diligently working on her images. "I have become a miner with a hard hat, a big head light, and a drill. I'm cleaning my ducts. I think it's helping. I do feel better." She still had pain, but she felt less depressed and less desperate.

Celia believed she had gained increased control over her situation. Although her illness was not cured and other problems still existed, she required less pain medication and felt she had a new skill that allowed her respite from a demanding environment.

vigor, less stress, and improved functional and social quality of life. Both imagery and support improved coping, attitudes, and perception of support.

Chronic Illnesses

Imagery has been utilized and studied as an intervention in numerous chronic illnesses. Hand-warming visualization has been a useful intervention in selected populations. In this technique, the individual imagines his or her hands warming as a result of putting them in front of a blazing fire and sitting in warm water. People suffering from migraine headaches and fibromyalgia have experienced symptomatic relief from the application of this technique.[21]

In an investigation funded by the Office of Alternative and Complementary Medicine of the National Institutes of Health, researchers attempted to learn whether imagery relieves the experience of asthma.[22] Patients who used imagery described increases in a

BOX 8–3
How to Use Imagery as a Therapeutic Technique

Assess
- Assess the person; gain an understanding of the problem.
- Listen to the description of the problem.
- Determine the answers to these questions:
  - How does the person image the problem?
  - What is the metaphorical representation of the problem?
  - What are the future implications of the problem?
  - What sort of imagery—for example, visual, aural, kinesthetic—does the person use now?

Plan
- Discuss any concerns about the intervention.
- In conjunction with the client, devise a plan for using therapeutic imagery.

Intervene and Evaluate
- Implement the imagery plan.
- Incorporate suggestions for continued success.
- Encourage practice outside of the therapeutic encounter (e.g., at home).
- Evaluate the intervention together.
- Plan for future practice or interventions.

Many intriguing and engaging imagery techniques are available and relevant to a variety of health-care needs. The numerous ways in which imagery can be used for healing are limited only by our own capacity for creative imagination.

sense of mastery and control, an awareness of the process of asthma in their bodies, and a hope of overcoming asthma. In this controlled study, 47 percent of those in the imagery group decreased or discontinued their medication. Only 18 percent of those in the control group decreased their medication, and none discontinued it.

In a controlled study of patients with multiple sclerosis, Maquire[23] examined the effects of mental imagery on their moods and attitudes. Patients' drawings of themselves and their illness were used to measure how images of themselves and their illness changed over the course of treatment. The treatment group experienced a significant decrease in anxiety over time. The sense of internal control among those in the imagery group remained stable, whereas that among the control group decreased. The imagery group also experienced a significant increase in a positive perception of their illness.

Healthy Populations

Imagery has been studied in healthy populations as well. A goal of imagery interventions in health care and in athletics is a reduction of stress and an increase in competence. A study of elite athletes found that 99 percent of them used imagery techniques to enhance performance.[24] Two studies of new nursing mothers who used imagery also demonstrate its effectiveness.[25,26] In a study of 55 mothers of premature infants, Feher and colleagues[27] found that the 30 women who listened to a 20-minute relaxation/imagery tape produced 63 percent more milk than the 25 women who did not. (See Box 8–3.)

Summary

Throughout our lives, we use a kaleidoscope of images that changes form and color as we move in our environments and as our perceptions change. Imagery offers an easily accessible and potentially powerful tool in an overall plan of helping oneself and others to heal.

Clearly a mind-body-spirit holistic phenomenon, imagery has the potential to both cause and alleviate distress and disease. Many intriguing and engaging techniques are available and relevant to a variety of health-care needs. They are limited only by an individual's imagination.

REFERENCES

1. Epstein, G: Healing Visualizations: Creating Health through Imagery. Bantam Books, New York, 1989, p 3.
2. Horowitz, MJ: Controls of Visual Imagery and Therapeutic Intervention. In Singer, JL, and Pope, KS (eds.): The Power of Human Imagination. Plenum, New York, 1978, p 43.
3. Achterberg, J: Imagery in Healing: Shamanism and Modern Medicine. New Science Library, Boston, 1985.
4. Achterberg, J, Dossey, B, and Kolkmeier, L:. Rituals of Healing: Using Imagery for Health and Wellness. Bantam Books, New York, 1994.
5. Zahourek, RP: Relaxation and Imagery: Tools for Therapeutic Communication and Intervention. WB Saunders, Philadelphia, 1988.
6. Kosbab, P: Imagery techniques in psychiatry. Archives of General Psychiatry 31:283, 1974.
7. Achterberg, Dossey, and Kolkmeier: Rituals of Healing.
8. Dossey, BM: Imagery. In Dossey, BM (ed): Core Curriculum for Holistic Nursing. Aspen Publishing, Gaithersburg, Md., 1997.
9. Horowitz, MJ: Image Formations and Psychotherapy. Jason Aronson, New York, 1983.
10. Sheikh, AA, and Sheikh, KS: Healing East and West: Ancient Wisdom and Modern Psychology. Wiley, New York, 1996, pp. 491–495.
11. Ashen, A: Eidetics: An overview. Journal of Mental Imagery 1:5–38, 1977.
12. Achterberg, J, and Lawlis, GF: Imagery of Cancer: A Diagnostic Tool for the Process of Disease. Institute for Personality and Ability Testing, Champaigne, Ill., 1978.
13. Trestman, RL: Imagery, Coping, and Physiological Variables in Adult Cancer Patients. Doctoral dissertation, University of Tennessee, Knoxville, 1981.
14. Achterberg, J, and Lawlis,GF: Imagery and Disease. Institute for Personality and Ability Testing, Champaign, Ill., 1984.
15. Achterberg: Imagery in Healing, pp 115–116.
16. Simonton, OC, Mathews-Simonton, S, and Sparks, TF: Psychological intervention in the treatment of cancer. Psychosomatics 21(3):226, 1980.
17. Seigel, B: Love, Medicine, and Miracles. Harper & Row, New York, 1986.
18. Spiegel, D, et al: Effect of psychological treatment on survival of patients with metastatic breast cancer. Lancet 2:888–891, 1989.
19. Gruber, BL, et al.: Immunological responses of breast cancer patients to behavioral interventions. Biofeedback and Self-Regulation 18:1, 1993.
20. Richardson, MA, et al: Coping, life attitudes, and immune responses to imagery and group support after breast cancer treatment. Alternative Therapies in Health and Medicine 3(5): 62, 1997.
21. Albright, GL, and Fischer, AA: Effects of warming imagery aimed at trigger-point sites on tissue compliance, skin temperature, and pain sensitivity in biofeedback trained patients which chronic pain: A preliminary study. Perceptual and Motor Skills 71:1163, 1990.
22. Epstein, G, et al: Alleviating asthma with mental imagery: A phenomenologic approach. Alternative and Complementary Therapies 3(1):42, 1997.
23. Maquire, BL: The effects of imagery on attitudes in multiple sclerosis patients. Alternative Therapies in Health and Medicine 2(5):75, 1996.
24. Orick, T, and Partington, J: Mental links to excellence. Sport Psychology 2:105, 1988.
25. Feher, SDK, et al: Increasing breast milk production for premature infants with a relaxation/imagery audiotape. Pediatrics 83:1, 1989.
26. Rees, BL: Effect of relaxation with guided imagery on anxiety, depression and self-esteem in primiperas. Journal of Holistic Nursing 13:255, 1995.
27. Feher et al: Increasing breast milk production.

CHAPTER 9

Nutrition

Neil S. Orenstein

Neil S. Orenstein, PhD, is a nutritional biochemist whose background includes staff appointments at Massachusetts General Hospital, Harvard Medical School, and Beth Israel Hospital. Dr. Orenstein, who has coauthored two books on nutrition, is an internationally recognized leader in educating health-care professionals, students, and the general public. He maintains a private practice in Lenox, Massachusetts, as a consultant in nutritional biochemistry, working with individuals to re-establish biochemical balance.

Nutrition is one of the most talked about subjects today. The media are filled with news about the latest studies warning us of the dangers of one food, reminding us of the virtues of another. Should we eat more of it? Less of it? Different types of it? It all depends on what you read and whom you ask. Deciding what to eat to ensure health and longevity has become a daunting feat.

This chapter helps take the mystery out of good nutrition and presents an overview that goes beyond fad and fashion. To help you make sound choices that are right for you, we include information gleaned from current science, historical wisdom, and clinical experience. Rather than overwhelming you with reams of material, we provide key highlights of today's hottest topics:

Dietary nutrients
Traditional versus modern diets
Degeneration of soil and crops
Nutrient density
The ideal diet
Carbohydrate-protein balance
Trigger foods and allergies
Supplementation

Dietary Nutrients

The purpose of the digestive process is for our body to extract everything of nutritive value from the foods we eat. After these nutrients are digested and broken down to component parts, the body absorbs and uses them in several different ways.

Structural Components

First, nutrients serve as structural components of our body. These are the building blocks from which all our body cells and biochemical processes are created. Some of these nutrients are termed "essential," which means that our body cannot make them from other nutrients. They must be eaten in sufficient daily quantities; otherwise a deficiency occurs.

The major essential macronutrients are categorized as either essential amino acids or essential fatty acids (EFAs). Amino acids are necessary for the body's complete synthesis of protein and other tissue constituents. The body requires approximately 22 amino acids in specific patterns to make human protein. All but nine of these are produced within the body. These nine are called "essential" because they must be supplied in the diet: histidine, isoleucine, leucine, lysine, methionine (and cysteine), phenylalanine (and tyrosine), threonine, tryptophan, and valine.

Fatty acids come from the storage of fats from the energy-yielding nutrients of carbohydrates, proteins, and fats in the body. There are three EFAs that cannot be made from the breakdown of body constituents and therefore must come from the diet. The essential fatty acids have traditionally been defined as linoleic, linolenic, and arachadonic acids. In times of metabolic stress and biochemical imbalance, the body may require other fatty acids, such as gamma linolenic acid (GLA) and eicosapentaenoic acid. In some circumstances in certain individuals these latter may be considered to be essential for optimum body function and health.

Functional Components

The second use of dietary nutrients is functional. EFAs and small peptides (strings of amino acids not yet large enough to be called proteins) that are contained in food and released by the digestive process have major functional roles. In addition, numerous phytonutrients (contained in plant foods that we eat) have direct functional roles in the body.

The role of EFA metabolites illustrates the functional role of dietary nutrients. GLA, for example, is a fatty acid that, under some circumstances, can be classified as essential. GLA is found in (among other places) seed oils and seed oil supplements, such as the oil of evening primrose, borage, and black currant. GLA is converted via a two-step process into prostaglandin E_1. This is an eicosanoid control hormone that has both anti-inflammatory and mood-elevating effects.

The mineral calcium is another example of a functional dietary nutrient. In addition to its obvious structural role in bone health, calcium is a major functional nutrient. There are many more calcium molecules outside the cell, in the intracellular space, than inside the cell. This concentration gradient is the basis for one of calcium's most important functional roles as a messenger molecule.

If one of a large variety of cell surface receptors is activated by external triggers, such as a pollen antigen, calcium channels in this cell surface open and calcium (because of its higher concentration outside of cells) floods into cells. This stimulates a variety of actions, such as an asthmatic attack.

Calories

A third function of digested foods is to provide calories (the amount of heat required to raise the temperature of 1 kilogram of water 1°Celsius). Pure protein and pure carbohydrate release four calories per gram, and fats release nine calories per gram.

Traditional versus Modern Diets

There is much to learn about healthy eating from the nutritional habits of our early ancestors. Traditional diets contained no processed foods, had more essential food ingredients than processed foods have, and had fewer toxins than does the modern-day diet of processed foods.

TABLE 9–1   Comparison of the Late Paleolithic Diet, the Current
American Diet, and U.S. Dietary Recommendations
for a More "Ideal" Diet

	LATE PALEOLITHIC DIET	CURRENT WESTERN DIET	SENATE SELECT COMMITTEE RECOMMENDATIONS
Total Dietary Energy (%)			
Protein	34	12	12
Carbohydrate	45	46	58
Fat	21	42	30
P:S Ratio (Polyunsaturated/ Saturated Fat)	1.41	0.44 to 0.02	1.00
Cholesterol (mg)	591	600	300
Fiber (g)	45.7	19.7	30–60
Sodium (mg)	690	2300–6900	1100–3300
Calcium (mg)	1580	740	800–1200
Vitamin C (mg)	392.3	87.7	45

Modified from Eaton and Konnor, Paleolithic nutrition: a consideration of its nature and current implications. New England Journal of Medicine 312: 283–289, 1985, with permission.

The concept of paleolithic nutrition, first seriously discussed by Eaton and Konner, gives us a broad understanding of the difference between traditional and modern diets. In an article in the *New England Journal of Medicine*, Eaton and Konner[1] detailed the types of food that humans ate thousands of years ago. (See Table 9–1.) The natural diet for humans thousands of years ago contained far greater amounts of essential nutrients, particularly EFAs, than does our modern diet of processed foods. In addition, the paleolithic diet contained much less sugar and more vitamins and minerals in general. The amount of EFAs in a paleolithic diet compared to a modern one is also striking. Carcass meat of free-ranging animals thousands of years ago contained an abundance of omega-3 fatty acids, found also in flaxseed, flaxseed oil, deep cold water fish, fish oils, green plants, and algae. Omega-3 fatty acids help keep skin and other tissues youthful and healthy by preventing dryness.[2]

Omega-3 makes up a high percentage of the oil in green vegetation, but the total amount of oil—and therefore the absolute amount of omega-3 oil—in green plants is low. The land-based animals of the paleolithic period had body fat that resembled fish oil. This can be explained by the fact that omega-3 oils are produced by the plant kingdom, not by animals. (Fish get omega-3 oils from algae and then process them and modify the fatty acids.) Several thousand years ago four-legged land-based animals, which were food sources for humans, ate an abundance of greenery both by grazing on grasses and eating leaves off trees. These free-ranging animals had a much higher concentration of omega-3 fatty acids in their carcasses than do current cattle, which are raised on concrete feed lots and fed corn (which provides abundant omega-6 but very little omega-3 fatty acids).

Degeneration of Soil and Crop-Growing Conditions

Modern agriculture depends on synthetic, manufactured fertilizers to keep soils productive. The major nutrients in these fertilizers—sodium, potassium, and phosphorus (NPK)—are the same three used in typical lawn fertilizer. These three nutrients cause plants to look healthy, grow tall, and hold a lot of water (increased turgidity), the point of which is to make them appear succulent. The effects of NPK fertilizer can be observed on lawns: grass grows faster and fuller. Similarly, when these fertilizers are used in agriculture, crops will look healthy but will lack other key nutrients essential for health.

When other soil nutrients are not replaced (because of economic considerations), the soil becomes increasingly depleted with each new crop generation. These nutrients, which are not annually replaced and are not needed for the simple growth of plants, are absolutely necessary for the health of people who eat those plants. Plants need to contain them to be good sources of food. Depleted nutrients include selenium, magnesium, manganese, and a wide range of trace minerals.

Nutrient Density

The density of a specific nutrient is equivalent to the amount of that nutrient in 100 calories of a particular food. Picture two 1-inch cubes, one made of foam rubber, the other of wood. Which cube, the rubber or the wood, is denser? Obviously, the wood cube is denser than the foam cube. Now picture two 1-ounce pieces of bread: a 100-calorie piece of whole wheat bread and a 100-calorie piece of white bread. Which piece contains more nutrients? Again, the answer is obvious. The whole wheat bread contains more nutrition than does the white bread. Whole wheat bread is therefore more nutrient dense than white bread. What do these two examples have in common? They both illustrate the concept of density. Nutrient density is the amount of nutrition in a given portion of food and can be compared to the amount of nutrition in the same-size portion of a different food. This enables us to determine which food is more nutritious. With a diet low in nutrient density, we can consume too many calories and be undernourished at the same time.

Nutrient density is extremely useful because many of us do not eat adequate quantities of one or more nutrients. Understanding the concept of nutrient density will enable us to make more healthful food choices and increase our dietary intake of nutrients to as high a level as possible. As an example, let us examine the nutrient intake of a woman who is 5 feet 6 inches tall, walks for 1 hour each day, and bicycles for an additional one-half hour each day. This is a significant amount of daily exercise that results in burning 450 exercise calories per day. As a rule of thumb for people with a normal metabolic rate, women burn 11 calories per pound of body weight (plus exercise calories) and men burn 12 calories per pound of body weight (plus exercise calories).

130 pounds × 11 calories per pound = 1430 calories per day
Walking plus biking each day = 450 calories per day
1880 total calories needed

The woman in this example, who exercises every day for 1½ hours, still can only eat 1880 total calories per day. If she eats more than this, she will gain weight. For instance, if she eats 200 calories over the 1880 total each day, she will consume 73,000 extra calories in a year, with a weight gain of more than 20 pounds! The challenge (or at least one of them) is to get optimal quantities of all necessary nutrients in the daily allotment of calories. This requires that we eat the foods most packed with nutrients.

How do we know whether foods are loaded with nutrition? By checking the food's nutrient density. This information can usually be found on the food package. Table 9–2 illustrates the wide range of nutrient density in different foods. Foods with high nutrient density are good food choices. The higher the amount of each nutrient per 100 calories of the particular food, the higher the nutrient density. Dark-green vegetables such as spinach, broccoli, and kale are extremely good sources of important nutrients. For example, a large salad with at least 2 cups of these vegetables provides more than 600 mg of calcium and at

TABLE 9–2 Nutrient Density (Nutrients per 100 Calories)

NUTRIENT	SPINACH	KALE	BROCCOLI	BEEF	BACON	BIG MAC
Calcium (mg)	358	471	322	3	8	28
Magnesium (mg)	338	97	57	8	2	6
Potassium (mg)	1808	837	1191	117	46	43
Iron (mg)	11.9	5.8	3.4	0.9	0.9	0.7
Vitamin C (mg)	196	329	353	none	4	trace
Protein (g)	12.3	11.1	11.3	5.4	1.5	4.6
Fiber (g)	2.3	3.4	4.7	none	none	0.1
Fat (g)	1.2	2.1	0.9	8.6	10.4	5.9
Fat/protein	10.7	5.3	2.0	0.1	0.8	

least 9 mg of iron. This provides more calcium than 2 cups of milk and more iron than one-half pound of beef.

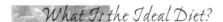 ## *What Is the Ideal Diet?*

What should a healthy diet consist of? There is no one ideal diet for all persons. The food guide pyramid provided by the U.S. Department of Agriculture (*www.nal.usda.gov:8001/ py/pmap.htm*) is based on the government's published "Dietary Guidelines." Although it is an improvement over previously published guidelines, it leaves much to be desired. (See Table 9–3.)

A better alternative was developed jointly by Oldways (a nonprofit educational organization) and the Harvard School of Public Health (*www.oldwayspt.org/html/ meet.htm*). The Oldways approach details several different food pyramids, each based on traditional, endogenous diets from around the world. These include a vegetarian diet pyramid, an Asian diet pyramid, a Latin-American diet pyramid, and a Mediterranean diet pyramid. All these healthy dietary food plans emphasize plant foods over animal-based diets.

Because of the substantial amount of published material on the health benefits of the Mediterranean diet, we will use this food pyramid as an example. Dietary data from populations in the Mediterranean region have been correlated with health, longevity, and well-being. This diet is based mostly on plant (as opposed to animal) food sources. A significant part of the health benefits of the Mediterranean diet no doubt stems from the use of traditional, rather than modern, agricultural techniques. As previously discussed, modern agricultural techniques can deplete the soil of micronutrients.

The Mediterranean diet contains abundant micronutrients. Sugar and other refined food products are used infrequently. Additionally, locally grown fruits and vegetables are eaten with minimal cooking and processing. According to Oldways (*www.oldwayspt.org./ hmtl/pmed4.htm*), there are 10 characteristics of a traditional healthy Mediterranean diet:

1. The majority of food is from plant sources, including fruits, vegetables, potatoes, grains (breads), legumes, nuts, and seeds.
2. Foods are minimally processed.
3. Olive oil is the main dietary fat.
4. Total fat intake is between 25 and 35 percent of calories consumed (saturated fat in not greater than 8 percent of total calorie intake).
5. There is low dairy consumption.
6. Fish is the primary high-protein food, with relatively low weekly consumption.
7. Desserts are mainly fresh fruit (meaning very little refined sugar in the diet).
8. Red meat consumption limited to 16 oz per month.
9. Regular physical activity (exercise) is the norm.

TABLE 9–3   Changes in Food Consumption 1970
to 1995 (Lower Nutritional Value
of Refined Food)

| FOOD | GALLONS PER PERSON PER YEAR* | |
	1970	1995
Soda	24	53
Tea	7	8
Coffee	33	23
Fruit juice	6	9
Bottled water	2 (1975)	13
Total milk	32	24
2% milk (reduced fat)	3	8
Skim milk (fat free)	1	4
Sugar (and other sweeteners)	123	154
Artificial sweeteners	5	24
Total added fats	52	66
Salad and cooking oils	15	28
Margarine	11	9
Butter	5	4
Shortening	17	21
Meat, poultry, fish	177	195
Total flour and grains	136	200
Cheese	11	28
Fresh fruit	101	134
Fresh vegetables	92	135
Canned vegetables	100	106

Source: Center for Science in the Public Interest, Washington, D.C.
(www.cspinet.org), with permission.

*Rounded to nearest whole number.

10. Moderate wine consumption is enjoyed. (Oldways points out that wine consumption should be considered optional and avoided when it would put theindividual or others at risk.)

For some people, however, the Mediterranean diet will not contain enough meat protein. Some individuals actually thrive on high-protein, low-carbohydrate diets. There are two primary reasons for this phenomenon. First, high-carbohydrate diets contain a large quantity and a large variety of grain antigens. (Antigens are exogenous substances that trigger the immune system and thus are allergenic). Consequently, wheat, corn, and possibly other grains cause allergies or sensitivities in some people. Second, some people have developed reduced insulin sensitivity. These people seem to be better able to lose weight and maintain constant, healthy blood-sugar levels by reducing carbohydrates and increasing dietary protein in their diets.

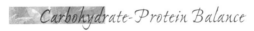 *Carbohydrate-Protein Balance*

Current Controversies

Defining the most healthful carbohydrate–protein balance is the subject of a current controversy in nutrition. One extreme position is a Pritiken-type diet, which is almost exclusively composed of complex carbohydrates, with dietary fat reduced to 10 to 12 percent of calorie intake. By definition, this is a low- to moderate-protein diet. It is very difficult for a low-fat diet to be simultaneously high in protein (without using fat-free processed protein powder of vegetable origin). The other extreme position is an Atkins-type diet, a high-protein, low-carbohydrate regimen that can reduce dietary carbohydrate intake to as little as 10 to 20 g per day. Somewhere in the middle is Peter D'Adamo's "For Your Type Diet,"[3] an attempt to overcome the "one size fits all" dietary guidelines. This approach, which matches a person's diet to his or her blood group (O, A, B, or AB), is an example of the variations possible in optimizing nutrition plans.

Clearly, different people have different nutritional requirements. Different genetics, different biochemistry, and intermediary metabolism may require different "substrates" (food breakdown products) for optimal health. For example, Rudin,[4,5] states that individuals with northern genetic roots require more omega-3 oils than people with southern genetic roots. These super-polyunsaturated omega-3 oils act as antifreeze in plant and animal life in very cold climates. They stay liquid at very low temperatures compared to either omega-6 polyunsaturated oils or less saturated dietary oils.

How to Determine the Optimum Diet

To determine their personal optimal dietary ratio of carbohydrate to protein, individuals may have to experiment with various healthy foods. One useful approach is as follows. First, start with a whole-food diet (i.e., one that relies on fresh, unprocessed foods) high in complex carbohydrates and reasonably low in fat. Complex carbohydrates are found predominantly in unrefined cereal grains such as oatmeal and unrefined whole-grain breads. Additionally, legumes such as chickpeas and lentils are very high in complex carbohydrates. In determining an individual's optimal food plan, it is essential to emphasize unprocessed foods. The fewer times foods are taken apart and put back together, the more healthful they are. Additionally, because of the emerging awareness of the importance of environmental and food-borne toxins, it is useful to consume as much organic food (which has not been exposed to pesticides and other toxins) as possible.

By starting with a diet high in complex carbohydrates and low in fat, individuals can assess whether or not they are doing the following:

1. Holding excess water
2. Consuming a reasonable number of calories without gaining weight (i.e., maintaining a healthful weight)
3. Maintaining a high energy level.
4. Showing no sign of food allergy or sensitivity.
5. Having no gastrointestinal complaints (which would indicate possible food intolerance).

If all these criteria are met and the foods are high in nutrition (i.e., they have high nutrient density and are both healthful and relatively free of toxins), a diet that is high in carbohydrates and moderate to low in fat and protein is a good starting point. If, however, these criteria are not met, the next step might be to eliminate common trigger foods that cause allergic or sensitivity-type reactions. The most common trigger foods are corn, wheat, citrus, dairy (all milk-containing and milk-derived products), wheat, chocolate, alcohol, sugar, peanuts, and yeast (including risen dough products and all fermented foods, such as soy sauce and vinegar). If avoiding all these common immune system triggers (allergens) allows an individual to meet the five criteria, the offending food(s) can be identified by adding the trigger foods back one at a time at 3- or 4-day intervals. If the criteria are not met and elimination of common trigger foods does not help, it might be useful to consider a high-protein, low-carbohydrate food regimen (such as an Atkins-type diet). These guidelines are simply an example to show how daily food intakes can be tailored to an individual's requirements to get away from the "one size fits all" recommendation.

TABLE 9–4   **Migraine-Producing Foods in Study by Egger and Colleagues**

FOOD	% OF CHILDREN AFFECTED
Cow's milk	27
Eggs	24
Chocolate	22
Orange	21
Wheat	21
Benzoic acid (preservative)	14

Source: Egger, J, et al: Is migraine food allergy? A double-blind controlled trial of oligoantigenic diet treatment. Lancet 2:865–869, 1983.

Trigger Foods and Allergies

According to the chairman of the Food Allergy Committee of the American College of Allergists, of the 108 million people who have allergies, 30 million of them suffer from food allergies. In *Basics of Food Allergies*, James C. Breneman[6] states that allergies to food are the second most common type of ingestant allergy. The foods that account for the great majority of allergies—some of them mentioned previously—include cow's milk, eggs, chocolate, citrus (such as orange), wheat, preservatives (benzoic acid), yeast, and corn. The fact that only a relatively few kinds of food are implicated makes the job of detecting food allergies easier.

The development of a food allergy is related to incomplete protein digestion. If food protein is not properly digested and is not broken down into small enough component parts, the larger-than-optimal breakdown products of these food proteins are absorbed and misinterpreted by the immune system as a foreign substance (antigen). Repeated exposure to these food antigens sensitizes the immune system, which then becomes "immunized," resulting in food sensitivity and food allergy.

The way we experience the symptoms of food allergy is largely determined by our genetic makeup. For instance, an allergy to wheat may be expressed in one person as a headache, in another as abdominal cramps, or in yet another as a skin rash. Egger and colleagues[7,8] studied 88 children who suffered from severe migraine headaches that were not relieved by drugs. The children were placed on a simplification-type diet, and their symptoms were continually monitored. When foods to which the individual children were allergic were removed from their diets, an amazing 93 percent were cured of headache. This study showed that only a few foods are responsible for the vast majority of the allergy-produced headaches. (See Table 9–4.)

In addition to showing that migraines could result from eating foods to which one is allergic, this study demonstrated something that may be even more important. The simplification-type diet that reduced headaches also reduced abdominal pain in 87 percent of the children, aches in limbs in 83 percent, chronic running nose in 56 percent, vaginal discharge in 91 percent, asthma in 7 percent, eczema in 50 percent, and seizures in 86 percent. Similar results have been reported in studies with adults as well as children.

Supplementation

Basic supplementation is considered a nutritional insurance policy. For an individual who is otherwise healthy and very well nourished, a high-quality multiple vitamin plus omega-3 essential fatty acids can be adequate. (See Table 9–5.) The multiple vitamin needs to contain a wide range of vitamins, minerals, and antioxidant nutrients. The key antioxidant nutrients are vitamin C, vitamin E, beta-carotene, and the mineral selenium.

Additionally, natural bioflavanoids are important cofactors for healthy utilization of vitamin C. The omega-3 oils are important to make up for what is an epidemic deficiency of omega-3 essential fatty acids in the typical diet. Even though most people get sufficient omega-6 dietary oils (most vegetable oils), omega-3 components are often at low levels in a typical diet. Good sources for supplemental omega-3 EFAs are flaxseed, flaxseed oil, and fish oil. Using flaxseed oil as part of a salad dressing could profoundly improve a family's essential fatty acid intake. Alternatively, fish oil, such as emulsified mint-flavored cod liver oil (which is usually well accepted by youngsters), and fish-oil capsules can both provide omega-3 essential fatty acid supplementation.

The basic multiple vitamin is designed to provide relatively small quantities of a broad range of nutrients to make up for occasional dietary deficiencies. However, seriously and chronically low intake of food nutrients requires (in addition to a reassessment of food intake) more potent daily vitamin supplementation. If there is a possibility of serious dietary nutrient deficiency, a range of clinical chemistry tests can be useful.

Some minerals are best measured intracellularly, where their natural levels are high in the body. Determining red blood cell levels of magnesium, zinc, copper, selenium, and manganese can also be helpful, although testing for serum levels (which represent extracellular fluid) of these substances is generally more available. Serum levels of vitamin B_{12}, folic acid, and vitamin A are also useful markers of vitamin nutritional status. If essential fatty acid deficiency is clinically suspect, red blood cell membrane essential fatty acid analyses are available.

**TABLE 9–5 Multiple Vitamin/
Mineral Supplements**

This moderate-dose formula is designed as a nutritional insurance policy.

VITAMIN/MINERAL	AMOUNT
Beta-carotene	15,000 I.U.
Vitamin E	400 I.U.
Vitamin C	750 mg
Bioflavonoids	100 mg
Vitamin B_1	15 mg
Vitamin B_2	10 mg
Vitamin B_3	10 mg
Vitamin B_3	50 mg
Vitamin B_5	25 mg
Vitamin B_6	10 mg
Vitamin B_{12}	200 mcg
Folic	400 mcg
Biotin	200 mcg
Vitamin A	5,000 I.U.
Vitamin D	100 I.U.
PABA	15 mg
Calcium	250 mg
Magnesium	250 mg
Zinc	25 mg
Copper	3 mg
Chromium	200 mcg
Selenium	200 mcg
Manganese	5 mg
Molybdenum	25 mcg
Vanadium	10 mg
Iodine	150 mcg

In addition to basic supplementation with a multiple vitamin and omega-3 essential fatty acids, the following may be useful under varying circumstances.

Fiber

Dietary fiber used to be called "roughage." It is neither digested nor absorbed but rather passes through the gastrointestinal tract, ultimately ending up in stool. Some fiber is used as food by intestinal microbes (gut flora). Adequate dietary fiber has been shown to do all the following:

* Improve blood-sugar problems
* Relieve constipation
* Increase stool bulk
* Reduce stool transit time
* Prevent diverticular disease and irritable bowel syndrome
* Increase bile salt excretion (with lowering of blood cholesterol)
* Lower blood triglyceride levels
* Reduce the risk of certain types of cancer
* Increase feeling of "fullness"
* Promote greater fecal loss of dietary fat.

The intake of fiber has changed drastically over the millennia. Our paleolithic ancestors consumed a diet that was 60 to 70 percent vegetable. This vegetable diet contained between 40 and 50 g of fiber per day. Some cultures in various parts of the world consume even more than this, perhaps up to 80 or 90 g per day in some cases. Compare this to the current Western diet of less than 20 g per day of fiber. Various estimates of currently unsupplemented U.S. fiber consumption are even lower, sometimes in the range of 8 to 15 g per day.

Lactobacillus acidophilus and *Lactobacillus bifidus*

Lactobacillus acidophilus and *Lactobacillus bifidus* are examples of intestinal flora (good bacteria), microbial organisms that live in a healthy human gastrointestinal tract. Several hundred species inhabit the healthy human gut, totaling more than 2 pounds of microbes per person.

These "good" intestinal microbes have been shown to inhibit or kill pathogenic intestinal microbes such as *Salmonella, Shigella, Klebsiella, Pseudomonas, Vibrio,* and *Candida* (yeast). Additionally, these "good" bacteria produce anticancer agents, reduce blood cholesterol levels, and assist in the digestion of food. Other benefits attributed to healthy flora are partial relief from lactose intolerance, production of B-complex vitamins such as vitamin B_{12}, and control of bad breath and body odor.

Manufacturers of intestinal flora products claim that taking one or more capsules (usually *L. acidophilus*) will relieve conditions caused by intestinal microbe imbalances. Gastrointestinal symptoms such as diarrhea, constipation, and gas are also relieved by their use.

In 1908 Metchnikoff, the famous Nobel Prize–winning microbiologist, published a book advocating the use of naturally fermented dairy products for health enhancement.

Antioxidants

Oxygen is a double-edged sword. It is absolutely necessary for life, but an excess—either naturally produced or caused by radiation and certain environmental toxins—stimulates the body to produce supercharged oxygen molecules (free radicals). These free radicals are normally present in the body and play a useful role as potent antibiotics, destroying harmful bacteria. However, when there is too much supercharged oxygen, or when we are not sufficiently protected with antioxidants, it can destroy polyunsaturated oils and "good" high-density lipoprotein cholesterol, causing severe damage to the affected body tissue. The process is very similar to burning oil in the bottom of a frying pan when cooking. The dark, hard film of burnt cooking oil is oxidized. Spoiled or rancid foods contain oxidized oils, which impart the characteristic rancid odor and taste.

The antioxidant nutrients beta-carotene, vitamin C, and vitamin E prevent damage to body tissue because they themselves, instead of body tissue, are oxidized. Supercharged oxygen attacks and destroys the antioxidant nutrients, and our body tissues remain undamaged. In the process we "use up" antioxidant nutrients. For continued protection, these important nutrients, which are depleted as they work to protect us, must be replaced on a daily basis.

Antioxidants Reduce Cancer Risk

A report by the National Academy of Sciences entitled "Diet, Nutrition and Cancer," as well as hundreds if not thousands of articles in the medical literature, conclude that cancer risk is in part reduced by the antioxidants beta-carotene, vitamin C, and vitamin E. These nutrients also help lower the risk of heart disease.

Antioxidant nutrients reduce the risk of cancer by neutralizing this overabundance of supercharged oxygen. (See Table 9–6.) They do this by being themselves destroyed. They are appropriately called "sacrificial antioxidants," because they are sacrificed to protect healthy cells from damage by the free radicals. These are the same antioxidant nutrients that are also necessary for a strong immune system, which is susceptible to oxidative injury.

In a study of Japanese quail, whose arteries are very similar to those of humans, Donaldson[9,10] found that the antioxidant nutrient vitamin E protected quail arteries from damage. Without vitamin E, the animals had oxidized cholesterol, which produced (1) high blood cholesterol levels and (2) increased atherosclerotic lesions in their artery walls. When they were protected with vitamin E, their blood cholesterol levels dropped and they had less plaque on their artery walls.

More recently, studies by Manson[11–14] of more than 87,000 nurses found that the women whose vitamin E intake was in the upper 20 percent had a 35 percent lower risk of heart disease and those whose beta-carotene was in the upper 20 percent had a 22 percent lower risk of heart disease than did others in the study. Many other studies support these findings. Grundy,[15,16] one of the leading researchers in this area, maintains that beta-carotene, vitamin C, and vitamin E have the ability to block the oxidation of low-density lipoproteins.

In summary, the antioxidant nutrients beta-carotene, vitamin C, and vitamin E protect us from both heart disease and cancer by protecting us from the damage caused by supercharged oxygen. In the process of protecting our cells, antioxidant nutrients are used up and must be replaced. The most effective way to replace them is to take a daily multiple vitamin with high antioxidants and to eat foods high in antioxidant nutrients. They prevent us from rusting from the inside out, the biological equivalent of Rustoleum paint.

TABLE 9–6 **Foods High in Antioxidant Nutrients (Beta-Carotene, Vitamins C and E)**

Carrots	Kale	Apricots
Collards	Sweet potatoes	Parsley
Spinach	Broccoli	Watercress
Wheat germ	Mangoes	Sunflower seeds
Wheat germ oil	Almonds	Red peppers
Brussels sprouts	Cauliflower	Squash
Barley	Whole wheat bread	Brazil nuts
Garlic	Guavas	Pumpkins

Echinacea

Echinacea, discovered by the Indians of North America, is a natural remedy that has achieved wide acceptance and is possibly the most popular natural remedy being used today. A large volume of high-quality research shows that echinacea stimulates immune system cells to increase antiviral, antibiotic, and antitumor activity. The upper part of the plant and the roots of *Echinacea* species (*E. purpurea, E. angustifolia,* and *E. pallida*) are typically used. Various active components have been isolated (polysaccharides and phenolic compounds).

Astragalus

Astragalus has been used for thousands of years in China, where it is also known as Huang Qi. Various species and variants of the genus *Astragalus* are used in herbal medicine. Astragalus is a very potent "adaptogen," considered by many to be at least as powerful and maybe even more potent than ginseng. Adaptogenic herbs normalize physiological imbalances. Historically, astragalus has been used to strengthen the immune system as well as to relieve congestive heart failure. The root of the plant contains the active ingredients, which include bioflavanoids, choline, and a peptide called Astragalan B. Astragalus root extracts are potent free-radical scavengers (antioxidants), with activities that appear similar to those of superoxide dismutase.

Iron

Iron supplements should only be used if a specific need can be demonstrated. Iron overload is a very real concern because it can contribute to immune system dysfunction. Iron is capable of catalyzing free-radical production, with subsequent tissue damage. Clinical documentation of iron deficiency includes, but is not limited to, a complete blood count test for serum iron and serum ferritin.

Summary

It is now well established that nutritional factors are of major importance in the pathogenesis of many illnesses, including atherosclerosis and cancer, the two leading causes of death in Western countries.[17] Research on the importance of balanced nutrition reflects what our bodies tell us: when we eat the foods that are right for us, we feel better, have more energy, can think more clearly, can enjoy life, and have fewer health problems.

This chapter provides a basic overview of the nutritional components of a healthy diet, from which the health-care practitioner can develop a broader knowledge base that will inform his or her holistic care. Nutrition is more than ingestion of food for health. Food is an intrinsic part of our daily lives as individuals, families, and cultures. It is associated with comfort, identity, and pleasure as well as a state of physical health. Social and psychological factors affect dietary habits as much as does knowledge about healthy eating.

In addition, our fast-paced, stressed lifestyles, as well as the questionable nutritional quality of the commercially grown and processed foods that comprise most Americans' diets, provide barriers to the sound nutritional base that can support optimal wellness.

REFERENCES

1. Eaton, SB and Konnor, M: Paleolithic nutrition: A consideration of its nature and current implications. N Engl J Med 312:283–289, 1985.
2. Simopoulos, AP, Leaf, A, and Salem, N, Jr.: Essentiality and recommended dietary intakes for omega 6 and omega 3 fatty acids. Ann Nutr Metab 43(2):127–130, 1999.
3. D'Adamo, PJ: Eat Right for Your Type. Penguin, New York, 1997.

4. Rudin, D: The major psychoses and neuroses as omega-3 essential fatty acid deficiency syndrome: Substrate pellagra. Biological Psychiatry 14(9):837–850, 1981.

5. Rudin, D: The three pellagras. Journal of Orthomolecular Psychiatry 12(2):91–110, 1983.

6. Breneman, JC: Basics of Food Allergy. CC Thomas, Springfield, Ill., 1978.

7. Egger, J, Stolla, A, and McEwen, LM: Controlled trial of hyposensitization in children with food-induced hyperkinetic syndrome. Lancet 339(8802):1150–1153, 1992.

8. Egger, J, et al: Is migraine food allergy? A double-blind controlled trial of oligoantigenic diet treatment. Lancet 2(8355):865–869, 1983.

9. Donaldson, WE: Atherosclerosis in cholesterol-fed Japanese quail: Evidence for amelioriation by dietary vitamin E. Poult Sci 61:2097–2102, 1982.

10. Donaldson, WE: Effect of cholesterol feeding on serum lipoprotein and atherosclerosis in atherosclerosis-susceptible and atherosclerois-resistant Japanese quail. Poult Sci 61:2407–2414, 1982.

11. Manson, JE: A prospective study of dietary glycemic load, carbohydrate intake, and risk of coronary heart disease in US women. Am J Clin Nutr 71(6):1455–1461.

12. Manson, JE: Dietary saturated fats and their food sources in relation to the risk of coronary heart disease in women. Am J Clin Nutr, pp 1001–1008, 1999.

13. Manson, JE: Wholegrain consumption and risk of coronary heart disease: Results from the Nurses' Health Study. Am J Clin Nutr, pp 412–419, 1999.

14. Manson, JE: Dietary intake of alpha-linolenic acid and risk of fatal ischemic heart disease among women. Am J Clin Nutr 69:890–897, 1999.

15. Grundy, SM, et al: Lipoprotein-cholesterol responses in healthy infants fed defined diets from ages 1 to 12 months. J Lipid Res, pp 1178–1187, 1995.

16. Grundy, SM: Individual responses to a cholesterol-lowering diet in 50 men with moderate hypercholesterolemia. Arch Intern Med 154(3):317–325.

17. Werback, MR: Nutritional Influences on Illness: A Sourcebook for Clinical Research. Keats, New Canaan, Conn., 1988.

CHAPTER 10

Herbs through the Ages

Gary A. Holt and Samir Kouzi

Gary Holt, PhD, MEd, RPh, is a medical writer and former adjunct, assistant, and associate professor of pharmacy at the Universities of Oklahoma, Wyoming, Stamford, and Louisiana, respectively.

Samir Kouzi, BSc, PhD, is an associate professor at the School of Pharmacy and Health Sciences, University of the Pacific, Stockton, California.

Contemporary Americans tend to view medicine in terms of prepared medications, technogadgets, and the gripping human drama of television doctors. Yet the magic of science associated with modern medicine is a late development in the history of humankind. People have always had limited resources for treating their ailments and injuries. Even today, self-care represents the largest component of health care in the United States. Herbs represent the most continuous and universal form of treatment throughout human history and have been used by every recorded culture. The history of herbals parallels the evolution of medicine and provides a foundation for understanding modern attitudes regarding health, medicine, and, especially, alternative care.

Herbal practices have their roots in prehistoric times.[1] For example, 60,000-year-old ritual burials of Neanderthal humans contain seeds and pollen of medicinal herbs that are still used today.[2] Herbal knowledge probably emerged from trial and error. Many plants consumed as nutrients had pharmacologic activity, both desirable and undesirable, from which valuable lessons were learned.

Ancient Greeks and Romans were clearly aware of the use of herbals for medicinal purposes. Asclepius, the legendary first physician of ancient Greece (ca. 1500 BC), achieved fame through his mastery of surgical skills and a knowledge of the curative powers of plants. At his spa at Epidaurus overlooking the Saronic Gulf, the names of 400 herbs are engraved on a stone slab that can be seen today.[3] In most historical representations, he is accompanied by two maidens, Hygeia and Panakeia. Panakeia was a true healing goddess who utilized her knowledge of natural medicines (e.g., herbs). Her philosophy is reflected in our unending search for drug panaceas.[4] Hygeia was a goddess who guarded the health of Athens and was likely a personification of Athena, the goddess of reason. Her name was derived from a word meaning "health" and is the source of our contemporary word *hygiene*. She was not actually involved in the treatment of the sick, but instead symbolized a belief that people can remain well if they live wisely.[5]

Little is actually known about Hippocrates as an individual. Many of the writings attributed to him may have been written by others, including his students. Even so, he established the foundations for many contemporary medical and health beliefs. He advocated the use of herbs in combination with fresh air, rest, and proper diet to help the body's life force to restore health. He promoted rational thinking based on knowledge rather than myths and supernatural influences.[6] Ancient physicians were students of the natural order of things and sought to promote healthy environments and lifestyles.

During the Middle Ages a great deal of information was preserved by monks of the various monasteries, who hand-copied manuscripts. These monasteries became repositories of information, and their herb gardens provided folk treatments for many health problems.[7]

There were few formally trained physicians in the colonial era of America. Hospitals and medical schools as we know them did not exist for 200 years following the arrival of the first colonists, since formally trained physicians were reluctant to leave the civilization of Europe for a new land characterized by uncertainties and a lack of traditional medical supplies. Native-American medicines were important to the early colonists, especially during the winter months when few ships came from Europe. Squaws sold herbs in the colonial settlements and often assisted with healing efforts.[8] More than 200 Native-American herbs were included in the first edition of the *U.S. Pharmacopoeia* in 1820 and later in the *National Formulary* in 1888. Thousands more were used unofficially by both professional and nonprofessional healers.[9]

In early American society, the family was the center of both social and economic life. Because the care of babies was a natural role for mothers, women became the caregivers for the entire family—and often for other families as well. In the fall, women collected and preserved medicinal herbs, just as they did foods. Successful healing skills and recipes were valued and handed down from one generation to another.[10,11] Home remedies and self-care were not merely conveniences for early Americans, but were essential for survival.[12] Most communities had at least one woman who was experienced with the use of herbs and other simple remedies. Even after doctors began to appear, self-care remained the most common form of health care. Doctors were sought only when the problem was considered to be too serious for self-care.[13]

Anyone with knowledge of or experience in dealing with illness and injury was in great demand. For example, Samuel Thompson achieved considerable success as a healer.[14,15] His book, *Thompson's New Guide to Health*, became the foundation for botanical societies, mostly rural, throughout New England and New York, which held conventions and published journals (much like AMWAY, Shaklee, and other groups today). The Thompsonian movement was not restricted to healing; it also reflected political and philosophical orientations that appealed to the laity. It promoted common sense, a faith in the simplicity and accessibility of valid knowledge, and a belief that an educational aristocracy and a privileged order are hostile to ordinary people. The Thompsonians were opposed to the manner in which priests, lawyers, and doctors controlled their knowledge and kept it from common people.[16]

Movements such as the Thompsonians, homeopaths, and naturopaths were a cultural expression of political upheaval that continues today. The organized medical community has always insisted that regulations are necessary to protect the public from quacks. Yet American society was founded on principles of freedom. During the 18th and 19th centuries, there was much concern that licensure was more an expression of favor than of competence and that medical societies and boards had created a type of monopoly.[17]

The success of legitimate folk and professional healers has always been hampered by quacks (e.g., medicine shows, patent medicines). By the end of the 19th century, these charlatans had discouraged many people from using natural products. A decline in the popularity of medicinal plants and folk medicine also occurred because of an increasing emphasis on scientific medicine.[18]

From the Pages of History

Written records of medical herb use date back 5000 years to the Sumerians. Chinese herb guides from about 2700 BC list 365 medicinal plants and their uses.[19] The Egyptian Ebers Papyrus (1500 BC), found by the Egyptologist George Ebers, is one of many documents that describe medicines used by the ancient Egyptians.[20] A collection of hymns from before 1000 BC includes more than 1000 healing herbs, many of which are still used in Ayurvedic medicine.[21] Even the Old Testament mentions the use of mandrake, vetch, caraway, wheat, barley, and rye.

The first and most famous early European treatise on the medical use of herbs, *De Materia Medica* (Concerning Medical Matter), was written by the Greek botanist–physician Pedanios Dioscorides in the first century AD. It discussed more than 500 plant, animal, and mineral products and remained an authoritative reference for more than 1500 years.[22–24]

A Chinese drug encyclopedia, *Pen-ts' ao kang mu*, was compiled by Li Shih-Chen and published in 1596 AD. It listed more than 2000 natural products used for healing purposes. As many as 5000 native plants remain in use in China today.

John Wesley, the founder of Methodism, published a widely read book of medical advice in 1747 called *Primitive Physic*, which provided a listing of ancient cures and promoted individual autonomy in the care of illnesses.[25] The rise of Methodism reflected a growing trend in English society toward personal autonomy and self-direction. Wesley was extremely critical of physicians, who were being elevated to a superhuman status by society.

Because of the absence of traditional medicines and practitioners in colonial America, almanacs and newsprints became a resource of Old World recipes and medical information for the general public. By the late 18th century some physicians had begun to publish medical guides for the layperson. The intent was to demystify medicine and to promote self-care practices.[26,27]

Herbs and Modern Science

It is estimated that there may be as many as one million drug products in the United States.[28] The myriad bottles on the shelves of local pharmacies as well as grocery, convenience, and other stores disguise the natural origins of many commercial products. Aspirin serves as an example.

Ancient physicians (e.g., Hippocrates) had discovered that willow bark could be used to reduce pain and fever. It was not until 1829 that a French pharmacist, H. Leroux, isolated salicin from willow bark (it has since been discovered in other plants as well). Salicin is a pro-drug that is converted by the intestines and liver to the active drug, salicylic acid (also called sodium salicylate). Salicylic acid has excellent anti-inflammatory, analgesic, and antipyretic activity. However, it causes mouth, esophagus, and stomach irritation with long-term use. The aspirin we know, acetylsalicylic acid, was prepared by Felix Hoffman, a chemist with the Bayer Company in Germany, and introduced to the world in 1899. Because it is effective and better tolerated, Hoffman gave it to his elderly father, who suffered from rheumatism but could no longer take salicylic acid. The name is thought to be derived from *Spiraea*, the plant genus from which salicylic acid was once prepared.[29,30]

A hundred years of research have resulted in the identification of many new substances derived from the chemical manipulation of salicylic acid. Many proved to be no more effective or to have greater risks than aspirin. For example, acetanilide is too toxic; phenacetin is carcinogenic; acetaminophen is a useful pain and fever medication but does not have anti-inflammatory activity; the newer nonsteroidal anti-inflammatory drugs (NSAIDs) have activity similar to aspirin's but tend to have less blood-thinning activity.[31] Even so, some of the newer NSAIDs have unique benefits (e.g., naproxen is unusually effective for treating symptoms of premenstrual syndrome in many women). Table 10–1 summarizes other familiar drugs with plant origins.[32]

Over time, three divisions of pharmaceutical science that addressed natural products emerged: (1) pharmacognosy (natural products), (2) pharmacology (drug actions and effects in living systems), and (3) medicinal chemistry (synthetic medicines). The term *pharmacology* was first used by J. A. Schmidt in 1811 in Vienna to describe the study of medicinal plants and their properties.[33] Today, pharmacologists are not particularly concerned with the source of medicines, but rather with their activities. All three of these pharmaceutical specialties are very active today as the search for new drugs continues.

Historically, natural medicines have had four important roles in modern medicine: (1) as a source of drugs that are difficult to produce synthetically (e.g., some narcotics; ergots; cardiac glycosides, such as digitalis; many antibiotics; many serums and vaccines); (2) as a natural source of compounds that can be modified to create more effective or less toxic medicines (e.g., many synthetic narcotic pain medications); (3) as chemical models for synthetic development of new medicinals that possess pharmacologic activities similar to the natural product, but with greater efficacy or less toxicity; and (4) as the starting materials (with little or no pharmacologic activity) that can be utilized to synthetically create useful medications (e.g., hydrocortisone and related steroids occur in small amounts in nature but can be produced in large quantities from the synthetic modification of stigmasterol, which occurs abundantly in soybean oil).

Most Americans misunderstand synthetic drug manufacturing. Herbs usually contain numerous chemicals, some of which are useful and some of which are harmful or useless. Even potentially useful chemicals may be present in inappropriate quantities. Synthetic isolation and production allow for precise dosages to be given to the patient. In many

TABLE 10–1   Examples of Contemporary Medicines from Plant Sources

DRUG	SOURCE	MEDICAL USE
Atropine	Belladonna	Anticholinergic
Caffeine	Coffee shrub	Stimulant
Cocaine	Coca leaves	Local anesthetic
Colchicine	Autumn crocus	Gout
Digoxin	Digitalis	Cardiac glycoside
Emetine	Ipecac	Emetic
Ephedrine	Ephedra herb	Decongestant, hypotension
Ergotamine	Ergot	Migraine
Kawain	Kava	Anxiety
Morphine	Opium poppy	Pain
Penicillin	*Penicillium* species	Antibiotic
Physostigmine	Calabar bean	Cholinesterase inhibitor
Pilocarpine	Jaborandi leaves	Glaucoma
Quinidine	Cinchona bark	Arrhythmias
Quinine	Cinchona bark	Malaria
Reserpine	Rauwolfia	Hypertension
Salicylate	Willow bark	Pain, fever, inflammation
Scopolamine	*Datura* species	Anticholinergic
Theophylline	Tea shrub	Bronchial dilator

Source: Schulz, V, Hansel, R, and Varro, T: Rational Phytotherapy. Springer-Verlag, Berlin, 1998, with permission.

cases, the amount of drug found in commercial products is far less than the amount found in the natural source. For example, the concentration of digitoxin in commercial tablet products is only about 10 percent of that found in the original digitalis leaf.[34] Products such as deadly nightshade are well known for their toxicity, whereas commercial products containing carefully controlled amounts of these same chemicals have been safely and effectively used for decades.

Ironically, our scientific achievements have blurred the distinctions between "natural" and "synthetic" medicines. The American public has a tendency to incorrectly view every commercially produced product as "artificial" and every herbal as "natural." Problems in our understanding of natural versus synthetic medicinals are further compounded by American free enterprise. Drug manufacturers cannot obtain exclusive patent rights for most known herbals (and the ingredients they contain), because these products are classified as in the public domain. Since the costs of research and development for most common herbals far exceed the potential profits that can be earned, most major drug companies are searching for exotic plants in remote areas of the world (e.g., rain forests) in the hope of obtaining exclusive patent rights and greater profit potentials.

A Rationale for Herbs

Self-care refers to *anything* that we do for ourselves or others to promote or improve health. The demand for self-care is deeply rooted in American culture. Threats to cherished cultural values (e.g., freedom and independence) are deeply resented. Throughout most civilized history, health-care professionals have been criticized because of their control of desirable medications and health products. Even so, self-care practices can pose a significant problem when professional care is actually needed.

Americans experience two to three problems each week for which self-care can offer some benefit, and about 90 percent of consumers report minor health problems at some time during each month.[35] Self-care practices are learned early (e.g., the majority of children under age 2 have been given a nonprescription drug at least once). Most Americans have nonprescription drugs at home and often supplement prescription therapy with self-prescribed products. People tend to opt for self-care when they think that health problems are not serious.[36–39]

Nonprescription drugs are also known as *over-the-counter* (OTC) or *nonlegend* products. No one actually knows how many OTC products are available in the United States. In part, this is because some manufacturers and health fraud promoters distribute products without approval of the Food and Drug Administration. It is estimated that there are more than 300,000 OTC products available, manufactured by 12,000 firms. Despite the large number of products, there are only about 800 active ingredients for use in OTC products.[40–42] So, there are many duplications. Nonprescription drugs are considered to be safe and effective as long as people read and follow label directions and warnings.

Herbals represent a unique entity among self-care products because they are regulated as foods rather than as drugs. Yet they are clearly promoted for self-care purposes. The problem is compounded by the fact that many consumers erroneously view them as "natural" or as "God's medicines" and, therefore, as completely devoid of risks. The relative benefits and concerns regarding the use of herbals (and self-care practices in general) are summarized in Table 10–2.

Alternative health-care practices (especially self-care) have survived because they offer alternatives that are relatively simple in concept and seemingly more harmonious with life rather than antagonistic to it.[43] Indeed, people prefer simple answers for complex problems. The concepts of modern medicine are often far too complex to be explained in simple terms. So, the seeming simplicity of things "natural" finds increasing appeal in a culture bewildered by advances in medical knowledge and increasing health-care costs.

TABLE 10–2   The Pros and Cons of Self-Medicating with Herbals

ISSUE	PROS	CONS
Safety	Many herbs are relatively safe when used appropriately.	Many herbs are toxic or can be hazardous if not used appropriately. Potential herb/drug interactions.
Effectiveness	Many herbs are beneficial for their promoted uses.	Many herbals offer no benefits for their promoted uses. Self-care may weaken consumer trust in health-care professionals and decrease the demand for high-quality care.
Consumer education	Consumers are more educated today regarding health, medicine, and self-care.	Consumers often have misinformation and inaccurate beliefs regarding herbs. Consumers often lack the knowledge to make accurate clinical diagnoses and medical assessments or to select appropriate herbs for their actual needs. Herbs can be misused and abused. It can be difficult for people to think and act objectively on their own behalf or for significant others. Inappropriate use of medical references can lead to poor self-care decisions.
Cost	Self-care practices are less expensive than professional care (e.g., time and money).	Competition in an aggressive market can actually increase the costs of self-care products. Inappropriate self-care can result in increased health problems and costs. Ineffective self-care is not economical.
Convenience	Self-care is convenient and available.	Convenience and availability can discourage consumers from seeking professional care when it is truly needed.
Self-responsibility	Self-care practices may reinforce responsibility for self and others. Self-care is perceived to be an inalienable right.	Overconfident and uninformed consumers are often willing to accept responsibility for self-care at times when it is not advisable. Demands for self-care products and practices often involve unreasonable therapeutic expectations.
Self-awareness	People are more aware of their bodies and how they feel than they can usually describe to a health-care professional.	How people feel may not always correlate accurately to their actual health status.
Concerns and emotions	Self-care practices allow people to avoid disappointments, anxieties, suspicions, concerns, and embarrassments that may be associated with professional care.	Individuals may avoid professional health care at times when they truly need it.
Professional manpower	Self-care practices reduce the demand for professional manpower.	Lower demands for professional manpower could have a negative impact on cultural efforts to insure that professional health care is readily available.

Problems with Herbs

1   Herbal products lack regulations to guarantee the safety and efficacy required for other health-care products. They may vary in their makeup, may be adulterated with other substances, and may lack standards regarding cultivation and preparation techniques utilized by herbal manufacturers and distributors. In short, there is no quality control.[44] Increasingly, health officials are recommending regulation of the herbal industry.[45]

2   Understanding herbals can be confusing because of the many names that are associated with any given plant. In early U.S. publications, native plants were often described by their uses or by some obvious physical characteristic. In some cases, a given name can refer to several species of plants, which may have considerable variations in chemical and pharmacologic makeup (e.g., "dye weed" can refer to dozens of distinctly different plants used as a dye).[46] Even within the scientific community there is often a lack of agreement regarding the formal names of a given plant. As a result, an herb may be associated with numerous common and scientific names.

Many aspects of herbal pharmacology remain unknown (e.g., drug–herbal interactions; impact of chronic use; use by specific patient groups, such as pregnant or lactating women, the elderly, or children; adverse effects). Because most herbals contain numerous components, it can be difficult to tailor products to specific symptoms or health problems without the occurrence of adverse effects. These problems can vary because of the season during which an herb was collected or as a result of other cultivation and preparation techniques.[47,48]

Problems with herb use include not only the actions of the varied individual ingredients they contain but also interactions with traditional drug products. Table 10–3 lists examples of potential herb and drug interactions. It is intended as neither an exhaustive nor a definitive listing, but rather as a sample of the types of interactions that have been reported in the medical literature. This list grows daily as these products are researched and better understood by medical science. The interested reader is encouraged to review other resources for a more in-depth discussion of the pharmacological and chemical basis for herb–drug interactions.

Many medical authorities prefer to categorize these interactions according to the mechanism of action involved (e.g., pharmacodynamic versus pharmacokinetic). A simple definition of these concepts is that pharmcodynamics is concerned with what the drug does to the body, whereas pharmacokinetics involves what the body does to the drug. Pharmacodynamics considers drug action on biochemical, physiological, or molecular functions in the body and the mechanisms of action by which the drug or herb in question is able to achieve its effects.

Pharmacokinetics examines factors that affect drug or herb administration, absorption, biotransformation, distribution, and excretion, especially the rate at which these processes occur. For example, pharmacokinetics is interested in the time required for onset of drug action after the drug is administered in some way. It would also examine how long it takes for the drug to be excreted, since this would affect dosing schedules.

Obviously, some herb–drug interactions operate by pharmacodynamic processes (e.g., taking an herb and drug that both cause sedation, so that additive or synergistic sedation occurs), whereas other interactions operate by pharmacodynamic mechanisms (e.g., the herb may increase or decrease normal elimination of the drug, possibly resulting in drug levels that are too high or too low). Table 10–3 does not attempt to distinguish herb–drug interactions according to these categories, since the objective is merely to provide examples of the types of herbs and drugs that may be involved in interactions. Even so, it can be readily seen that both types are present, and an awareness of this may prove useful in our efforts to prevent, modify, or treat adverse outcomes due to interactions.

TABLE 10–3   Examples of Potential Drug-Herb Interactions

DRUGS OR THERAPEUTIC SCENARIO	HERBS AND INTERACTION	
Anesthetics	Increased sympathomimetic activity; disturbances of heart rhythms.	
	Ma huang	
Anticholinergics	Anticholinergic activity; potentiation of drug with anticholinergic activity.	
Amantadine	Deadly nightshade	Scopolia
Antihistamines	Henbane	
Anticholinergics		
Phenothiazines		
Procainamides		
Quinidine		
Tricyclics		
Anticoagulants	Coagulant activity; antagonize anticoagulants.	
	Agrimony	Mistletoe
	Goldenseal	Yarrow
Aspirin	Anticoagulant activity; potentiaton of anticoagulants.	
Warfarin	Alfalfa	Gingko biloba
	Angelica	Ginseng
	Aniseed	Green tea
	Arnica	Horse chestnut
	Asafoetida	Horseradish
	Bogbean	Licorice
	Boldo	Meadowsweet
	Buchu	Melilot tea
	Capsicum	Nettle
	Cassia	Papain
	Celery	Parsley
	Chamomile	Passion flower
	Chinese red sage	Poplar
	Clove	Prickly ash
	Danshen	Quassia
	Echinacea	Red clover
	Fenugreek	Tonka bean tea
	Feverfew	Wild carrot
	Fucus	Wild lettuce
	Garlic	Woodruff tea
	Ginger	
	Anticoagulant interference.	
	Co Q 10	
Anticonvulsants	Lower seizure threshold.	
	Black cohosh	Evening primrose
	Borage	
Carbamazepine	Decreased drug effects via cytochrome P 450 induction by herb.	
Phenobarbital	St. John's wort	
Phenytoin		
Phenytoin	Decreases phenytoin levels and activity.	
	Shankapulshpi	
Antihistamines	Causes histamine release.	
	Mistletoe	

continued

TABLE 10–3 Examples of Potential Drug-Herb Interactions continued

DRUGS OR THERAPEUTIC SCENARIO	HERBS AND INTERACTION	
Blood pressure	Hypertensive activity.	
	Bayberry	Gentian
	Blue cohosh	Ginger
	Brewer's yeast	Ginseng
	Broom	Licorice
	Capsicum	Vervain
	Cola	Yohimbe
	Coltsfoot	
	Hypotensive activity.	
	Agrimony	Hawthorn
	Asafoetida	Horehound
	Avens	Horseradish
	Black cohosh	Mistletoe
	Calamus	Nettle
	Celery	Parsley
	Cornsilk	Pokeroot
	Cowslip	Prickly ash
	Devil's claw	Psyllium
	Elecampane	Sage
	Fenugreek	Shepherd's purse
	Fucus	Squill
	Fumitory	St. John's wort
	Garlic	Vervain
	Ginger	Yarrow
	Ginseng	
Guanethidine	Increased sympathomimetic activity.	
	Ma huang	
Calcium salts	Calcium activity and adverse effects increased.	
	Oleander	Strophanthus
Cardiac drugs	Bradycardia, hypotension, cardiac arrest.	
	Delphinium	
	Cardiac depressant activity.	
	Broom	Wild carrot
	Cardioactive; increased activity and adverse reactions.	
	Devil's claw	Horehound
	Fenugreek	Pleurisy root
	Fumitory	Quassia
	Ginger	Shepherd's purse
	Ginseng	Squill
	Goldenseal	
	Cardiotonic amine (contains tyramine).	
	Hawthorn	
	Contain caffeine; increases in heart rate and blood pressure.	
	Cola	Maté
	Guarana	
	Negative ionotropic effect.	
	Mistletoe	
	Vascular congestion	
	Parsley	

continued

TABLE 10–3   Examples of Potential Drug–Herb Interactions continued

DRUGS OR THERAPEUTIC SCENARIO	HERBS AND INTERACTION
Antiarrhythmics	Promote potassium excretion; increased arrhythmia risk.
	Aloe Cascara sagrada
	Buckthorn
Beta blockers	Decreased activity of drugs metabolized by the cytochrome P450
Cardiac glycosides	pathway via enzyme induction by the herb.
Diltiazem	St. John's Wort
Nifedipine	
Beta blockers	Antagonism of beta blockers; increases heart rate and blood pressure.
	Licorice
	Decreased drug effects via cytochrome P450 induction by herb.
	St. John's wort
Calcium channel blockers	Antagonism of calcium channel blocker activity; increased sodium and lowered potassium levels.
	Licorice
	Antagonism of drug activity; mechanism not specified.
	Yohimbe
	Calcium channel blocker activity; potentiation of calcium channel blocker activity.
	Coltsfoot
	Decreased drug effects via cytochrome P450 induction by herb.
	St. John's wort
	Interference with liver metabolism of drug; potentiation of drug activity and adverse effects.
	Grapefruit
Cardiac glycosides	Cardiac glycoside activity; potentiation of cardiac glycosides, increase risk of adverse reactions (e.g., bradycardia, arrhythmmias).
	Figwort Kyuwhin
	Motherwort Rauwolfia
	Ginseng Uva ursi
	Cardioprotective; decreases plaque formation on blood vessels.
	Licorice
	Disturbances of heart rhythm.
	Ma huang
	Interference with digoxin pharmacodynamics and monitoring.
	Hawthorn Psyllium
	Licorice Uzara root
	Laxative activity; increased potassium losses; increased activity and adverse reactions of cardiac glycosides.
	Aloe Castor bean
	Black cohosh Castor oil
	Buckthorn Rhubarb
	Cascara sagrada Senna
	Potassium losses; potentiation of cardiac glycoside activity and adverse effects.
	Goldenrod Juniper
	Horsetail Squill
Methylxanthines	Increased risk of cardiac arrhythmias.
Quinidine	Digitalis Squill
Sympathomimetics	Foxglove
Phosphodiesterase inhibitors	Increased risk of cardiac arrhythmias.
	Digitalis Squill

continued

TABLE 10–3   Examples of Potential Drug–Herb Interactions continued

DRUGS OR THERAPEUTIC SCENARIO	HERBS AND INTERACTION
Quinidine	Increased quinidine activity, including adverse effects. Oleander Strophanthus
Chemotherapy Cyclophosphamide Etoposide Tamoxifen Taxol	Decreased drug effects via cytochrome P450 induction by herb. St. John's wort

Cholesterol and lipid modifers	Cholesterol and/or lipid lowering activity; potentiaton of cholesterol and/or lipid lowering drugs.
	  Alfalfa Licorice
	  Artichoke Psyllium
	  Fenugreek Scullcap
	  Garlic Tansy
	  Ginger

Central nervous system (CNS)
Alcohol
Alprazolam
Antidepressants
Antipsychotics
Barbiturates
Benzodiazepines
CNS depressants
Phenothiazines
Sedatives
Sleeping medications
Tricyclics
	Central paralyzing effect.
	  Delphinium
	CNS depression, potentiation of CNS depressant drugs.
	  Balm plant Kava
	  Black cohosh Lavender
	  Calamus Nettle
	  Catnip Passion flower
	  Celery Rauwolfia
	  Chamomile Sage
	  Couchgrass Scullcap
	  Elecampane Shepherd's purse
	  Goldenseal St. John's wort
	  Hops Valerian
	  Hydrocotyle Wild carrot
	  Jamaica dogwood
	Decreased activity of drugs metabolized by cytochrome P450 pathway via enzyme inducation by herb.
	  St. John's wort

Alcohol	Increase in motor skill impairment. Raulwofia
Antidepressants	Interference with drug absorption. Fiber
Amoxapine Amitriptyline Imipramine	Decreased drug effects via cytochrome P450 induction by herb. St. John's wort
Levodopa	Decreased levodopa activity; increase in extrapyramidine effects. Rauwolfia
Neuroleptics	Synergism of neuroleptic activity. Rauwolfia

Selective serotonin reuptake inhibitors
  Sertraline
	Serotonin syndrome (potentially serious); fever, sweating, dizziness.
	  St. John's wort

Psychoactives	Psychoactive activity; potentiation of psychoactive effects and adverse effects (e.g., nervousness, insomnia anxiety). Nutmeg Yohimbe

continued

TABLE 10–3   Examples of Potential Drug–Herb Interactions continued

DRUGS OR THERAPEUTIC SCENARIO	HERBS AND INTERACTION
Corticosteroids	Additive effects, including adverse reactions.
	Ginseng
	Increased potassium excretion.
	Aloe Licorice
	Buckthorn Senna
	Cascara sagrada
	Immunostimulant; antagonism of immunosuppression.
	Echinacea Ginseng
Diabetics	Hyperglycemic activity.
	Devil s claw Hydrocotyle
	Elecampane Licorice
	Figwort Marshmallow
	Ginseng
	Hypoglycemic activity.
	Alfalfa Garlic
	Aloe Ginger
	Burdock Ginseng
	Celery Goat's rue
	Cornsilk Juniper
	Dimiana Myrrh
	Elecampane Nettle
	Eucalyptus Sage
	Fenugreek Tansy
	Fiber
	Interference with diabetic therapy.
	Bilberry Dandelion
	Coffee Karela
Insulin	Insulin dose may need to be decreased; mechanism not specified.
	Psyllium
Diuretics	Diuretic activity; mechanism not specified.
	Agrimony Dandelion
	Artichoke Elder
	Boldo Guaiacum
	Broom Juniper
	Buchu Pokeroot
	Burdock Shepherd's purse
	Celery Uva ursi
	Cornsilk Yarrow
	Couchgrass Yohimbe
Potassium-depleting drugs	Potassium depletion via laxative activity.
Furosemide	Aloe Rhubarb
Thiazides	Buckthorn Senna
	Cascara sagrada Squill
	Castor bean
	Potassium depletion via diuretic activity.
	Goldenrod Juniper
	Horsetail

continued

TABLE 10–3 **Examples of Potential Drug–Herb Interactions** continued

DRUGS OR THERAPEUTIC SCENARIO	HERBS AND INTERACTION
Gastrointestinals	GI irritation (e.g., nausea, vomiting, hemorrhagic diarrhea); can become severe.
	Colocynth Yohimbe
	Sarsaparilla
Iron	Interference with iron absorption; herb contains tannic acid.
	Saw palmetto St. John's wort
Glucocorticoids	Increased levels, activity and adverse effects.
	Licorice Strophanthus
	Oleander
Hepatotoxics	Hepatotoxic activity; increased hepatotoxicity risk when taken with drugs that are hepatotoxic.
	Borage Licorice
	Coltsfoot Petasites
	Echinacea Rhubarb
	Hound's tongue Senecio
	Hydrocotyle
HIV therapy	Decreased activity of drugs metabolized by the cytochrome P450 pathway via enzyme induction by the herb.
Non-nucleoside reverese Transcriptase inhibitors	St. John's wort
Delaviridine	
Efavirenz	
Nevirapine	
Protease inhibitors	
Amprenavire	
Indinavir	
Nelfinavir	
Retonavir	
Sequinavir	
Hormones	
Estrogen	Estrogenic activity.
	Alfalfa Pleurisy root
	Aniseed Red clover
	Black cohosh Saw palmetto
	Ginseng Wild carrot
	Licorice
Ethinyl estradiol	Decreased activity; via herb induction of the cytochrome P450 pathway.
	St. John's wort
Gonadotropins	Gonadotropic inhibition activity.
	Vervain
Oxytocin	Oxytocic; increased risk of adverse reactions (e.g., hypertension.
	Ma huang Motherwort
Thyroid	Hyperthyroid activity.
	Bladder wrack Kelp
	Hyper- and Hypothyroid activity.
	Fucus
	Thyroid depression activity.
	Horseradish

continued

TABLE 10–3   Examples of Potential Drug–Herb Interactions continued

DRUGS OR THERAPEUTIC SCENARIO	HERBS AND INTERACTION	
Immunomodifiers	Immunodepressants.	
	Drosera	Licorice
	Immunostimulants; antagonize immunodepressant therapy.	
	Boneset	Ginseng
	Calendula	Mistletoe
	Drosera	Periwinkle
	Echinacea	Saw palmetto
	Eleutherococcus	
Laxatives	Laxative activity; potentiation of laxative effects including adverse effects.	
	Adonis	Lily of the valley
	Aloe	Milk thistle
	Buckthorn	Psyllium
	Cascara sagrada	Rhubarb
	Castor bean	Senna
	Eyebright	Squill
	Frangula	Strophanthus
	Horehound	Yellow dock
	Ispaghula	
Many drugs	Interference with drug absorption (e.g., laxative activity, GI irritation, etc.)	
	Aloe	Flaxseed
	Buckthorn	Psyllium
	Cascara sagrada	Rhubarb
	Castor bean	Senna
	Coffee	Slippery elm
	Flax	
	Increases liver metabolism; decreased drug activity of drugs that undergo liver metabolism.	
	Naiouli	
	Decreased activity of drugs metabolized by cytochrome P450 pathway via enzyme induction by herb.	
	St. John's wort	
Monoamine oxidase inhibitors (MAOIs)	Antagonism of MAOI activity.	
	Yohimbe	
	Potentiation of MAOI activity and adverse effects; hypertensive crisis.	
	Broom	Passion flower
	Ginseng	Scotch broom
	Ma huang	St. John's wort
Phenelzine	Interaction suspected; headache, trembling, and manic behavior.	
	Ginseng	
Migraine therapy	Contain caffeine, migraine trigger.	
	Cocoa	Maté
	Guarana	
NSAIDs	Interferes with migraine therapy of herb.	
Aspirin	Feverfew	
Salicylates		

continued

TABLE 10–3   Examples of Potential Drug-Herb Interactions continued

DRUGS OR THERAPEUTIC SCENARIO	HERBS AND INTERACTION
Mineralocorticoids	Mineralcorticoid activity; potentiation of mineralcorticoid drug activity; sodium and fluid retention. Bayberry Licorice
NSAIDs	Contain salicylates; potentiation of drug activity and adverse effects. Willow species Contain salicylates; GI irritation. White willow bark Willow species
Organ transplant antirejection therapy Cyclosporine Rapamycin Tacrolimus	Decreased activity of drugs metabolized by the cytochrome P450 pathway via enzyme induction by the herb. St. John's wort
Photosensitizers	Photosensitizers; increased risk of photosensitivity. Angelica Rue Bishop's weed St. John's wort Celery
Pregnancy	Abortifacients (esp. with high doses). Angelica Nutmeg Mugwort Saffron
Radioisotopes	Interferes with diagnostic procedures using radioisotopes. Bugleweed
Respiratory	Curare-like effect on respiration. Delphinium
Saluretics	Increased activity (e.g., sodium losses) and adverse effects. Oleander Strophantus Squill
Stimulants	Contain caffeine Cola Maté Ginseng
Weight control products Acutrim Dexatrim	Excessive stimulation, dizziness, agitation, confusion. St. John's wort
Sympathomimetics	Sympathomimetic activity; potentiation of sympathomimetic activity. Aniseed Parsley Capsicum Pleurisy root Digitalis Rauwolfia Foxglove Vervain
Thrombocytopenics	Increased risk of thrombocytopenia when combined with other drugs that cause this problem. Cinchona
Urinary	Kidney damage, cystitis Colocynth

Interactions are difficult to assess because the interaction depends greatly on the product selected and the amount taken. Herb products are not regulated like other nonprescription drug products. Herbal labels are often inaccurate regarding the actual contents. Even when the label is accurate, consumers are usually given inadequate instructions for use. Unfortunately, many consumers believe strongly in the "more is better" principle—if one will do some good, just think what 10 would do!

Herbs are promoted as "natural" substances that are "nondrugs" and have no adverse effects. This simply is not true. These products fit the definition of drugs and medicines relative to their actions and proposed uses.[49]

Attempts to Regulate Herbs

The German Experience: Commission E Reviews

In countries such as Germany, herbal use is widely accepted by both medical professionals and the laity. As many as 700 plants (singly or in various combinations) are sold in Germany for medicinal purposes. The majority of physicians prescribe herbals and government health insurance programs pay for some herbal therapy. Because of their popularity, the German government developed a quality assurance program to help ensure public safety. This program is unique and merits review since it may serve a model for other countries.

In 1978, an expert committee was established to evaluate herbal remedies. This committee, which has come to be known as "Commission E," consisted of health professionals (e.g., physicians, pharmacists, pharmacologists, toxicologists), representatives of the pharmaceutical industry, and laypersons. The data collected by the commission included clinical trials, field studies, single case reports, scientific literature, standard reference works, and medical expertise. This program did not demand the safety and efficacy standards required of U.S. drugs, but it was a less costly process. The commission justified this approach on the grounds that the degree of safety and efficacy that it sought was adequate for these products.[50]

Following commission review of an herb, a monograph was published that indicated a favorable or unfavorable assessment (see examples in Table 10–4). Monographs on more than 300 herbs had been completed by 1993. Of these, roughly two-thirds were found to be favorable (i.e., considered to be safe and effective), whereas one-third were found to be unfavorable (i.e., unsafe, ineffective, or both). Because of a lack of quality controls, any of these products can be marketed in the United States.[51,52] The Commission E monographs are considered to represent the most authoritative herbal evaluations currently available, even though they do not provide standards for the quality and purity of herbal products.[53] Additionally, not all health authorities are in total agreement.[54] It is clear that despite efforts to establish guidelines for safe and effective use of herbals, much remains to be learned about the use of these products as medicinal agents, and, certainly, professional judgment is imperative.

Herbs and the Food and Drug Administration

Many people believe that U.S. herbal regulations should be as liberal as those in European countries. Yet America is unique in the world in many regards. Our culture is characterized by the most aggressive retail competition in the world and, probably, the most greed. The average American watches more than 7 hours of television and is exposed to more than 1500 advertisements daily. The majority of attorneys in the world currently practice in this country. The United States currently has a $100 billion health fraud industry (i.e., products and services promoted that have not been demonstrated to be safe or effective). As of 1980, there were more than 5500 self-help books available to American consumers,

TABLE 10–4 Examples of Herbs (Un)Approved by the German Commission E

Approved Herbs
( ) = approved uses

Agrimony (diarrhea)
Aloe (appetite loss, GI spasms, flatulence)
Angelica root (anorexia, GI spasms, flatulence)
Anise seed (dyspepsia, catarrh)
Arnica flower (external treatment of injury)
Artichoke leaf (dyspepsia)
Asparagus root (UTI, kidney stone prevention)
Autumn crocus (gout)
Belladonna (GI and bile spasms)
Bilberry fruit (diarrhea)
Birch leaf (UTI)
Bitter orange peel (anorexia, dyspepsia)
Black cohosh root (PMS, dysmenorrhea, menopause)
Blackberry leaf (diarrhea)
Blackthorn berry (oropharyngeal inflammation)
Blessed thistle herb (anorexia, dyspepsia)
Boldo leaf (GI spasms, dyspepsia)
Buckthorn bark, berry (constipation)
Butcher's broom (venous insufficiency, hemorrhoids)
Calendula flower (oropharyngeal inflammations)
Camphor (hypotonic circulation, catarrh)
Caraway oil, seed (dyspepsia, bloating, fullness)
Cascara sagrada bark (constipation)
Chamomile, German flower (GI spasms and inflammation)
Chaste tree fruit (PMS, menstrual irregularities, mastodynia)
Cinnamon bark (anorexia, dyspepsia, GI spasms, bloating, fullness, flatulence)
Cloves (oral inflammation, dental anesthetic)
Cola nut (fatigue)
Coltsfoot leaf (cough, hoarseness, catarrh)
Comfrey herb, leaf, root (externally: bruises, strains, sprains)
Coriander seed (anorexia, dyspepsia)
Couch grass (UTI)
Dandelion herb (anorexia, dyspepsia, bloating, fullness)
Devil's claw root (anorexia, dyspepsia, locomotor disorders)
Dill seed (dyspepsia)
Echinacea herb (colds, flu, chronic respiratory infection, UTI)
Elder flower (colds)
Ephedra (respiratory diseases)
Eucalyptus leaf, oil (catarrh)
Fennel oil, seed (peptic discomfort, catarrh)
Fenugreek seed (anorexia)
Fir needle oil, shoots (catarrh)
Flaxseed (constipation, irritable colon, gastritis, enteritis, diverticulitis, age-related vascular changes)
Gentian root (digestive disorders)
Ginger root (dyspepsia, motion sickness)
Gingko biloba leaf extract (organic brain syndrome, vertigo, tinnitus, peripheral arterial occlusive disease)
Ginseng root (fatigue, declining work capacity)
Goldenrod (lower UTI)

continued

TABLE 10–4 Examples of Herbs (Un)Approved by the German Commission E continued

Approved Herbs continued
( ) = approved uses

Haronga bark, leaf (dyspepsia, pancreatic insufficiency)
Hawthorn leaf, flower (decreased cardiac output)
Henban leaf (GI spasms)
Hops (mood and sleep disturbances, anxiety)
Horehound herb (anorexia, dyspepsia, bloating, flatulence)
Horsechestnut seed (venous insufficiency)
Horseradish (catarrh, UTI)
Horsetail (edema, lower urinary inflammation)
Iceland moss (anorexia, oropharyngeal irritation)
Indian snakeroot (mild hypertension)
Ivy leaf (catarrh)
Jambolan bark (acute diarrhea)
Java tea (lower urinary inflammation)
Juniper berry (dyspepsia)
Kava kava (anxiety, stress)
Kidney bean pod (urinary difficulty)
Lady's mantle (diarrhea)
Lavender flower (mood disturbances, insomnia)
Lemon balm (nervous sleep disorder, GI complaints)
Licorice root (catarrh, ulcers)
Lily of the valley herb (mild cardiac insufficiency)
Linden flower (colds, cough)
Lovage root (lower urinary inflammation)
Mallow flower, leaf (dry, irritating cough)
Manna (constipation)
Marshmallow leaf, root (GI mucosal irritation)
Maté (mental, physical fatigue)
Meadowsweet (colds)
Milk thistle fruit (dyspepsia, liver damage)
Mint oil (flatulence, GI and gallbladder disorders, catarrh)
Mistletoe herb (joint inflammation and degeneration, malignant tumors)
Motherwort herb (nervous cardiac disorders, hyperthyroid)
Mullein flower (catarrh)
Mustard, white seed (external: respiratory and degenerative diseases)
Myrrh (oropharyngeal inflammation)
Niaouli oil (catarrh)
Nettle, stinging, leaf (kidney stones, rheumatic ailments, lower urinary inflammation)
Nettle, stinging, root (urinary difficulty caused by BPH)
Nettle, white dead, flower (catarrh)
Nightshade, woody, stem (eczema)
Oak bark (diarrhea;; oropharyngeal, genital, anal inflammation)
Oat straw (external: seborrhea, skin problems, itching)
Onion (anorexia, atherosclerosis)
Orange peel (anorexia)
Paprika, cayenne (external: muscle spasms)
Parsley herb, root (flushing of urinary tract)
Passion flower herb (nervous restlessness)
Peppermint leaf, oil (spasms of GI, gallbladder, bile duct; irritable colon, catarrh, oral mucosal inflammation)
Peruvian balsam (external: wound healing)

continued

TABLE 10–4   Examples of Herbs (Un)Approved by the German Commission E continued

Approved Herbs continued
( ) = approved uses

Petasites root (urinary spasm, especially with stones)
Petentilla (dysmenorrhea, diarrhea, oropharyngeal inflammation)
Pine needle oil, sprouts (rheumatism, neuralgia, muscle pain, catarrh)
Pheasant's eye (mild heart impairment)
Pimpinella root (catarrh)
Plantain (catarrh)
Pollen (anorexia, feebleness)
Poplar bud (skin injuries, hemorrhoids)
Primrose flower, root (catarrh)
Psyllium seed (constipation, irritable bowel, hemorrhoids, anal fissures)
Pumpkin seed (bladder irritation, BPH micturation problems)
Radish (peptic disorders, catarrh)
Rhubarb root (constipation)
Rose flower (oropharyngeal mucosal inflammation)
Rosemary leaf (dyspepsia)
Sage leaf (dyspepsia, excessive perspiration)
Sandalwood (lower UTI)
Sandy everlasting (peptic discomfort)
Sanicle (catarrh)
Saw palmetto berry (urinary difficulty caused by BPH)
Scopolia root (spasms: GI, bile, urinary tract)
Scotch broom herb (cardiovascular disorders)
Senega snakeroot (catarrh)
Senna leaf, pod (constipation)
Shepherd's purse (menorrhagia, metrogghagia)
Soapwort root (catarrh)
Soy lecithin, phospholipid (hypercholesterolemia)
Spiny restharrow root (lower urinary inflammation, kidney stone prevention)
Squill (mild heart insufficiency, diminished kidney capacity)
St. John's wort (depression, anxiety, nervous unrest)
Star anise seed (catarrh, peptic discomfort)
Sundew (cough)
Sweet clover (chronic venous insufficiency)
Thyme (bronchitis, whooping cough, catarrh)
Tolu balsam (catarrh)
Tormentil root (diarrhea, oropharyngeal inflammation)
Tumeric root (dyspepsia)
Turpentine (purified) oil (chronic respiratory distress, rheumatism, neuralgia)
Uva ursi leaf (urinary inflammation)
Uzara root (diarrhea)
Valerian root (restlessness, sleep disorders)
Walnut leaf (external: skin inflammations, perspiration)
Watercress (catarrh)
Witch hazel leaf, bark (external: skin and mucous injury and irritation, hemorrhoids, vericose
    veins)
Wormwood (anorexia, dyspepsia, biliary dyskinesia)
Yarrow (anorexia, dyspepsia, GI spasms)
Yeast, brewer's (anorexia, chronic acne, furunculosis)

continued

TABLE 10–4 Examples of Herbs (Un)Approved by the German Commission E continued

Unapproved Herbs continued
( ) = problems associated with herb

Angelica herb, seed (photosensitivity)
Ash bark, leaf (lack of efficacy)
Asparagus herb (lack of efficacy)
Barberry (lack of efficacy)
Basil herb (mutagenesis)
Bilberry leaf (intoxication with high or chronic doses)
Bishop's weed fruit (allergy, photosensitivity)
Bitter orange flower (lack of efficacy)
Blackberry root (lack of efficacy)
Blackthorn flower (lack of efficacy)
Bladder wrack (hyperthyroidism)
Borage (numerous risks)
Buchu (lack of efficacy)
Burdock root (lack of efficacy)
Calendula herb (lack of efficacy)
Cat's foot flower (lack of efficacy)
Celery (allergy, lack of efficacy)
Chamomile, Roman (allergy)
Chestnut leaf (lack of efficacy)
Cinnamon flower (allergy)
Citronella oil (toxic alveolitis)
Cocoa (allergy, migraines)
Coltsfoot (hepatotoxicity)
Damiana leaf, herb (lack of efficacy)
Delphinium flower (cardiovascular and respiratory problems)
Dill weed (lack of efficacy)
Elecampane root (contact dermatitis, mucosal irritation)
Ergot (numerous problems cited)
Eyebright (lack of efficacy)
Figs (lack of efficacy)
Gingko biloba leaf (lack of efficacy)
Goat's rue herb (hypoglycemic effects)
Hawthorn berry, flower, leaf (lack of efficacy)
Hibiscus (lack of efficacy)
Hollyhock (lack of efficacy)
Horse chestnut leaf (lack of efficacy)
Hyssop (lack of efficacy)
Jimsonweed leaf, seed (anticholinergic poisoning, lack of efficacy)
Kelp (hyperthyroidism)
Lady's mantle, alpine, herb (lack of efficacy)
Lemongrass oil (toxic alveolitis)
Linden leaf, wood, charcoal (lack of efficacy)
Linden, silver, flower (lack of efficacy)
Liverwort herb (skin, mucous irritation)
Marjoram (risks unclear, potential hazards)
Marsh tea (toxicity)
Milk thistle herb (lack of efficacy)
Monkshood (various risks)
Mugwort (abortifacient)
Muira puama (lack of efficacy)

continued

TABLE 10–4   Examples of Herbs (Un)Approved by the German Commission E continued

Unapproved Herbs continued
( ) = problems associated with herb

Nutmeg (psychoactive, abortifacient)
Nux vomica (CNS action of strychnine)
Oat herb (lack of efficacy)
Oats (allergy, lack of efficacy)
Oleander leaf (poisoning)
Olive leaf, oil (lack of efficacy)
Oregano (lack of efficacy)
Papain (clotting disorders)
Paprika species low in cayenne (allergy, lack of efficacy)
Parsley seed (vascular congestion; smooth muscle contraction, e.g., bladder, GI, uterus)
Pasque (Pulsatilla) flower (skin, mucosa irritation)
Peony flower, root (lack of efficacy)
Periwinkle (immune suppression)
Raspberry leaf (lack of efficacy)
Rhododendron, rusty-leaved (poisoning)
Rose hip, seed (lack of efficacy)
Rue (phototoxicity, mutagenesis, liver and kidney damage)
Sandalwood, red (lack of efficacy)
Sarsaparilla root (gastric irritation, kidney impairment)
Scotch broom flower (contraindicated in MAOI therapy and hypertension)
Senecio herb (hepatotoxicity)
Soapwort, red, herb (mucous membrane irritation)
Spinach leaf (lack of efficacy)
Strawberry leaf (lack of efficacy)
Sweet woodruff (lack of efficacy)
Tansy flower, herb (poisoning)
Unsea (oropharyngeal inflammation)
Verbena herb (lack of efficacy)
Walnut hull (mutagenesis)
Yohimbe bark (nervousness, tremor, insomnia, anxiety, hypertension, tachycardia, nausea, vomiting)

GI = gastrointestinal, UTI = urinary tract infection, PMS = premenstrual syndrome, BPH = benign prostatic hyperplasia, MAOI = monoamine oxidase inhibitor.

Source: The Complete German Commission E Monographs—Therapeutic Guide to Herbal Medicines. Integrative Medicine Communications, Boston, 1998, with permission.

many of which lacked credibility and were written by authors with no expertise.[55] Nowhere else in the world does there exist such potential for misuse, abuse, and fraud as regards the sale of health-care products for profits. So, the desire for herbal alternatives must be balanced with appropriate regulations to protect the public from disreputable manufacturers and promoters.

The view of naive self-help books, uninformed consumers and legislators, and a great many self-serving health product promoters is that the U.S. drug approval process is slow, cumbersome, and pointless. It is even suggested that the Food and Drug Administration (FDA) callously prevents the availability of "valuable" and even "miracle" products. Yet the FDA is a consumer protection agency. U.S. drug laws require that all drugs marketed in this country must be proven to be safe and effective for their promoted uses. Consider, for example, that there were an estimated 600 to 700 plant species available in herbal products in the United States in 1990—yet only 100 of these plants appear to have medical or economic merit.[56]

In the early 1970s, the FDA began an extensive review of nonprescription drug products. This review eliminated many unsafe or ineffective ingredients, allowed some prescription drugs to be sold without a prescription, and resulted in greater quality control of self-care products. It is a process that continues today. This review process initially regarded all OTC ingredients in use at the time as "old" drugs. As such, they were treated more leniently than "new" ingredients, which require extensive and expensive clinical trials to demonstrate safety and effectiveness. The FDA only considered U.S. ingredients to be eligible for "old" drug status. This excluded most herbals, which were being used primarily in European countries as self-care products. In response, a group of European and American companies filed a petition with the FDA through the European-American Phytomedicines Coalition to include "old" drugs from Europe and to establish an expert panel for their review. The rationale for this petition was based on European experience with herbal products. To date, the FDA has not responded to this petition. In the interim, the FDA has taken the position that herbals consumed primarily for their taste, aroma, or nutritional value may be sold as foods. If they are promoted for medicinal effects, they are drugs—and therefore must be tested as drugs. Without a mechanism for these products to be reviewed as "old" drugs, they would have to undergo the time-consuming and expensive clinical trials required of all "new" drugs.[57,58]

The increasing popularity of herbals has not escaped the attention of U. S officials. Literally millions of letters, faxes, and phone calls from Americans in support of legislation to increase access to herbal products resulted in the creation of the Dietary Supplement and Education Act of 1994, which currently allows labels of herbal products to communicate potential safety problems, side effects, special warnings, and contraindications that are appropriate for some users. Labels can also make statements about how the product can affect the structure and function of the human body (i.e., statements of nutritional support). However, labeling cannot make claims that the product is useful for the diagnosis, treatment, cure, or prevention of disease (i.e., labels cannot promote herbal for a "drug" purpose). The Nutrition Labeling and Education Act of 1990 (NLEA) allows for statements on the labels of food or nutrient products that describe the relationship between the nutrient(s) involved and specific diseases or health-related conditions. However, the NLEA guidelines do not apply to herbal products.[59] Thus herbal products seem to be suspended between the domains of traditional food versus drug products.

Even though labels cannot promote the use of an herbal as a drug, this does not prevent disreputable promoters and authors from making outrageous claims in the form of books, pamphlets, or other literature, which are often placed next to herbal products in retail settings.[60] Because of their deceptive promotional practices, it has been relatively easy to dupe the public into believing that herbs represent a veritable smorgasbord of magical, mystical, but absolutely harmless healing substances that have been ignored by traditional medicine because they pose a significant threat to professional profits.

Herbal advocates insist that feasible models for regulatory reform exist in European countries, where phytomedicines have been accepted and integrated into traditional medical practices (e.g., Commission E). Yet because of sociocultural differences, the regulatory guidelines of other countries may not function in the same way in our culture.

Back to Nature in the United States

Although Americans may fail to exercise wisdom in their fads, their enthusiasm is never lacking. In the last quarter of the 20th century, the marvel and mystery of the plant have been rediscovered as if for the first time. Much of this trend can be traced to a growing dissatisfaction with modern medicine or to the enticements of "natural" products. This "green revolution" has achieved incredible popularity, and there appears to be no limit to the number and variety of herbal products that will crowd retail shelves in the foreseeable future. The total amount of herbs sold in mass-market outlets (grocery stores, pharmacies, mass merchandiser retail stores) increased by 79.5 percent between 1996 and 1997. This amount is still increasing, with the result that these products represent a significant and growing component of U.S. health care and economics.[61-63]

Even though these products are not labeled as drugs, consumers use them for the treatment and cure of health problems, to prevent disease, and as proactive agents to maintain health and wellness. Additionally, they are often added to conventional therapies. Some health insurance companies cover herbs as "alternative therapies," and herb products are being considered for use by some managed care organizations.

The Role of Health Professionals

The health-care professions seek to provide safe, effective, appropriate, and necessary care for the sick.[64] Unfortunately, cultural changes, increasing health-care costs, and advances in medical technology during the 20th century have tended to create a rift between physicians and patients, with the result that many Americans are seeking alternatives to traditional medicine.[65,66]

As herbal use by the public increases, it is important for health-care professionals to better understand these products (e.g., their botany, chemistry, pharmacology) and their use in popular self-care practices.[67] Not all herbs are safe and effective. Herbals, like all medicinals, must be used in proper doses, in appropriate formulations, and for appropriate lengths of time in order for their benefits to occur. It is important to know which conditions can be treated with self-care practices and which ones require professional medical care. For example, herbals are rarely effective for use in emergencies or acute care situations.[68,69] Consumers need advice about the rational use of all health-care products.[70] Table 10–5 lists representative references that are considered to be reputable resources for herbal therapeutics.

Professional responsibilities regarding herbals extend beyond merely understanding what is now known about natural products. (See Table 10–6.) Additional research is absolutely essential to better understand these products and their legitimate role in contemporary health care and to identify new drug products. Finally, regulations are needed to ensure that herbal products are prepared in accordance with safe manufacturing practices and that labeling and product information are accurate.

The Future of Herbals

The contribution of plants to human well-being and medicine is beyond question. Unfortunately, neither is the tendency of humans to "soil their own nest" by the selfish and greedy exploitation of natural resources. Rain forests, whose natural resources are largely undiscovered, are being destroyed at an alarming rate. Finding these resources has become a race against time. It is clear that Americans will opt for herbal alternatives more and more as problems with traditional medicine and third-party payers continue to plague our culture. Therefore these products merit appropriate investigation in order to avoid therapeutic misadventures and economic fraud—and also because many may offer valid therapeutic alternatives.

Herbals are here to stay. Ironically, they are actually far more traditional as medications than the processed tablets and capsules that we commonly refer to as "traditional." In coming years, their use will inevitably increase. The accountability demanded from the manufacturers and promoters of these products should be no different from that de-

TABLE 10–5   Examples of Reputable Herbal References for Health-Care Professionals

Complete German Commission E Monographs, The—Therapeutic Guide to Herbal Medicines. Integrative Medicine Communications, Boston, 1998.

DerMarderosian, A (ed): The Review of Natural Products. Facts and Comparisons, St. Louis, 1999.

Leung, AY, and Foster, S: Encyclopedia of Common Natural Ingredients, ed. 2. John Wiley & Sons, New York, 1996.

McGuffin, M (ed): Botanical Safety Handbook. CRC Press, Boston, 1997.

Newall, CA, Anderson, LA, and Phillipson, J D: Herbal Medicines—A Guide for Health Care Professionals. Pharmaceutical Press, London, 1996.

PDR for Hebal Medicines. Medical Economics, Montvale, N.J., 1998.

Robbers, JE, Speedie, MK, and Tyler, VE: Pharmacognosy and Pharmacobiotechnology. Williams & Wilkins, Baltimore, 1996.

Robbers, JE, and Tyler, VE: Tyler's Herbs of Choice—The Therapeutic Use of Phytomedicinals. Haworth Press, New York, 1999.

Schulz, V, Hansel, R, and Tyler, V: Rational Phytotherapy. Springer-Verlag, Berlin, 1998.

Tyler, VE: The Honest Herbal. Pharmaceutical Products Press, New York, 1993.

TABLE 10–6   Summary of Responsibilities of Health Professionals Regarding Herbals

- Increase knowledge of herbs:
  - administration
  - adverse effects
  - contraindications
  - dosage
  - duration of therapy
  - efficacy
  - interactions (drugs, foods)
  - mechanism of actions
  - risks, warnings, precautions
  - safety
- Prevent destruction of natural resources
- Promote quality assurance practices and regulations
- Promote research

manded from other medical products. And health professionals should commit themselves to an understanding of these products, just as they do for other health-care products and practices.

Because human beings prefer simple answers for complex problems, it is far more desirable to classify herbs either as "miraculous" or "worthless." Yet, in reality, they are neither. Their merit, as is the case with all health-care products, is absolutely dependent on rational use. For health-care professionals, this demands an objective exploration of their merits and limitations.

The psychologist–philosopher Abraham Maslow once said, "When the only tool you have is a hammer . . . you tend to treat everything as if it were a nail." To refuse to better understand these products or to ignore their potential merits deprives us of potential medical "tools." At the very least, a continued avoidance of these products only serves to further alienate health-care providers from a public that is increasingly committed to their use.

REFERENCES

1. Lust, J: The Herb Book. Bantam Books, New York, 1974.
2. Dawson, AG: Using herbs wisely. In Albright, P, and Albright, B (eds): Body, Mind and Spirit. Stephen Greene Press, Brattleboro, Vt., 1980.
3. Ibid.
4. Dubos, R: Mirage of Health. Harper Torchbooks, New York, 1959.
5. Holt, GA, et al: Extend Your Lifespan. Mancorp Publishing, Tampa, Fla., 1997.
6. Lust: The Herb Book.
7. Ibid.
8. Meyer, C: American Folk Medicine. Meyerbooks, Glenwood, Ill., 1973.
9. Hastings, A, Fadiman, J, and Gordon, J (eds): Health for the Whole Person. Westview Press, Boulder, 1980.
10. Meyer: American Folk Medicine.
11. Starr, P: The Social Transformation of American Medicine. Basic Books, New York, 1982.
12. Holt et al: Extend Your Lifespan.
13. Lust: The Herb Book.
14. Meyer: American Folk Medicine.
15. Starr: The Social Transformation of American Medicine.
16. Ibid.
17. Ibid.
18. Hastings, Fadiman, and Gordon: Health for the Whole Person.
19. Lust: The Herb Book.
20. Stetter, C: The Secret Medicines of the Pharaohs—Ancient Egyptian Healing. Quintessence Publishing, Chicago, 1993.
21. Robbers, JE, Speedie, MK, and Tyler, VE: Pharmacognosy and Pharmacobiotechnology. Williams & Wilkins, Baltimore, 1996.
22. Lust: The Herb Book.
23. Robbers, Speedie, and Tyler: Pharmacognosy and Pharmacobiotechnology.
24. Schulz, V, Hansel, R, and Tyler, V: Rational Phytotherapy. Springer-Verlag, Berlin, 1998.
25. Starr: The Social Transformation of American Medicine.
26. Schulz, Hansel, and Tyler: Rational Phytotherapy.
27. Starr, P: The Social Transformation of American Medicine.
28. Holt et al: Extend Your Lifespan.
29. Gilman, AG, et al (eds): Goodman and Gilman's The Pharmacological Basis of Therapeutics. Pergamon Press, New York, 1990.
30. Robbers, Speedie, and Tyler: Pharmacognosy and Pharmacobiotechnology.
31. Ibid.
32. Schulz, Hansel, and Tyler: Rational Phytotherapy.
33. Robbers, Speedie, and Tyler: Pharmacognosy and Pharmacobiotechnology.
34. Schulz, Hansel, and Tyler: Rational Phytotherapy.

35. Health Care Practices and Perceptions—A Consumer Survey of Self-Medication. Prepared for the Nonprescription Drug Manufacturers Association by the Harry Heller Research Corp. (HHR #72792), Washington, D.C., 1984.

36. Holt, GA., Beck, D, and Williams, MM: Interview Analysis Regarding Health Status, Health Needs and Health Care Utilization of Ambulatory Elderly. Unpublished study sponsored by Warner Lambert and the National Council on Aging. College of Pharmacy, University of Wyoming, Laramie, 1991.

37. Maiman, LA, Becker, MH, and Katlic, AW: How mothers treat their children's physical symptoms. Journal of Community Health 10(3): 1985.

38. Much geriatric drug use is inappropriate. American Druggist, August. 1991.

39. Wolinsky, FD: The Sociology of Health: Principles, Professions and Issues. Little, Brown, Boston, 1980.

40. Esmay, JB, and Wertheirmer, AI: A review of over-the-counter drug therapy. Journal of Community Health 5(1):54–66, 1979.

41. Gossel, TA, and Wuest, JR: Over-the-counter: The trend to self-medication. U.S. Pharmacist, September 1981, p 14.

42. Young, FE (ed): A Theme in Three Parts: Science, Society, the Economy. Self-Care, Self-Medication in America's Future—A Symposium. The Nonprescription Drug Manufacturers Association in cooperation with the FDA, Washington, D.C., 1988.

43. Lust: The Herb Book.

44. Robbers, Speedie, and Tyler: Pharmacognosy and Pharmacobiotechnology.

45. The Complete German Commission E Monographs—Therapeutic Guide to Herbal Medicines. Integrative Medicine Communications, Boston, 1998.

46. Meyer: American Folk Medicine.

47. Otto, HA, and Knight, JW (eds): Dimensions in Wholistic Healing. Nelson-Hall, Chicago, 1979.

48. Hastings, Fadiman, and Gordon: Health for the Whole Person.

49. Fink, JL, Vivian, JC, and Cacciatore, GG (eds): Pharmacy Law Digest. Facts and Comparisons, St. Louis, 1998.

50. The Complete German Commission E Monographs.

51. Ibid.

52. Robbers, JE, and Tyler, VE: Tyler's Herbs of Choice—The Therapeutic Use of Phytomedicinals. Haworth Press, New York, 1999.

53. The Complete German Commission E Monographs.

54. Robbers and Tyler: Tyler's Herbs of Choice.

55. Holt: Extend Your Lifespan.

56. The Complete German Commission E Monographs.

57. Ibid.

58. Holt, Gary: Extend Your Lifespan.

59. The Complete German Commission E Monographs.

60. Tyler, VE: The Honest Herbal. Pharmaceutical Products Press, New York, 1993.

61. The Complete German Commission E Monographs.

62. Robbers, Speedie, and Tyler: Pharmacognosy and Pharmacobiotechnology.

63. Schulz, Hansel, and Tyler: Rational Phytotherapy.

64. Ibid.

65. Ibid.

66. Wolinsky: The Sociology of Health.

67. Tyler: The Honest Herbal.

68. Schulz, Hansel, and Tyler: Rational Phytotherapy.

69. Robbers and Tyler: Tyler's Herbs of Choice.

70. Newall, CA, Anderson, LA, and Phillipson, JD: Herbal Medicines—A Guide for Health Care. The Pharmaceutical Press, London, 1996.

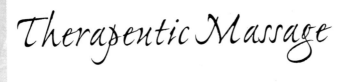

CHAPTER 11

Therapeutic Massage

Valerie Vaughan

Valerie Vaughan, BA, MLS, MST, is cofounder and former instructor at the Stillpoint Center School of Massage, Amherst, Massachusetts.

Massage is one of the oldest known forms of healing. Throughout the world, diverse cultures have developed traditional practices of massage, and there are numerous references to it in the medical literature from ancient Egypt, Persia, Greece, and Rome. Hippocrates, the "father of Western medicine," advocated the therapeutic use of massage. In medieval and renaissance Europe, it was practiced as an important part of folk medicine, although practitioners were often persecuted by the Church. Research shows that Chinese acupressure massage dates back thousands of years, and it continues to be a valued tradition in Oriental medicine today.

In the early 19th century, the modern Western practice of Swedish massage was systematized by Per Heinrik Ling, and some American physicians began to use massage in their treatment programs. In the late 19th century, massage came under the critical eye of the scientific community, scandals erupted over "massage parlors," and there was widespread questioning of massage as a legitimate medical practice. Even though massage was practiced in some hospitals, a wide gap between established medicine and massage was created by advances in surgery and drug therapy as well as differences in terminology.

During the 20th century, many attempts were made to discover the scientific basis of massage through controlled clinical tests, and practitioners began to organize professional groups. In the 1960s and 1970s, the human potential movement fostered a revived interest in massage, and several non-Western practices were introduced and popularized in the United States. During the 1980s and 1990s, therapeutic massage gained respect, professional status, and popularity, and it is now included in many insurance plans. According to a 1997 survey, Americans spend about $3 billion annually on 75 million visits to massage therapists—a quarter of the total spent on alternative health care every year.

How Massage Works

In order to understand how massage affects the body as a whole, some of the physiological effects need to be examined. Massage is known to increase the circulation of the blood and the flow of lymph. The direct mechanical effect of rhythmically applied manual pressure and movement in massage can increase the rate of blood flow, and the stimulation of nerve

161

receptors causes the blood vessels to dilate (by reflex action), which also facilitates blood flow. Lymphatic fluid, which carries impurities and waste away from tissues, does not circulate like blood but depends on muscle contractions for movement. When people are inactive because of injury or illness, their lymphatic system is not stimulated to flow, but massage can aid in this process. (See Fig. 11–1.) The basis for the physiological effectiveness of massage is simple. Massage employs mechanical methods, which directly affect the soft muscle tissue or move bodily fluids, and reflexive methods, which stimulate the nervous system, chemical system, and endocrine system. The manual techniques are specific according to mode of application (pressing, rubbing, pulling) and speed or depth of pressure (sustained, staccato, light touch, deep tissue), and these have been tested in studies that validate the effects of massage.

Increases in the blood and lymph circulation are the most widely recognized physiological effects of massage therapy. Compression of tissue increases capillary blood flow and stimulates the release of vasodilators; the increase in blood flow has a bodywide effect. Both mechanical and reflexive styles also influence the subtle energy levels of the body, but these energy effects are more difficult to measure and validate with current scientific research and evaluative methods.[1]

There is a fair amount of research into the effects of massage on blood flow and composition, connective tissue, muscle, and the nervous system.[2] Research has shown that the oxygen capacity of the blood can increase between 10 and 15 percent after massage. Massage is also known to affect muscles throughout the body, helping to loosen contracted, shortened muscles and stimulating weak, flaccid muscles. Such muscle balanc-

FIGURE 11-1   Massage Client in Sitting Position, Clothed

Massage helps to loosen contracted, shortened muscles and stimulates weak, flaccid muscles.

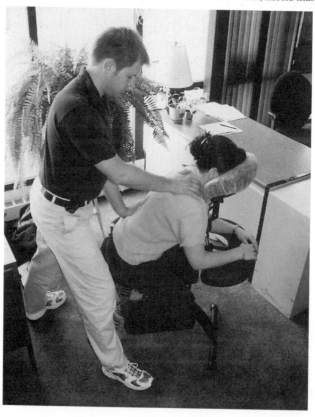

FIGURE 11-2   Massage Client in Reclining Position, Unclothed and Draped

Massage can speed recovery from the fatigue that occurs after exercise.

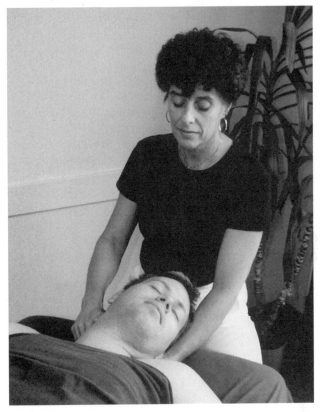

ing can assist with posture and promote more efficient movement. Massage can also speed recovery from the fatigue that occurs after exercise. (See Fig. 11–2.)

Another effect of massage is to increase the body's secretions and excretions. There is a proven increase in the production of gastric juices, saliva, and urine, as well as increased excretion of nitrogen, inorganic phosphorus, and sodium chloride. This suggests that the metabolic rate increases with massage, improving the utilization of absorbed material by the body's cells. Massage also affects the internal organs. By directly or indirectly stimulating nerves that supply internal organs, blood vessels of these organs dilate and allow greater blood supply to them. Massage affects peristaltic action and aids elimination. Manipulation of the skin and subcutaneous tissues can have a beneficial effect on tissues remote from the area of treatment. These effects appear to be mediated by neural reflexes that cause an increase in blood flow.[3]

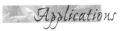

Applications

Massage is indicated for musculoskeletal discomfort, circulation enhancement, relaxation, stress reduction, and conditions for which analgesics, anti-inflammatories, and muscle relaxants are prescribed. Massage therapy has been used successfully to treat a variety of pathological conditions, including spinal deformities (lordosis, kyphosis, and scoliosis), brachial neuralgia, tendinitis, chondromalacia patellae, bursitis, sciatica, and temporomandibular joint (TMJ) syndrome.[4]

Massage can play an important role in the preparation for and recovery from exercise. Athletes can benefit from sports massage during training, during warm-up, and following competitive events.[5] Massage is often helpful for the patient with repetitive strain injury, such as carpal tunnel syndrome, trigger finger, shoulder impingement, tennis elbow, thoracic outlet syndrome, and myofascial pain disorders.[6]

Pregnant women experience physical and emotional changes that can be greatly assisted by massage therapy, and some massage techniques are particularly appropriate for labor and birth.[7] Pregnancy conditions relieved by massage are leg edema, backache, intestinal gas, leg cramps, and constipation.

Women who have undergone cosmetic breast surgery frequently experience over-stretching of the pectoralis groups by placement of the implants under the muscle. Because of the interconnection of the anterior and posterior muscle groups, pain is experienced in the midthoracic and lumbar regions as the muscle strives for the appropriate balance.[8] Hypertrophic scar formation can be reduced by gentle and frequent massage of the scar tissue, thus avoiding the disruption of the normal breast contour.[9]

Lymphedema can result from surgical interventions as well as pathological states.[10] Postmastectomy or pelvic surgeries often remove or damage nodes of the lymphatic system, leaving the area without adequate drainage.[11] Light massage can relieve the edema and resulting pain and limited motion of this condition.[12] The effects of the massage can be enhanced by gravitational assistance in positioning during the massage.

Methods of Massage

There is a core body of knowledge that all massage therapists use, but there is also a wide variety of applications. Many of these methods are named for their founders, such as Rolfing and the Rosen Method, and some are named for the key concept embodied by the style, such as Cranial-Sacral Therapy and Reflexology. Because massage is a universal form of healing and has developed in diverse areas of the world, some methods have indigenous names or are referred to by their place of origin, such as Swedish massage, shiatsu, and Do-In. Discussed here are the approaches that are most familiar to practitioners in the United States.

Swedish Massage

The most well-known bodywork method practiced today is Swedish massage, so called because of its Swedish founder, Per Heinrik Ling. Its techniques form the foundation for many other contemporary massage practices. Swedish massage works primarily to induce general relaxation while improving circulation, the functioning of the lymphatic system, flushing of wastes such as lactic acid, and restoring flexibility and range of motion. The five basic strokes are effleurage (touching lightly, a gliding stroke), petrissage (kneading), tapotement (tapping), vibration (shaking), and friction (rubbing).

Effleurage is a light, gliding stroke that focuses the pressure horizontally in the direction of the muscle fibers. Petrissage (kneading) applies a vertical lift to the muscle tissue as the pressure is applied to the muscle body. Tapotement (tapping, cupping) is application of a downward vertical pressure with an abrupt release. The technique of vibration (shaking) focuses the pressure down, then back and forth in place. Friction (rubbing) applies the pressure transverse or cross-fiber to the normal lay of the tissue.

Sports Massage

Sports massage is a specialized form of Swedish massage that assists the body in achieving maximum physical results. Athletes, performing artists (dancers, violinists, actors, etc.), construction workers, and others whose occupations require physical exertion can benefit from this type of massage. As with Swedish massage, pressure and movement are the basic ingredients of sports massage. Other techniques, such as cross–fiber massage, are also used, and the style is often vigorous and swift, concentrating on the muscles that are pertinent to the athlete's particular sport. Muscles that are constantly used "learn" a state of continual contraction, which makes them less efficient as well as exhausted and susceptible to injury.[13] Sports massage aims to loosen and warm up muscles prior to athletic events and to relax muscles and relieve soreness and stiffness between workouts. It is also designed to relieve the typical problems encountered by the athlete, such as "pulled muscles," sprains, and bruises. Many professional sports teams employ massage therapists.

Myofascial Release

Myofascial release seeks to restore balance to the body by releasing tension in the soft connective tissues known as fasciae. This technique is different from Swedish massage and sports massage, which focus on the muscle rather than on the fasciae and attachments. Because of their various layers and characteristic interweaving of tissue fibers, fasciae are dense and lack elasticity. This allows movement of the fasciae in all directions and support for the connecting muscle as well.

Fasciae can become constricted due to trauma such as illness and physical stress. When the fasciae are tight, they can pull muscles and bones out of place, resulting in pain and lack of mobility. Myofascial release uses trigger point release, strumming, and generalized as well as specific muscle stretching techniques to remove this tightness. This is a modality that requires careful work by the therapist because the pressure and stretching are performed at the edge of the client's tolerance. Practitioners believe that myofascial release produces wider, more long-lasting effects than muscle massage because fasciae surround, support, and interweave every muscle, organ, and bone in the body.[14]

Shiatsu Massage

There is a long tradition of massage methods in Asia. This category of healing bodywork encompasses practices originating in China, India, Japan, Korea, and Thailand. In general, these methods are philosophically based on the vital life-force energy that practitioners believe invigorates the human body. If this energy is disturbed, an imbalance occurs that results in ill health or disease.

Through physical manipulation, the different Asian methods attempt to balance the flow of this force, which is variously called *chi*, *ki*, or *prana*. Most of these systems are offshoots of traditional Chinese medicine.

Shiatsu, which means "finger pressure," was developed in Japan but traces its origins to a form of traditional Chinese medicine that is several thousand years old. Pressure is applied to specific points throughout the body that lie along channels of energy called "meridians." The meridians are closely associated with the blood pathways of the body and are named after the major organ through which they course (e.g., gallbladder, spleen, kidney). There are 7,000 to 12,000 points along the meridians, depending on the system of identification that is used.[15]

The pressure points are thought to be areas of chi concentration and are the same places where needles are inserted in the Eastern practice of acupuncture. Shiatsu is intended to open the flow of chi and support the natural healing of the body. As with other modalities, it is valuable for reintegrating the body, mind, and spirit, and assisting with both specific symptoms and the general energy level of the body. Feelings of deep relaxation and increased vitality are common benefits of a shiatsu treatment.[16]

Reflexology

Reflexology is the technique of massage that promotes unblocking of a terminal nerve reflex in order to improve functions associated with that particular reflex pathway. In this modality, the feet and hands, which contain accessible nerve endings, are the focus of bodywork. Reflexology uses strokes such as kneading, compression, and tissue rolling. This therapy is based on the work of William Fitzgerald at St. Francis Hospital in Connecticut. Fitzgerald found that by massaging the terminal point of the nerve reflex, the corresponding body parts are affected, possibly through the extensive interconnection of these nerve endings with the spinal cord and brain.[17] Fitzgerald's work was furthered by Eunice Ingram, who developed the present "map" of the body parts (including organs) on the feet and hands.

Ingram proposed that the body is represented on the foot, with the toes corresponding to the head, the balls of the feet to the shoulders and thoracic area, and the heels to the pelvic area and legs. The feet are a natural focus for healing, being one of the most innervated and complex surface areas of the body, with 7000 nerve endings, 33 joints, 19 muscles, 107 ligaments, and 26 bones in each foot. There also appears to be some relationship between the reflex zones and the acupressure meridians. Research has shown that manipulating the reflex zones stimulates the same energy balancing that occurs using acupuncture points.[18] Reflexology has been used successfully to treat premenstrual syndrome (PMS), hypertension, anxiety, and pain.

Research

Massage can assist in relieving the physical and emotional growing pains experienced by infants, children, and adolescents. Studies in medicine, animal behavior, and anthropology have shown that nurturing touch is essential for life. Tests have proved that baby animals and humans grow faster and develop greater immunity to disease when they are raised with touch-contact.[19] One study showed that premature infants who were massaged regularly gained almost 50 percent more body weight than unmassaged infants,[20] and another study showed that massaged infants were hospitalized for 6 fewer days than their unmassaged counterparts, maintained their weight advantage long after discharge, and exhibited greater motor and mental skills.[21]

Massage therapy has also been found effective for infants who have been exposed to cocaine or HIV, as well as those with depressed mothers. Massage has been shown to result in lower anxiety and improved clinical course for children with a variety of conditions, including asthma, autism, diabetes, bulimia, rheumatoid arthritis, and psychiatric problems.[22] Massage is also one of the preferred initial treatments for pseudotumor of infancy and congenital muscular torticollis.[23]

The elderly have unique health disruptions that benefit from massage. Massage can provide relief for problems created by the aging process, such as decreased muscle tone, osteoarthritis, and poor circulation. Massage has been proven to be a useful modality in the rehabilitation of the elderly patient with arthritis[24] and is moderately effective in the treatment of lymphedema, a rare complication of rheumatoid arthritis.[25] Massage can also address sleep disturbance, a common problem for the elderly patient hospitalized in a critical care unit.[26,27] Human touch can provide a tender balance to the harsh effects of technology. Therapeutic massage can improve the experience of critically ill patients in a high-technology environment, thus helping them cope with the impersonality and unfamiliarity of intensive care units.[28]

Chronic diseases and terminal illnesses are conditions for which massage can offer rehabilitation and comfort. Massage has been shown to be effective for the muscular pain of the terminally ill.[29] Chronically debilitating diseases that respond well to the short-term relief of massage include Parkinson's disease, multiple sclerosis, lupus, rheumatoid arthritis, fibromyalgia, AIDS, chronic fatigue syndrome, and disk problems resulting in back or neck pain. Therapeutic massage has also been shown to be a successful intervention that modifies anxiety and alleviates the perception of pain in hospitalized cancer patients.[30]

Additionally, it has proven useful in the treatment of neuropathic pain syndrome in cancer patients.[31]

Massage offers a therapeutic touch to those who have experienced physical, sexual, or emotional abuse, including children, and it is particularly beneficial for people with physical and mental disabilities, mood disorders, and those recovering from chemical or alcohol addiction.[32]

Massage has also proven effective when combined with other treatments. In the emergency treatment of heatstroke, the use of cold water immersion with skin massage is effective in rapidly lowering body temperature and in avoiding severe complications or death.[33]

The specific therapeutic effects of massage are often accompanied by pleasurable feelings of relaxation and well-being. Relaxation is promoted through the release of endorphins and enkephalins, neurochemicals that have been called "the body's natural opiates." The tactile and neurochemical effects of massage interrupt patterns of stress that are held in the body. They induce a state of deep rest from which the recipient can emerge feeling more balanced, relaxed, and energized.

Summary

The operative principle in effective massage is assisting the flow of sensory information to the mind. Practiced massage not only delivers sensory impressions but also can convey the possibility for wider experience, openness to a whole new way of sensing, and, ultimately, self-awareness. It helps us learn to assess our own condition more accurately, to identify habitual patterns, and to resolve stress. This heightened awareness leads in turn to greater health, for until we feel something more pleasurable, complete, and balanced, we cannot know or envision how to be more complete, balanced, and healthy. In this regard, massage is sensory education toward a positive attitude of self-healing.

Massage offers ways in which we can manage the results of disease and injury, slow down the process of degeneration, avoid pitfalls in the course of chronic illness, and make recoveries more complete. Therapeutic massage is helpful in any situation in which control over conditioned response and heightened self-awareness might be of constructive use.

RESOURCES

American Massage Therapy Association.
820 Davis St., Suite 100
Evanston IL, 60201-4444
www.amtmassage.org

Board of Massage Therapy
825 N. Capital St.
NE Room 2224
Washington, DC 20002
(202) 442-4764
www.dchealth.com

Massage Therapy Journal, published by American Massage Therapy Association

REFERENCES

1. Cawley, N: A critique of the methodology of research studies evaluating massage. European Journal of Cancer Care (English-language ed.) 6(1):23–31, 1997.

2. Goats, GC: Massage: The scientific basis of an ancient art. Physiological and therapeutic effects. British Journal of Sports Medicine 28(3):153–156, 1994.

3. Goats, GC: Connective tissue massage. British Journal of Sports Medicine 25(3):131–133, 1991.

4. Claire, T: Bodywork. William Morrow, New York, 1995, p 38.

5. Cafarelli, E: The role of massage in preparation for and recovery from exercise. Sports Medicine 14(1):1–9, 1992.

6. Sheon, RP: Repetitive strain injury: Diagnostic and treatment tips on six common problems. Postgraduate Medicine 102(4):72, 1997.

7. Stillerman, E: Mothermassage: A Handbook for Relieving the Discomfort of Pregnancy. Delacorte, New York, 1992.

8. Nettina, SM (ed): The Lippincott Manual of Nursing Practice, ed. 6. JB Lippincott, Philadelphia, 1996.

9. Field, DA: Cosmetic breast surgery. Am Fam Physician 45(2):711–719, 1992.

10. Bullock, B, and Henze, R: Focus on Pathophysiology. JB Lippincott, Phildelphia, 1999.

11. Ibid.

12. Nettina: The Lippincott Manual of Nursing Practice.

13. Cash, M: Sports and Remedial Massage Therapy. Edbury Press, London, 1996.

14. Barnes, J: Myofascial Release. Presented at the Myofascial Release Seminars, 1990.

15. Ellis, A, et al: Fundamentals of Chinese Acupuncture. Paradigm Publishing, Brookline, Mass., 1991.

16. Stevenson, C: The role of shiatsu in palliative care. Complementary Therapies in Nursing and Midwifery 1(2):51–58, 1995.

17. Klein, L. Reflexology: The healing art of "sole" searching. Massage 40:62, 1992.

18. Burton Goldberg Group (compiler): Alternative Medicine; the Definitive Guide. Future Medicine Publishing Co., Pullyallup, Wash., 1994.

19. Montagu, A: Touching: The Human Significance of the Skin. Harper & Row, New York, 1986, pp 23, 238–239.

20. Field, T: Tactile-kinesthetic stimulation effects on preterm neonates. Pediatrics 7:654–658, 1986.

21. Knaster, M: A new dimension in intensive care: Premature infants grow with massage. Massage Therapy Journal 30(3):50, 1991.

22. Field, T: Massage therapy for infants and children. Journal of Developmental & Behavioral Pediatrics 16(2):105–111, 1995.

23. Porter, SB: Pseudotumor of infancy and congenital muscular torticollis. American Family Physician 52(6):1731–1736, 1995.

24. Daly, MP: Rehabilitation of the elderly patient with arthritis. Clin Geriatr Med 9(4):783–801, 1993.

25. Joos, E: Lymphatic disorders in rheumatoid arthritis. Seminars in Arthritis and Rheumatism 22(6):392–398, 1993.

26. Richards, KC: Sleep promotion in the critical care unit. AACN Clinical Issues 5(2):152–158, 1994.

27. Richards, KC: Sleep promotion. Critical Care Nursing Clinics of North America 8(1):39–52, 1996.

28. Hill, CF: Is massage beneficial to critically ill patients in intensive care units? Intensive and Critical Care Nursing 9(2):116–121, 1993.

29. Urba, SG: Nonpharmacologic pain management in terminal care. Clin Geriatr Med 12(2):301–311, 1996.

30. Ferrell-Torry, AT: The use of therapeutic massage as a nursing intervention to modify anxiety and the perception of cancer pain. Cancer Nursing 16(2):93–101, 1993.

31. Martin, LA: Neuropathic pain in cancer patients. Journal of Pain and Symptom Management 14(2):99–117, 1997.

32. Hilliard, D: Massage for the seriously mentally ill. J Psychosoc Nurs Ment Health Serv 33(7):29–30, 1995.

33. Costrini, A: Emergency treatment of exertional heatstroke and comparison of whole body cooling techniques. Med Sci Sports Exerc 22(1):15–18, 1990.

RECOMMENDED READING

Chasnov, M: Healing Sports Injuries: A Hands-On Guide to Restorative Massage and Exercise. Fawcett Columbine, New York, 1988. [sports massage]

Chinese Massage Therapy: A Handbook of Therapeutic and Preventative Massage. Hartley & Marks, New York, 1987. [Oriental methods]

Fritz, S: Fundamentals of Therapeutic Massage. Mosby Lifeline, 1995.

Juhan, D: Job's Body: A Handbook for Bodywork. Station Hill Press, 1987.

Lawrence, DB: Massageworks: A Practical Encyclopedia of Massage Techniques. Putnam, New York, 1983.

Leboyer, F: Loving Hands: The Traditional Art of Baby Massage. Newmarket, 1997. [infant massage]

Tappan, F: Healing Massage Techniques: Healing, Classic, and Emerging Methods. Appleton & Lange, 1988. [Swedish massage]

Thomas, C: Bodywork. William Morrow, New York, 1995.

CHAPTER 12

Therapeutic Touch

Mary Anne Bright

Mary Anne Bright, RN, CS, EdD, the editor of this book, is an associate professor at the University of Massachusetts–Amherst School of Nursing. She teaches courses in holistic healing and mental health nursing, conducts research on Therapeutic Touch, and is a member of the International Institute of Bioenergetic Analysis and of the American Holistic Nurses Association.

Therapeutic Touch is a contemporary interpretation of several ancient healing practices and is a conscious process of directing or modulating energies.[1] The practice of Therapeutic Touch is distinguished from other subtle energy healing practices through its research base and its widespread use in health-care settings. This method of healing is based on knowledge of human energy fields, conscious focusing to a centered state, and the influence of intention in healing.

The Human Energy Field

Human beings are complex energy fields that are embedded in internal and external environmental processes. Just as the weather both results from and influences earth and atmospheric dynamics, the human energy field interfaces with all with which it comes into contact. The existence of the human energy field has been reported around the world and for thousands of years. Many cultures have concepts of, language about, and treatments of the energy field that have only recently become known in the West.

The human energy field, also referred to as the aura and the etheric body, has electromagnetic properties. The energy field can be detected around the physical body, yet in reality it interpenetrates every cell. Bendit and Bendit[2] described its qualities:

> Indeed, the body can be looked at as a consolidation of dense matter inside the auric field . . . the etheric or vital aura is the matrix in which the body grows, just as the embryo does in the womb; but this womb is not hollow; it is filled with the energy counterparts of every organ, every cell, every cell nucleus, molecule, chemical atom and subdivision of these atoms, in a series of energy levels. Thus, if we consider the physical body alone, it consists of a structure of lines of force or energy patterns more or less fixed, anchored to the physical matter of the tissues. The converse is also true, that the tissues exist as such only because of the vital field behind them.

The energy field is a blueprint or template, a pattern of vibration finer than the physical body. It interpenetrates the physical body, extends 2 to 6 inches beyond the surface of the skin, and has a shape similar to its palpable, visible counterpart. The physical body is energetically connected and dependent on the energy field; without the energy body, the physical body could not exist. This subtle energy body functions as a road map for

BOX 12–1
Energetic Assumptions about Health and Healing

1. Human beings are open, complex, and pandimensional energy systems.
2. In a state of health, life energy flows freely through the organism in a balanced, symmetrical manner.
3. Human beings are capable of both transformation and transcendence.
4. Healing is an intrinsic movement toward order that occurs in living organisms and can be facilitated by practitioners. Life energy follows the intent to heal.

Source: Nurse Healers—Professional Associates International, Inc. Cooperative Connections 13(3):1, 1992, with permission.

development in health and cellular repair in disease. Like weather changes that affect the terrain beneath, the state of the energy field is intrinsically connected to the well-being of the physical body. (See Box 12–1.)

Clairvoyant healers who have the capacity to visualize the energy body describe how disruptions in it can precede the appearance of illness in the physical body as well as reflect disease already present in organs and tissues.[3] As such, it is possible not only to treat existing physical disease but also to prevent the manifestation of disease in the body through intervention at the level of the energy field. Manipulation of the energy field through electrical or magnetic interventions has demonstrated results on the physical level.

The electric nature of the human energy field was described by neuroanatomist Harold S. Burr in the 1940s.[4] He measured electrical fields around salamanders and seeds that reflected the shape of the adult organism; he then postulated that the electrical field influenced growth and development of the physical bodies of animals and plants. Burr called this field the "field of life," or "L-field," and thought that latent illnesses could be detected in the field before bodily symptoms appeared. Although the instrumentation required to investigate the energetic manifestations of the human field is in a rudimentary stage of development, scientific evidence of their existence is building. Several researchers have demonstrated the existence of a bioelectromagnetic field.[5–9] Through sophisticated instrumentation, a relationship between the electric and magnetic aspects of bioenergy fields, their reactivity to environmental electromagnetic fields, and patterns of field coherency and anticoherency in human health and illness have been observed.[10] For example, cancerous and noncancerous tissue can be differentiated in the electromagnetic field through Kirlian technology imaging.[11]

Becker and Selden[12] have advanced the understanding of energy healing though their pioneering research on tissue regeneration. Their experiments include salamander limb regeneration, suspension of mitosis in fibrosarcoma cells, and anesthesia induction through manipulation of electromagnetic fields. In addition to limb regeneration in animals, they have also proved that electrical stimulation of the energy field stimulates nerve, skin, and bone healing in humans. Magnetic therapy is an increasingly popularity and effective treatment of many health disruptions, from common acute sports injuries to chronic conditions such as treatment-resistant diabetic peripheral neuropathy.[13] There are also commonly used natural substances that are thought to balance the energy field, such as copper bracelets for joint pain and crystals for energy balancing.

The scientific community has gone beyond conventional dependence on the view that healing is a response to chemical interactions, an assumption now considered an incomplete explanation of the holistic nature of healing. Becker, Selden, and others have demonstrated, in the language of Western science, that there are observable intrinsic relationships among electromagnetic dynamics, healing, and life processes.

Vitalism

The concept of energy fields has also been associated with the idea of a life force that energizes and flows through the field in health but becomes decreased or blocked in illness. The idea of an all-pervasive energy has been held by many minds of the highest intellect. Around 500 BC, Pythagoras described a luminous body reflecting a vital force that he named "vital energy." Paracelsus, a 16th-century alchemist, described the aura and its effects on states of health and disease. This life force has been called by various names: *chi* in China, *ki* in Japan and Thailand, *prana* in India, *mana* in Hawaii, *vital elan* in Europe. This universal energy is considered the basic constituent and source of all life. Though called by different names, it is the same life force that underlies all energy healing practices.

Eastern scholars and clinicians base their healing techniques on vitalistic principles: acupuncture, shiatsu, acupressure, Qigong, Do-In, reiki, polarity therapy, and other techniques are based on an understanding of the energy field and the life force that flows through it. Western energy healing methods include Therapeutic Touch, Healing Touch, the Brennan Method, and Touch for Health. These methods are facilitated by specific preparation of the practitioner, a focused intention, and use of one's hands to interact with the vital force in the energy field. There are variations in the practice of these methods, but they are similar in that they are variations of "hand-mediated energetic healing," a term coined by Slater[14] that refers to all healing methods in which the practitioner's hands mediate energy.

Therapeutic Touch

Meehan[15] described Therapeutic Touch as a knowledgeable and deliberate patterning of the person–environment energy field process in which the practitioner assumes a meditative awareness and uses his or her hands as a focus for patterning of the energy field. Although the name of this healing technique implies tactile contact, no skin contact is necessary; rather, the interaction occurs between the energy fields of the practitioner and recipient. It should not be confused with "faith healing." To be effective, Therapeutic Touch does not require the recipient to have a specific belief system or to anticipate its effects.

Therapeutic Touch fosters the healing capacities present in every person. The practitioner does not do the healing. As Florence Nightingale so aptly observed, "only nature heals." The practitioner acts as nature's helper, using Therapeutic Touch to accelerate the healing process already inherent in the recipient. As such, it can be learned and used by anyone. However, its development as a therapeutic modality has occurred primarily within the context of professional nursing practice and research.

Therapeutic Touch was developed by Dolores Kreiger and Dora Kunz in the early 1970s. Kreiger's nursing research, combined with Kunz's clairvoyant healing abilities as a medical intuitive, evolved into the Kreiger/Kunz Method of Therapeutic Touch that is widely taught and practiced today. More than 70,000 health professionals have learned the method, which has been taught in 80 colleges and universities in the United States and more than 60 countries worldwide.

A growing number of U.S. and Canadian health-care facilities have incorporated Therapeutic Touch as a formal component of standard nursing practice. For example, the University of Colorado Hospital Medical Center has within its nursing organizational structure a department of energy, in which experienced practitioners offer treatments to patients and conduct research throughout the hospital. Therapeutic Touch is a noninvasive, cost-effective method that can be used as a primary or adjunctive treatment in any clinical or community setting, with clients of any age, and for a variety of health disruptions.

Therapeutic Effects

Kreiger[16] described three highly reliable clinical changes in the recipient during Therapeutic Touch. The first is a rapid relaxation response, usually within 2 to 4 minutes. The major operative factor may be concerned with a dampening of the autonomic nervous system—as evidenced by reduction in blood pressure, respiratory rate, and pulse—and a dilation of the vessels of the peripheral nervous system. The second clinical change is a significant reduction in pain, making it possible either to reduce the need for analgesic medications or to enhance their effects. It is not yet known with certainty how Therapeutic Touch alters pain perception, although it could be through endorphins. Therapeutic Touch enhances mood and fosters a sense of well-being—indications of endorphin release. The third major effect is an acceleration of the healing process, affecting both physical and psychological wounds.

How Does It Work?

Research has demonstrated more about the effects of Therapeutic Touch than about the processes that create its effects. To date, there is no definitive theory of how healing occurs in general or of how Therapeutic Touch works in particular. Rubik,[17] a biophysicist and founding director of Frontier Sciences at Temple University, observed:

> The evidence for therapeutic touch and other non-standard healing processes is too compelling for medical scientists to responsibly ignore. But how to explain these phenomena? Evidence for biophoton and other electromagnetic emissions is suggestive, but the data do not account for all the anomalies associated with "subtle energies."

Therapeutic Touch is thought to work on the level of energy field interactions, the phenomena of which are based on a shift of understanding from mechanistic (Newtonian) to quantum (Einsteinian) physics. This theoretical shift is evident in Rogers's Science of Unitary Human Beings.[18–20] Rogers, a nursing theorist, asserted that the human energy field is in open interaction with environmental energy fields, through which each coevolve through mutuality. Among the patterned manifestations of the human energy field are the physical body, the electromagnetic energy field, and the subtle energy field of the etheric body. Disturbances in energy field patterns are observed as disease in the physical body and as disruption of imbalance in the electromagnetic field and etheric body.

Kreiger associated healing with the phenomenon of universal energy. Universal energy underlies the organization of life processes and is taken in from the environment through breathing and nutritional assimilation. A healthy organism enjoys an abundance of this energy, whereas an ill organism suffers from its deficit, which results in loss of vitality and appearance of symptoms in both the physical body and the psyche. Therapeutic Touch is thought to facilitate the assimilation, circulation, and balance of universal energy within the energy field. In addition, the human field is reordered in its relationship to the environmental field in a more life-enhancing pattern of interconnectedness.

Straneva[21] described Therapeutic Touch as a form of energetic communication. She further asserted that Therapeutic Touch transcends the placebo effect, as evidenced by the healing response of unaware research subjects, unconscious persons, and children who do not have the cognitive capacity to develop an expectation of healing.

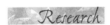

Research

Therapeutic Touch has been the subject of scientific inquiry for more than 20 years. Research studies have demonstrated a variety of beneficial effects:

- Increased hemoglobin in hospitalized adults[22]
- Decreased anxiety in hospitalized adult cardiovascular patients[23,24]

- Decreased anxiety in hospitalized psychiatric patients[25]
- Reduced pain and anxiety in burn patients[26]
- Stress reduction in hospitalized neonates, children, and adolescents[27–29]
- Reduction in tension headache pain[30]
- Accelerated wound healing[31]
- Relief from pain and increased function in persons with arthritis[32,33]
- Reduced agitation as well as increased comfort and relaxation among dementia patients[34–36]
- Enhanced well-being of HIV-infected children,[37] persons with terminal cancer,[38] and persons experiencing grief[39]

The energetic nature of Therapeutic Touch was demonstrated by Quinn and Stelkauskas,[40] who observed that it effects the giver as well as the receiver. They discovered that indices of enhanced immune function occurred in both the Therapeutic Touch practitioner and the clients who received treatments. This interesting research finding demonstrates energy field phenomena: both persons involved in the interaction of Therapeutic Touch are affected by the dynamic process of energetic reorganization.

In an integrative review and meta-analysis of Therapeutic Touch research, Winstead-Fry and Kijek[41] observed that the most often reported and validated treatment effect is the method's anxiety-reducing effectiveness. They described the strengths and weaknesses of this body of research and observed that, as with other complementary and alternative modalities, research needs to be broadened to include more randomized clinical trials, other outcome research methodologies, more discriminating operational definitions, and attention to issues of reliability and validity. However, even with a high degree of variation among existing Therapeutic Touch studies, the method has been demonstrated to have a moderate-sized effect. In addition to more finely tuned treatment outcome studies, research on *how* and *why* the method works is also needed.

The Method

The procedure involves five steps: centering, identifying intention, assessment, treatment, and evaluation. There is an overall sequence of stages, but the practitioner moves among the stages as the unique needs of the client become evident. Before treatment begins, the practitioner explains the procedure and elicits the client's participation, reflecting standards of ethics and conduct for the practice of Therapeutic Touch. (See Table 12–1.)

Centering is the first step in preparation for the Therapeutic Touch encounter. Centering is the way to the state of quietude, poetically reflected by Lao Tzu:

> *There is no need to run outside*
> *For better seeing,*
> *Nor to peer from a window, rather abide*
> *at the center of your being;*
> *For the more you leave it, the less you learn.*
> *Search your heart and see*
> *if he is wise who takes each turn:*
> *The way to do is to be.*

Centering is a process of focused attention that facilitates awareness of energy field phenomena. It involves bringing the body, mind, and emotions to a quiet, focused state of consciousness. It initiates the process of Therapeutic Touch and is maintained as a deliberately conscious process in which the nurse is engaged in every step of the technique. It allows the practitioner to be sensitive to his or her own process and energies, as well as how they are separate from those of the recipient's, and makes it possible to assess and treat the person with empathic clarity. Centering is a simple process to learn, and it has an immediate impact on the experience of the practitioner and of the client. (See Table 12–2.)

Intention, which occurs after the practitioner is centered, is focused on the client's intrinsic wholeness and on the restoration of harmony and order in the energy field. This step is the recognition that, as Florence Nightingale said, "Only nature heals; we put the person in the best condition for healing to occur." The practitioner does not "heal" the client. Rather, the practitioner takes responsibility for facilitating a more balanced energetic environment that supports the client's wholeness. Thus the practitioner's intention is expressed as a desire to facilitate an energetic reorganization, rather than an attempt to eliminate specific symptoms.

Assessment is the discovery of the client's energy field characteristics. The client remains fully clothed, either sitting or lying down, while the practitioner moves his or her hands, lightly and symmetrically, through the energy field 2 to 6 inches above the surface of the body. The assessment reveals differences within the field that indicate energy imbalance. A healthy person's energy field feels like a soft, vibrant warmth, with a quality of unbroken evenness in the practitioner's hands. Imbalances are felt in the hands as differences in temperature, fullness or emptiness, tingling, static, pulling or drawing, and pressure and/or pulsation.

Treatment is based on the assessment and on one or more for the following objectives:

- The facilitation of energy flow
- The stimulation of energy flow
- The mobilization of congestion or pressure in the energy field
- The dampening or quieting of energetic activity
- The synchronization of rhythmicity in the energy flow

TABLE 12–1   Statement of Ethics and Conduct for the Practice of Therapeutic Touch

1. I will practice Therapeutic Touch consistent with the process as developed by Dolores Kreiger, PhD, RN, and Dora Kunz, and as established by the Nurse Healers—Professional Associates International, Inc.
2. I will obtain the person's and/or family's permission and consent for Therapeutic Touch, whenever possible.
3. I will respect the person's rights and responsibilities in the Therapeutic Touch process.
4. I will inform people of my fees prior to practicing Therapeutic Touch.
5. I will provide Therapeutic Touch based upon people's unique needs and with respect for their individual differences.
6. I will keep my interactions with people nonexploitive and complementary to their care.
7. I will not market, by mail or in person, any other product or service without permission.
8. I will hold in confidence all information shared during Therapeutic Touch.
9. I will not incorporate other healing modalities into my Therapeutic Touch practice unless I have both the qualifications to do so and the person's permission whenever possible.
10. I will not discuss my personal problems or issues with those seeking my professional services.
11. I will strengthen my abilities to practice Therapeutic Touch through continuing practice, education, and/or mentoring.
12. I will practice Therapeutic Touch with integrity, always keeping the interests of the person foremost.

Source: Therapeutic Touch Network (Ontario) document, with permission from Nurse Healers—Professional Associates International.

TABLE 12–2   How to Center

1. Begin by sitting comfortably in a quiet place. Close your eyes if you feel excessively distracted. Inhale and exhale slowly and deeply. Feel the lower belly, soften and expand with a few deep breaths.
2. Allow your eyes, jaw, face, back of the neck, shoulders, arms, pelvic floor, legs, and joints to soften and relax. Move your body and exhale deeply to release any tensions of which you are aware.
3. Notice your breath. Breathe normally, then gradually let your breath slow down until it is quiet, even, and relaxed. Notice how slowing the breath induces a quiet, relaxed state.
4. Observe how your thoughts, sensations, and emotions continue in your experience. Allow them without becoming preoccupied with them. Gently return to your awareness of the breath when distracted.
5. Allow yourself to take in vital energy when inhaling and release deep tension when exhaling.
6. Maintain awareness of yourself as the center of your own experience, with your inner experience as the main focus. Observe sensation, stimulation, sounds, and thoughts from the external environment as peripheral to the center of your being.
7. Experience the sense of doing nothing but being with yourself. Allow yourself to enjoy any sense of relaxation, calm, and peacefulness that you might feel as you maintain your inner focus. Be aware of how your are breathing as you enjoy being with yourself.
8. As you relax, gradually allow your focus to expand to meet the external environment. Stay connected with your inner focus and bring it along with you as you re-engage in your professional role.
9. Approach your client with your sustained focus, and include your awareness of the client within it.
10. When you experience the inevitable distractions of the workplace, sustain your attention within the therapeutic relationship by bringing your attention back to your breathing and to your awareness of the client.

Source: Bright, MA: Centering: The path to healing presence. Alternative Health Practitioner 1(3):191–194, 1995, with permission.

Treatment occurs in three phases: the clearing away of congestion, the transfer of life energy into depleted areas, and the balancing of energy flow. The needs of the individual and the intuitive style of the practitioner will determine how these phases are expressed and modified to address therapeutic objectives. A feeling of relaxation is often experienced within the first 5 minutes of treatment. Average treatment time reported by advanced practitioners is 20 minutes and is dependent on the condition of the client and the ongoing evaluation of treatment effects.

Evaluation is the use of professional, informed, intuitive judgment to determine when to end the session. This is accomplished by reassessing the field and eliciting feedback from the client. Typically, a treatment ends when energy flow has been re-established and when the energy field feels more balanced in the hands of the practitioner. If possible, the client should be encouraged to rest after a treatment, which allows a fuller integration of the experience.

CASE STUDY 1

The Baby Can't Sleep

Two-year-old Jason was suffering from cold symptoms and had a difficult time falling asleep. At bedtime, he became restless, whiny, and clingy. Comfort measures that usually facilitated sleep—rocking, nursing, reading, and rubbing his back—were ineffective. After 2 minutes of Therapeutic Touch, Jason relaxed and fell asleep.

Discussion. This example demonstrates the effect of a single treatment. Relaxation is one of the major effects of this intervention. Therapeutic Touch is taught to parents as a comfort measure for various manifestations of children's distress, including anxiety, restlessness, and pain. Both child and parent benefit from this technique: the child experiences relief, and the parent enjoys an enhanced sense of competence in stressful circumstances when often "nothing else works" to comfort the child.

CASE STUDY 2
Too Tired

Jennifer, a 28-year-old graduate student, requested Therapeutic Touch for a condition her physician had diagnosed as chronic fatigue syndrome. For 2 years she had suffered from extreme exhaustion, frequent colds, sore throats, headaches, inability to sleep well or to concentrate, and persistent muscle weakness and pain. Her symptoms had forced her to resign from her job as a secretary, and her graduate studies had been delayed by her inability to complete her schoolwork. Jennifer found variable but incomplete and unsatisfactory symptomatic relief from the many remedies she had been prescribed, including antidepressant, nutritional, and chiropractic therapies.

Therapeutic Touch was administered weekly for 3 months. Jennifer experienced a deeply relaxed state after each session and was able to sleep much better on Therapeutic Touch treatment days. Treatments focused on decreasing energetic stasis and increasing the balance and vitality of her energy field. There was no immediate improvement, but after four sessions, Jennifer began to experience more energy and less muscle pain; she was also able to resume work on her graduate course papers. After the sixth session, she reported that a number of painful warts on the bottom of her feet, which had plagued her for 2 years, had disappeared without her using any treatments specific to them. She attributed the disappearance of her warts to Therapeutic Touch. Although Jennifer's overall health status did not return to the prediagnosis level, she attributed a gradual sense of strengthening, relaxation, and mental clarity to her 3-month course of Therapeutic Touch.

Discussion. Therapeutic Touch was a useful intervention, used adjunctively with other therapies, in the ongoing treatment of a complex and enigmatic constellation of health problems. Jennifer experienced many of the beneficial effects of Therapeutic Touch reported in the research literature: enhanced ability to relax, to concentrate, to sleep, and to heal. Remission of plantar warts suggested that Jennifer's immune system had begun to respond during the period of treatment with Therapeutic Touch, a clinical finding also demonstrated in research.

This example illustrates two points: (1) Repeated treatments over time have a cumulative effect and enhance the therapeutic outcome. (2) Therapeutic Touch is holistic in its effects. Not only were the presenting symptoms of fatigue, muscle pain, and sleeplessness relieved, but other signs of imbalance (plantar warts) were also ameliorated.

Summary

Therapeutic Touch is a contemporary energy healing intervention that promotes relaxation, healing, restoration of vitality, and enhancement of well-being. Knowledge of human energy fields, the nature of healing, and the mechanisms of energy healing is mounting through scientific investigations worldwide.

A holistic understanding of energy field phenomena is central to the practice of Therapeutic Touch. What is known as a person is the result of interaction among the many parts of the human energy field, observable in physical, psychological, emotional, and spiritual aspects of being. Although we often conceptualize these aspects as being separate components of experience, they are more aptly understood as different energy frequencies in continuous interaction, dynamically self-organized and fully expressed. The person is embedded within the context of the environment, with which the person maintains an energetic interchange necessary for growth, development, maintenance, restoration, reproduction, and, eventually, entropy decline. Through compassionate intuition, the practitioner of Therapeutic Touch helps a person to take the necessary steps toward vital reintegration and "enwholement" of his or her energy field.[42]

The capacity to heal, which literally means "to make whole," is an innate restorative tendency in all living things. Energetically, disease is a disorder of imbalance between the individual and the environment. Health and disease are mediated through exchanges in person–environment energy fields. Therapeutic Touch is effective because it facilitates the balanced energetic environment necessary for reestablishment and maintenance of health.

RESOURCES

Nurse Healers—Professional Associates International, Inc.
3760 S. Highland Drive, Suite 429
Salt Lake City, UT 84106
Phone: (801) 273-3399
Fax: (801) 273-3352
www.NHPAI.TherapeuticTouch.org

REFERENCES

1. Kreiger, D: The Therapeutic Touch: How to Use Your Hands to Help and Heal. Prentice-Hall, New York, 1979.
2. Bendit, LJ, and Bendit, PD: The Etheric Body of Man. Theosophical Publishing House, Wheaton, Ill.,1989, p 22.
3. Kargulla, S, and van Gelder Kunz, D: The Chakras and the Human Energy Fields. Theosophical Publishing House, Wheaton, Ill., 1989.
4. Burr, HS: The Fields of Life. Ballantine Books, New York, 1972.
5. Becker, RO, and Selden, G: The Body Electric: Electromagnetism and the Foundation of Life. William Morrow, New York, 1985.
6. Burr: The Fields of Life.
7. Hunt, VV: Infinite Mind: The Science of Human Vibrations. Malibu Publishing Company, Malibu, CA 1989.
8. Motoyama, H, and Brown, R: Science and Evolution of Consciousness: Chakras, Ki and Psi. Autumn Press, Brookline, Mass., 1978.
9. Kirlian, S, and Kirlian, V: Photography and visual observations by means of high frequency currents. Journal of Scientific and Applied Photography 6:145, 1961.
10. Hunt: Infinite Mind.
11. Mallikarjun, S: Kirlian photography in cancer diagnosis. Osteopathic Physician 26:30, 1976.
12. Becker and Selden: The Body Electric.
13. Weintraub, MJ: Magnetic bio-stimulation in painful diabetic peripheral neuropathy: A novel intervention—a randomized, double placebo crossover study. American Journal of Physiological Medicine 9:8, 1999.
14. Slater, VE: Toward an understanding of energetic healing, part I: Energetic structures. Journal of Holistic Nursing 13(3):209, 1995.
15. Meehan, TC: The Science of Unitary Human Beings and theory-based practice: Therapeutic Touch. In Barrett, EAM (ed): Visions of Rogers' Science-Based Nursing. National League for Nursing, New York, 1990.
16. Kreiger, D: Accepting Your Power to Heal: The Personal Practice of Therapeutic Touch. Bear & Company, Santa Fe, 1993.

17. Rubik, B: Life at the Edge of Science. Institute of Frontier Science, San Francisco, 1993.
18. Rogers, ME: An Introduction to the Theoretical Basis for Nursing. FA Davis, Philadelphia, 1988.
19. Rogers, ME: Nursing science and art: A prospective. Nursing Science Quarterly 5:27, 1992.
20. Rogers, ME: Nursing science in the space age. Nursing Science Quarterly 1:99, 1992.
21. Straneva, JE: Therapeutic Touch: Placebo effect or energetic form of communication? Journal of Holistic Nursing 9(2):41, 1991.
22. Kreiger, D: The response of in-vivo human hemoglobin to an active healing therapy by direct laying-on of hands. Human Dimensions 1:12, 1972.
23. Heidt, P: Effects of Therapeutic Touch on anxiety levels of hospitalized patients. Nursing Research 30(1):101, 1981.
24. Quinn, JF: An investigation of the effect of Therapeutic Touch done without physical contact on state anxiety of hospitalized patients. Dissertation Abstracts International 49:2367. (University Microfilms No. DA 82-26-788)
25. Gagne, D, and Toye, R: The effects of Therapeutic Touch and relaxation therapy in reducing anxiety. Archives of Psychiatric Nursing 3(3):184, 1994.
26. Turner, JG, et al: The effect of Therapeutic Touch on pain and anxiety in burn patients. Journal of Advanced Nursing 28(1):10, 1998.
27. Federouk, RB: Transfer of the Relaxation Response: Therapeutic Touch as a method for reduction of stress in premature infants. Dissertation Abstracts International 46:9788. (University Microfilms No. 85-09-162)
28. Kramer, NA: Comparison of Therapeutic Touch and casual touch in stress reduction of hospitalized children. Pediatric Nursing 16(5):483, 1990.
29. Hughes, PP, Meize-Grochowski, R, and Harris, CND: Therapeutic Touch with adolescent patients. Journal of Holistic Nursing 14(1):6, 1996.
30. Keller, E, and Bzdek, VN: Effects of Therapeutic Touch on tension headache pain. Nurs Res 35(2):101, 1986.
31. Wirth, D: The effects of non-contact Therapeutic Touch on the healing rate of full thickness dermal wounds. Subtle Energies 1(1):1, 1990.
32. Peck, SD: The effectiveness of Therapeutic Touch for decreasing pain in elders with degenerative arthritis. Journal of Holistic Nursing 15(2):176, 1995.
33. Peck, SD: The efficacy of Therapeutic Touch for improving functional ability in elders with degenerative arthritis. Nursing Science Quarterly 11(3):123, 1998.
34. Snyder, M, Egan, EL, and Burns, K: Intervention to decrease disruptive behaviors in persons with dementia. Minnesota Nursing Accent 65(9):1, 1993.
35. Snyder, M, Egan, EL, and Burns, CR: Interventions for decreasing agitation in persons with dementia. Journal of Gerontological Nursing 27(7):34. 1995.
36. Griffin, RL, and Nitro, E: An overview of Therapeutic Touch and its application to patients with Alzheimer's disease. American Journal of Alzheimer's Disease 13(4):211, 1998.
37. Ireland, M: Therapeutic Touch with HIV-infected children: A pilot study. Journal of the Association of Nurses in AIDS Care 9(4):68–77, 1998.
38. Giasson, M, and Bouchard, L: Effect of Therapeutic Touch on the well-being of persons with terminal cancer. Journal of Holistic Nursing 16(3):383, 1998.
39. Robinson, LS: The effects of Therapeutic Touch on the grief experience. Dissertation Abstracts International 50:1269. (University Microfilms No. 87-36-422)
40. Quinn, JF, and Stelkauskas, A: Psychoimmunologic effects of Therapeutic Touch on practitioners and recently bereaved recipients: A pilot study. Advances in Nursing Science 14(4): 13, 1993.
41. Winstead-Fry, P, and Kijek, J: An integrative review and meta-analysis of Therapeutic Touch research. Alternative Therapies 5(6):58, 1999.
42. Kreiger, D: Therapeutic Touch: Toward an understanding of human be-ness. Cooperative Connection 12(1):1, 1991.

Complementary Healing Practices

Naturopathic Medicine—Vis Medicatrix Naturae: The Healing Power of Nature

James M. Lemkin

James M. Lemkin, ND, maintains a private naturopathic practice with an emphasis on preventive medicine, clinical nutrition, homeopathy, botanical medicine, hydrotherapy, and psychospiritual healing.

In 1892, Benedict Lust, an ambitious 20-year-old from Germany, traveled to the United States to seek his fortune. But luck did not go his way—he developed tuberculosis. Despite medical care, he wasted away and decided he had only one option left: return to Germany to die. When he reached his native country, however, Benedict was inspired to try one last measure. He visited Sebastian Kneipp, a Bavarian priest with a growing reputation for treating peasants and emperors alike with hydrotherapy and herbal treatments. Soon after starting the "Kneipp cure," Lust began to improve. Within 8 months he had totally regained his health.

Lust's near brush with death and his miraculous cure so transformed him, he decided to devote the rest of his life to communicating the benefits of nature cures to others. In the years that followed, he created and developed the profession of naturopathy and became known as the father of modern naturopathic medicine.

What is naturopathy? It is the science, art, and practice of maintaining health by understanding and acting in accord with the profound ability of the body to heal itself. Practitioners view naturopathic medicine as a system of health care defined by six principles based on the laws of nature. These ageless laws, on which all life thrives, include, among other precepts, the importance of a healthful diet and lifestyle.

Naturopathic medicine recognizes that health and disease are not random conditions but, instead, are dependent on the many factors that affect the human organism's functioning. These factors can be discerned by observing nature and recognizing that many of the excesses of the modern lifestyle are detrimental to health. Health is considered a vital dynamic state that supports robust living in spite of environmental stresses and is the result of respecting these laws. Alternatively, many diseases, if not most, as well as much of the degeneration associated with "normal aging," are thought to be the result of ignoring these laws and the resulting unhealthy lifestyle—and may be avoidable.

BOX 13–1
The Naturopathic Lineage

While its therapeutic and philosophic roots come from many cultures and traditions, naturopathy has its immediate origins mainly in the nature-cure and water-cure traditions popularized by a number of 19th-century European practitioners.

Victor Preissnitz (1799–1852) established the foundations of modern water therapy. He used primarily cold water compresses, packs, showers, sprays, and sponge baths together with fresh air, exercise, and simple natural foods.

Johann Schroth (1798–1856) introduced warm water therapies and moist heat packs. Arnold Rickli (1823–1906) emphasized natural living and the atmospheric cure (ample exposure to light and air); he also integrated steam baths with other hot and cold water therapies. Louis Kuhne (1835–1901) further refined hydrotherapy and dietary therapy; he also advanced the theory of the unity of disease, which held that although people are afflicted by diseases with many different names, their illness can be attributed to one basic cause: diminished vitality and increased susceptibility.

Father Sebastian Kneipp (1824–1897), who cured Benedict Lust, became popular throughout Europe and North America. He treated hundreds of thousands of patients and wrote more than 20 books, including the classic *My Water Cure.*

The writings of Kneipp, Kuhne, and other nature-cure doctors greatly influenced Mahatma Gandhi. In 1946 Gandhi founded the first naturopathic school in India, envisioning an effective, low-cost and low-tech, decentralized health-care system for the thousands of poor villages in his country. The simple, natural treatments of nature cure were well suited to Gandhi's homespun political ethos. His dream, however, was never realized after his death in 1948.

As primary care practitioners, naturopathic physicians (Doctor of Naturopathic Medicine—ND) emphasize preventive and holistic medicine employing the philosophy, art, and science of *vis medicatrix naturae*—"the healing power of nature." For more than a century, naturopathic physicians have used virtually all methods and treatments that respectfully assist and support the innate healing processes. Contemporary naturopathic medicine draws both from modern scientific studies and from traditional healing arts. Regardless of origin, it uses treatments that honor an individual and do not inflict harm on his or her self-healing processes. Modern medical research in such areas as physiology, biochemistry, clinical nutrition, and public health is increasingly rediscovering and verifying the profound truths embodied in *vis medicatrix naturae.*

While many naturopathic physicians pursue postdoctoral training in natural childbirth, acupuncture, homeopathy, or other specialties, most serve as general practitioners emphasizing holistic and preventive medicine. Their role can be compared to that of the traditional family doctor; they are generalists or gatekeepers, the first health-care professional the patient seeks. Because naturopathic physicians are trained in both conventional and holistic medicine, they recognize what it is appropriate to treat by conservative, natural methods and what should be referred out for specialized medical or surgical care. Conversely, because naturopathic physicians have extensive training in preventive and natural approaches, both conventional medical doctors and other holistic healing professionals often refer patients to them.

Patients who choose naturopathic physicians are usually seeking alternatives—either as part of a committed philosophy of holism and prevention, or in reaction to the conventional medical care they regard as inadequate. (See Box 13–1.)

The Six Principles of Naturopathic Medicine

Six interdependent, fundamental principles form the basis of naturopathic philosophy and practice.[1,2] Based on these principles, the naturopathic physician is able to consider the patient, the process, and the protocol for treatment with objectivity and respect for the organism's self-healing process.

1. *The healing power of nature (vis medicatrix naturae).* The inherent healing process is ordered and intelligent. Each person, each organism, has the innate ability to establish, maintain, and restore health. The physician facilitates and augments this process by identifying and removing obstacles to recovery by supporting the creation of a healthful internal and external environment.

2. *Identify and treat the cause (tolle causam).* Illness does not occur spontaneously and without cause. The seeds of a disease process may have been sown months or years prior to the first noticed symptom. The task of the naturopathic physician is to discern, when possible, the underlying causes and center of gravity of the disease and assist the patient in removing them. Only then is complete recovery from an illness possible.

3. *First, do no harm (primum non nocere).* The physician must be ever mindful of the consequences and side effects of the treatment. Treatments that suppress or eliminate symptoms without addressing underlying causes should be avoided whenever possible because they often hinder the innate healing process and can lead to a deeper level of chronic disease. (See the later section "The Meaning of Disease.") Naturopathic physicians acknowledge, respect, and work with the individual's self-healing process, using the least force necessary to effectively diagnose and treat in order to minimize the risks of suppression and harmful side effects.

4. *Treat the whole person.* Every person is unique. Their health depends on the harmonious functioning of a complex interaction of physical, emotional, mental, psychospiritual, hereditary, social, and environmental factors. Achieving wellness may require a different set of treatments for each person, even though all may have the same named disease. The physician treats the whole person by integrating his or her unique expression of these factors into the healing process and by working with each person's innate healing abilities.

5. *Prevention is the best cure.* Prevention is the ultimate goal of naturopathic medicine. Through health education, assessment of risk factors, and promotion of healthy life-habits, the physician enables each patient to build health and vitality, decreasing susceptibility to disease to the fullest extent possible. Treatment and prevention go hand in hand. Often, removing the underlying causes of disease has two simultaneous benefits: it reduces or eliminates the presence of the disease while it also strengthens the patient, placing him or her in a more proactive, preventive status.

6. *Doctor as teacher (docere).* The original meaning of the word *doctor* is "teacher," from the Latin *docere*, "to teach." One of the major roles of the naturopathic physician is to educate and encourage each person to take responsibility for his or her health. The physician acts as a catalyst for healthy change, empowering and motivating the patient through an informed, respectful, caring professional relationship. The physician must inspire hope and understanding. The physician must also inspire trust by reflecting those qualities of good health, personal development, and compassion in his or her own life. In an open, mutually respectful relationship, the patient also educates the doctor, helping to deepen his or her appreciation of the subtlety and depth of the art and science of healing.

The naturopathic profession believes that part of the role of all healers should be to find ways to apply these six principles on a larger scale to address the psychosocial, environmental, and political ills that burden so many peoples of the world. This complex planet, Earth, is simply a larger body with the same abilities to return to health as the individual has if treated appropriately. The model for health is virtually the same.

FIGURE 13–1

Naturopathic medicine views health as existing along a continuum. (From: Lemkin, JM: Unpublished manuscript, 1996, with permission.)

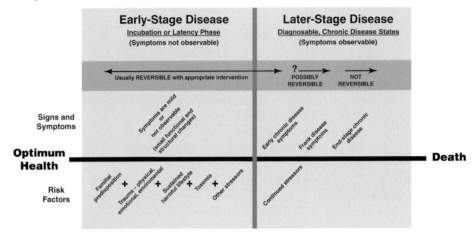

The Disease Continuum

Naturopathic medicine views health as existing along a continuum ranging from optimum health at one extreme to death at the other. (See Fig. 13–1.) Unlike the conventional biomedical model, which tends to view symptoms of chronic disease in isolation until they progress to a stage where they fit an established diagnostic pattern, the continuum model attempts to uncover the causation and its disturbances prior to the appearance of diagnostic symptoms.

The naturopathic physician can treat the person for the underlying precipitating factors of a disease before it perceptibly expresses itself. To this end, the doctor examines the patient's lifestyle for possible risk factors, such as poor life-habits, distressing mental and emotional states, nutritional deficiencies, and toxic accumulations, and observes subtle subclinical functional and structural changes.

The cumulative effect of small stressors or disturbances to the person's vitality, if untreated over time and/or augmented by hereditary predisposition, can propel an illness from incubation or latency to full-blown expression of chronic disease. Reversing the progress of disease becomes much more difficult when a condition becomes chronic and the healing ability is compromised.[3,4]

Philosophy and Theory of Naturopathic Medicine

The history and philosophy of naturopathic medicine may be viewed through two basic laws of nature. (1) Survival through the dynamic equilibrium of homeostasis is the constant goal of all living organisms. The organism naturally seeks to maintain or restore health when confronted with any condition that throws it out of balance. (2) The vitality of the whole organism—as measured by the strength of the innate homeostatic response to physical, emotional, and psychospiritual disturbance—together with its susceptibility to pathogenic influences (e.g., bacteria, viruses, antigens, environmental toxins, mental and emotional trauma, etc.) determine how or whether it becomes ill. Consequently, although pathogenic agents play a role in illness, their influence is directly related to the *vitality* and *susceptibility* of the individual. The primary roles of the naturopathic physician are to help enhance homeostasis by strengthening vitality and decreasing susceptibility and to remove the causes of disease.

Mechanism versus Vitalism

Western medicine, since at least the era of Hippocrates (c 460–377 BC), has followed two distinct, often diametrically opposed doctrines. The *mechanist school* (also called the rationalist school) has focused on the disease, or pathogen; the *vitalist school* (also called the empirical school) has focused on the susceptibility of the individual in whom the battle of health versus disease is played out.

The mechanist school views the human organism as a complex machine that breaks down when external or internal agents of disease (or wear and tear) disrupt the normal chemical and physical reactions in the body. These agents are either identifiable ones that must be controlled, or unknown ones that cause symptoms that must be suppressed. The goals of mechanistic medicine, then, are to conquer and remove the perceived causative agent(s) and/or suppress the symptoms. When the signs and symptoms of disease are gone, the treatment is deemed successful.[5,6]

In contrast, the vitalist doctrine, which naturopathic medicine embraces, maintains that the organism's vitality and susceptibility are just as important as, or more important than, the causes of disease. Vitalists value direct observation of the natural course of the disease and the body's response. Vitalists respect and rely on the body's inherent defense mechanisms (e.g., fever, inflammation, immune system reaction) and concentrate on removing the obstacles to healing while activating and augmenting the person's innate homeostatic resistance to the disease. This approach emphasizes wellness more than disease treatment, since the causes of disease are not always discernible but nonetheless exert an influence on the vitality of the person.[7]

Throughout history, vitalists have viewed healing as the shared responsibility of the patient and the doctor. The individual does the *healing*. The doctor and treatment only facilitate the process and, at best, can only stimulate the organism's self-healing. Vitalists recognize a treatment as *curative* only when it contributes to the organism's healing itself and recovering from the disease in a permanent manner. With all other outcomes, a treatment is either merely *palliative* (controlling symptoms but effecting little change in the general state of health) or, at worst, *suppressive* (controlling symptoms in a way that can make the whole individual progressively less healthy).

Although allopathic, or conventional, physicians have inherited the mechanistic model, recent changes in Western healing practices have softened and blended the sharp distinctions between these historically opposing doctrines. Naturopathic medicine and other vitalist healing practices have adopted certain aspects of the mechanistic model, such as modern diagnostic techniques, but are still vitalistically focused on the organism's innate healing (as opposed to mere palliation or suppression of symptoms), which takes place through the laws of nature.

The Meaning of Disease

It is the nature of a person or organism to heal. The doctor merely assists what nature provides. Healing occurs only when an organism accesses from within itself the conditions for health. In the view of naturopathic medicine, the disease agent itself does not directly cause the symptoms accompanying disease; rather, most symptoms are the result of the organism's intrinsic attempt to respond, defend, and heal itself.

An example of how the body responds to disturbances is inflammation. When a tissue is stressed over time, it may become irritated. Irritation can lead the body to produce an inflammatory response. Inflammation involves the release of chemicals from the injured or irritated tissue that initiate a cascade of events, such as widening of the blood vessels, increased flow of blood, and movement of white blood cells and other necessary healing substances into the affected area. Although the person may subjectively experience heat, redness, swelling, and pain, a symphony of homeostatic elements are all elegantly and efficiently working together to return the body to a healthier state. The body depends on this healing response. Suppression of this response under some circumstances can actually subvert and delay the healing process.

Four Types of Healing Responses

According to naturopathic philosophy, one of four different scenarios will be played out when a person's innate defense and healing system battles disease or any other pathogenic influence. The scenario depends on the vitality and susceptibility of the person and on the strength and complexity of the pathogenic influences. (See Table 13–1.)

Asymptomatic Response

The body-mind is capable of defending itself against pathogenic influences with no perceivable symptoms. This common reaction takes place in everyone countless times daily. Culturing the mouth of a healthy person will yield bacteria and other pathogens that without the silent vigilance of the immune system could easily overwhelm the body and lead to death. When the innate defense and healing systems are functioning normally, the response proceeds unnoticed and there is a quick resolution.

Acute Response—the "Healing Crisis"

As susceptibility increases or the strength of the pathogenic influences rises, a threshold is reached and symptoms become apparent. Usually the healing response is brief and vigorous, and the person returns to his or her normal state. Sometimes a discharge through the organs of elimination is noticed. Acute diseases and the common cold are simple examples of a spontaneous healing crisis. The organism has risen to the occasion, successfully reestablishing equilibrium after a few days of symptoms.

TABLE 13–1   Four Types of Healing Response

RESPONSE	MEANING
1. Asymptomatic	The organism easily defends itself against pathological or "disturbing" factors.
2. Acute response—healing crisis	The relative strength of disturbing factors and the organism are similar. Symptoms of the body in defending itself are apparent.
3. Acute, life-threatening crisis	Disturbing factors are stronger than the organism. Death will occur without intervention.
4. Chronic, smoldering symptoms —chronic disease	The healing response is feeble but adequate to maintain life. Progressive degeneration ensues.
A healing response that leads to cure is the opposite of symptom suppression.	Suppression may cause symptoms to diminish or disappear, but often the pathology is driven deeper into the organism, causing a more complex level of disease.

Source: Adapted from Bradley, R: Philosophy of naturopathic medicine. In Pizzorno, J, and Murray M (eds): A Textbook of Natural Medicine. Bastyr College Publications, Seattle, 1985. Revised by Lemkin, JM, 1999.

Acute, Life-Threatening Crisis

When a person's vitality is low and susceptibility is high relative to the strength of the pathogenic influences, the response of the organism may be insufficient to successfully return it to a normal state. Overpowered, the organism will die unless there is proper and timely therapeutic intervention. Major traumatic injury, acute bacterial meningitis, and severe suicidal depression often require prompt external intervention in order to reduce potential morbidity. When the organism's healing systems cannot mount an adequate defense, short-term suppressive treatments to control symptoms and to attack the immediate causative factors may be required. Natural therapies may still be useful as complementary treatments. It is important to note, however, that short-term use of a drug may have a beneficial, indeed a life-saving, effect and that naturopathic physicians support the use of such heroic treatments when necessary to save a life or to prevent a life-threatening disease from taking hold. But long-term drug use may suppress symptoms and weaken the constitution, further contributing to the organism's chronic degeneration; a drug should only be used when there is no equally effective natural substitute.

Chronic, Smoldering Symptoms—Chronic Disease

If the organism is weak or if the acute restorative process has been suppressed, a chronic disease response may emerge. It is as if the power to heal is stalled. The organism is barely able to hold its own. If disturbing factors such as harmful lifestyle, biochemical and emotional stressors, or drug suppression persist, they may cause an increasingly toxic state, diminished function, persistent inflammation, and structural or other changes. Left untreated, the disturbance penetrates deeper into the organism, producing increasingly graver symptoms. This progressive degeneration depicts most modern disease states. With supportive, naturopathic intervention, the physician assists the person in identifying and removing the causes of disease while strengthening resistance to stressors. If the person can be stimulated to produce a more vigorous healing response, he or she may be able to reverse this degenerative process and may undergo a healing crisis that was previously suppressed.[8,9] (See Box 13–2.)

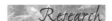

Research

Naturopathic therapies draw from wide-ranging sources: from the healing arts of traditional cultures of antiquity to the data of contemporary naturopathic physicians and an ever-increasing body of modern published scientific research. Each year, virtually thousands of clinical studies and governmental surveys worldwide give sound scientific verification and support to naturopathic methods and treatments. This research consists largely of peer-reviewed, clinical trials drawn from many disciplines, such as medicine, epidemiology and public health, clinical nutrition, botanical medicine, Eastern and Ayurvedic medicine, homeopathy, and psychology. Because of naturopathic medicine's inherently eclectic nature and relative freedom to adopt new treatment protocols, its practitioners are often the first to integrate effective natural treatments into their clinical practices.[10,11] (See Box 13–3.)

One recent example of a multifactorial treatment protocol that verifies naturopathic principles is the work of Dean Ornish and colleagues[12] on lifestyle and its effect on cardiovascular disease through the reduction of atherosclerotic blockage. This work was groundbreaking in its experimental design, examining the net effect of several natural therapeutic agents: diet combined with lifestyle alterations, physical and psychological exercises, and support groups. Integrated into one treatment protocol, they were shown collectively to reverse progressive coronary artery disease, a condition conventionally treated but not reversed with coronary artery bypass, angioplasty, and/or medications.

BOX 13–2
Birth of Modern Naturopathy

In 1896 Sebastian Kneipp sent 23-year-old Benedict Lust to New York City to disseminate the principles of water cure. A person of great vision, passion, and organizational skills, Lust taught this practice widely. Within 2 years, he had helped organize numerous Kneipp Societies throughout the United States and begun to publish a water-cure magazine. He opened a natural healing sanitarium, the Brooklyn Light and Water-Cure Institute, and created the first U.S. store to provide foods and materials for natural, drugless cures. It was aptly named Health Food Store.[1]

In the next few years Lust studied and became licensed in osteopathy and chiropractic, and in 1902 he opened the American School of Naturopathy in New York, the first naturopathic medical college. It grew quickly and by 1907 had moved to large quarters, housing a clinic, a hospital, and schools of chiropractic and massage. Tirelessly, he acquired degrees in homeopathy and eclectic medicine and received an MD license, all while teaching, writing, and publishing prolifically on naturopathic philosophy and therapy. He opened an estate-sized natural health sanitarium, Yungborn, in Butler, New Jersey, and later another in Florida. By 1918, Lust had organized the first professional national naturopathic organization, the American Naturopathic Association, and had published a 1400-page work, the *Universal Naturopathic Directory*, integrating the principles and practices of naturopathy.

Lust's program of naturopathic cure was based on three basic principles:

1. *Elimination of evil habits*, or the weeds of life, such as overeating; alcoholic drinks; drugs; tea, coffee, and cocoa, which contain poisons; meat; improper hours of living; waste of vital forces; lowered vitality; sexual and social aberrations; and worry
2. *Adoption of corrective habits*, such as correct breathing, correct exercise, the right mental attitude, and moderation in the pursuit of health and wealth
3. *Adoption of new principles of living*, such as proper fasting; proper selection of food; and use of hydropathy, light and air baths, mud baths, osteopathy, chiropractic and other forms of mechanotherapy, mineral salts obtained in organic form, electrotherapy, heliotherapy, steam or Turkish baths, and sitz baths[2]

Naturopathic medicine's lineage drew from the influences of water cure, nature cure, the hygienic movement, homeopathy, osteopathy, chiropractic, and the botanical medicine of the eclectic medical schools in the United States. These vitalistic traditions, all converging in the last years of the 19th century, afforded Lust and other early naturopathic pioneers the therapeutic tools and doctrinal perspectives to construct a profession that was based solely on holistic principles, broad in scope, and grounded in both nature and modern science.

Despite medicopolitical conflicts and harassment of naturopathic physicians in the first few decades of 20th century in the United States, the profession thrived. Numerous naturopathic medical colleges had produced a total of more than 10,000 physicians by the early 1920s. As the number of naturopathic practitioners increased, so did the attacks against them, primarily by the politically dominant medical profession and the American Medical Association (AMA). The influence of naturopathy and other vitalist professions diminished under this pressure. Only chiropractic emerged after World War II relatively unscathed. Osteopathy gave up many of its fundamental drugless therapies. Naturopathy, homeopathy, and eclectic medicine became seriously weakened as the number of professional schools decreased.

Several factors influenced this decline in the mid-20th century, including the increasing political clout of the AMA, which resulted in the passage of legislation that severely restrict the practice of alternative health care systems; the alliance of drug and chemical industries to support conventional medical schools; the discovery and popular appeal of so-called miracle drugs such as sulfa and antibiotics; the development of medical specialization and the cultivation of a mystique of authority; a cultural preoccupation with modernism and its accompanying technology; and the perception that natural, traditional medicines were "old fashioned" and not as effective as modern synthetic ones.[3]

By the mid-1960s, the number of naturopathic physicians in America had so declined that the survival of the profession was in question. There was only one 4-year, residential naturopathic medical school, the National College of Naturopathic Medicine, then in Seattle. But the convergence of several important societal changes began to have an influence. The ecology movement with its emphasis on living in harmony with nature, the women's rights movement's interest in self-care and empowerment,

continued

BOX 13–2 continued
Birth of Modern Naturopathy

and the 1960s value of questioning authority all combined with a growing realization of the limits of the conventional medical model to spur a rebirth of respect for and an interest in naturopathic medicine. Newly accredited naturopathic medical colleges were founded, and new licensing laws were passed in some states. In the last quarter of the 20th century, naturopathic medicine enjoyed a dramatic resurgence as awareness and utilization of holistic practices increasingly became integrated into mainstream American health care.

Although modern naturopathic medical training is based on the same model used originally by Lust, because naturopathic medicine is eclectic it has continued to evolve as new information and standards have evolved. It now incorporates the modern understanding of physiology, biochemistry, anatomy, microbiology, pathology, diagnostics, and the other basic and clinical sciences, as well as the educational standards expected of any program training doctors to function as primary care practitioners. Students entering the 4-year residential programs have at least an undergraduate degree, and many have advanced degrees. All students go through 2 or more years of supervised clinical training in general practice outpatient teaching clinics. Increasing numbers are going on to postgraduate residencies. As more integration with conventional medicine occurs, ever more students and residents are taking training in inpatient facilities.

A dark side of the growth in popularity of naturopathic medicine, and alternative medicine in general, is the proliferation of "ND" and other "doctoral" degrees by mail. It is clearly far below the standards of American higher education to offer a doctoral-level degree in health care through distance learning without rigorously supervised clinical training. But beyond failing to adhere to conventional educational standards, these programs are not accredited by federally recognized accrediting agencies, which means there is little accountability for the level of teaching or learning. Because naturopathic physicians are licensed only in 12 states, anyone can use the title in the other 38 states. As naturopathic medicine has gained more respect among the health-care community, media, and general public, the "ND" has become increasingly marketable. Without state regulation, these "mail-order doctors" may mislead the public as to their training (whether intentionally or not) and can create significant risk to the public's health.[4]

REFERENCES

1. Cody, G: History of naturopathic medicine. In Pizzorno, J, and Murray, M (eds): A Textbook of Natural Medicine. Bastyr College Publications, Seattle, 1985, p 1.
2. Ibid.
3. Ibid.
4. American Association of Naturopathic Physicians Website, *www.naturopathic.org*, 2000.

Naturopathic physicians frequently combine several treatments simultaneously, tailoring them to the specific needs of each patient. Treatment protocols vary from patient to patient, even when each may have the same named disease. These frequently complex protocols are based on the principle that treatments that complement each other and act through different mechanisms are likely to be more effective used together than any one of them used alone. Although testing of entire treatment protocols such as the Ornish program can be methodologically difficult, the benefits of such complex protocols may greatly exceed those of single-agent treatments.

Historically, most naturopathic physicians have chosen to be in clinical practice, with relatively few engaging in basic research. Since the mid-1980s, several naturopathic institutions and clinics have engaged in original research, stimulated by peer-reviewed naturopathic journals such as the *Journal of Naturopathic Medicine*. Topics range from the treatment of cervical cancer in situ by topical herbal preparations and nutrition intervention,[13] to clinical trials of hawthorn in the treatment of asthma,[14] to the study of a multifactorial naturopathic protocol in the treatment of HIV-infected men.[15]

Recently, a consortium of researchers at four naturopathic medical schools (National College of Naturopathic Medicine, Southwest College of Naturopathic Medicine, Cana-

BOX 13–3
The Vitalist Lineage

Maimonides (Rabbi Moshe ben Maimon, 1135–1204), Jewish legal scholar, philosopher, physician, and medical authority, stands out as visionary in the vitalist tradition. Centuries before the formal evolution of naturopathic medicine, he argued that, more important than drugs, the essential components of radiant health were diet, exercise, mental outlook, and respect for nature's laws. "The cause of most patient deaths is the treatment they receive from physicians who are ignorant of nature."[1] "The physician must keep in mind that the heart of every sick person is narrow and that every healthy person has an expanded soul. Therefore, the physician must remove emotional experiences that cause the shrinking of the soul. . . . One should select as attendants and caretakers those who can cheer up the patient. This is a must in every illness."[2]

Paracelsus (1493–1541), an iconoclastic physician and seeker of medical truth, implored doctors to rebel against unquestioned medical authority. In a famous act of defiance, he threw the widely accepted textbook of medieval medicine, the *Canon of Avicenna*, into a public bonfire in 1527. He sought to bring light to the neglected concept of nature's role in healing. "Nature is the physician, not you. From her you must learn, not from yourself; she compounds the remedies, not you."[3] While Paracelsus also introduced drugs derived from toxic metals such as arsenic and lead—drugs that were seriously abused by physicians in the 19th century—he nevertheless stands as a luminous point on the thread of vitalism that weaves its way through the history of Western medicine.

This thread of vitalism made its way through Europe, specifically through German-speaking countries, fully a century before it reached the Americas and was ardently articulated in the holistic practice of German physician, teacher, and writer Christoph Wilhelm Hufeland (1762–1836). In 1796, he published *The Art of Prolonging Human Life*, perhaps the first scientific work on holistic and preventive medicine and one of the most popular health books of the time. This book expresses most of the tenets embraced by a later generation of nature-cure doctors. Hufeland incorporated diet, exercise, emotional well-being, fasting, and other natural treatments that encourage the healing mechanisms of the body-mind. He spoke out against suppressing the natural healing reaction.

REFERENCES

1. Quoted in Greenbaum, A: The Wings of the Sun. Breslov Research Institute, Monsey, N.Y., 1995, p 40.
2. Quoted in Kirshfeld, F, and Boyle, W: The Nature Doctors: Pioneers in Naturopathic Medicine. Medicina Biologica, Portland, 1994, p 3.
3. Quoted in ibid, p 5.

dian College of Naturopathic Medicine, and Bastyr University) have embarked on a complex study around the question: What is the impact of 6 months of naturopathic care on a person's overall well-being? One intention of this consortium is to create new design models that faithfully respect naturopathic approaches to treatment while also scientifically testing the efficacy of a multifactorial approach to health care. (See Box 13–4.)

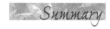 *Summary*

When practiced at its most fundamental level, naturopathic medicine attempts to address these questions:

- Do the practitioner, the patient, and the healing methods honor the universal laws of healing that are infinite, complex, and both precede and transcend human knowing?
- Who or what is being treated or healed?
- What and who are the agencies for healing?
- What are the underlying causes of the disease?
- What are the obstacles to healing?
- What is necessary to prevent the return of the disease and to minimize further disease?
- What constitutes the optimum possible health for this person?
- What are the least invasive yet the most effective methods of healing?

BOX 13-4
Case Study

Carole, a bright, hardworking 39-year-old journalist, tells her naturopathic physician of abdominal cramping, frequent loose bowel movements, and gas, a condition she has had since childhood but that now seems to be getting worse. Sometimes, Carole says, she is afraid to go to work in the morning for fear of being caught on the freeway without a restroom in sight. Her internist prescribed Imodium a year ago, but she said it did not help.

Carole has also been depressed for more than 2 years and often feels anxious for no particular reason. She has been taking Prozac, 20 to 30mg/day, for 2 years. A week before her monthly cycle begins, she also experiences extreme mood swings, bloating, and cramping in her lower abdomen. She takes Motrin to reduce the pain. Her cravings "go wild," she says. " I could eat a house if you put sugar on it."

Carole's lifestyle is a familiar story. Although her boss is kind and understanding, her job is filled with pressures. Working for a prestigious magazine, she wants to make the story right, fair, and on time. She works long hours with very few breaks. The coffee machine near her desk has become her constant companion, and she drinks five or more cups per day. She smokes about half a pack of cigarettes a day, and more as each deadline get closer.

Breakfast is usually a bagel with jam and coffee; lunch is at the local deli or on the run to an interview; dinner is at 8 or 9 PM—with a few glasses of wine to help her unwind. She exercises sporadically.

"I know my lifestyle is probably not helping any of these health problems," she says. "I feel like I'm stuck on a treadmill. If this is how I am at 39, what will my health be like when I'm 60 or 70 years old if I don't change something soon?"

Her naturopathic physician carefully notes Carole's entire health story, including physical, mental, and psychospiritual issues. She asks Carole about her family history of health problems, as well as physical and emotional traumas, and then details all the symptoms she would like help with. She reviews all medical records, medications, and nutritional supplements, as well as a 3-day diet record that Carole was requested to bring to the first visit.

The physician then gives her a complete physical exam, including a pelvic exam and a blood workup for a routine screening and for food allergies. Finally, Carole and her naturopathic doctor sit down to discuss the preliminary findings, the presumptive diagnoses, and the treatment strategy that will be followed in subsequent visits.

"It's likely that naturopathic methods can help relieve all your symptoms if you take an active part in the treatment," the doctor says, stressing dietary changes, exercise, stress-reduction techniques, and other self-initiated treatments. She explains that naturopathic medicine looks for a common thread or "center of gravity" that links symptoms to one another. There are usually multiple causes working together to produce disease states. By eliminating unhealthy lifestyle habits and other obstacles to health, and replacing symptom-suppressing treatments with medicines and treatments that support her innate healing processes, Carole will find that, over time, her symptoms will disappear or diminish and her level of vitality will increase. The naturopathic physician also explains to Carole that although one way of describing her health problems is to name them irritable bowel syndrome, depression, and premenstrual syndrome (PMS)—three seemingly separate conditions—there is a good deal of shared causality that can be addressed by treating the whole person.

The doctor explains that caffeine-sensitive people can experience anxiety, depression, bowel, and reproductive system problems. Food allergies and sensitivities can cause diarrhea and a host of other problems. Excess alcohol and sugar consumption can affect mood, blood-sugar levels, immune function, and the reproductive system, including PMS. Eliminating caffeine, alcohol, and sugar is the best way to assess the effects of these substances. The doctor says that Carole should notice a positive difference in 2 weeks. She also instructs Carole to perform a simple stress-reduction technique for 5 minutes twice a day, once at work and once in the evening before dinner. It consists of letting go of whatever worldly dramas are happening in the moment and progressively tensing and relaxing all the muscles and joints in her body, starting with her head.

Her doctor gives Carole an herbal and mineral formula composed of berberine (from Oregon grape root) and bismuth, both natural antimicrobials; Bentonite clay, which acts as a colloid to absorb endotoxins; licorice root extract, an anti-inflammatory to the digestive tract lining; and chamomile,

continued

BOX 13-4 continued

Case Study

rosemary, and peppermint extracts, which reduce spasms, pain, and gas in the digestive tract. Carole is also given betaine hydrochloric acid, a digestive aid that helps digest food proteins into smaller amino acid chains. Her doctor explains the long-term importance of healing the lining of the digestive tract, which can diminish future antigenic/allergic potential. Carole agrees to give all the recommendations a sincere try.

Two weeks later Carole returns to her naturopathic doctor. She is taking the supplements daily, has practiced the stress-reduction exercises every day at least once, and has reduced caffeine and alcohol consumption by about half. She no longer has intestinal urgency and cramping. "I also notice that the more alcohol I drink, the more depressed I get," she says. "And I am beginning to see that my body is tense most of the time, especially at work."

The food allergy test reveals possible strong sensitivities to milk, cheeses, wheat, rye, baker's yeast, strawberry, soybeans, cucumber, and dill. The other blood tests are normal except for moderately elevated triglyceride and low-density lipoprotein (LDL) cholesterol levels. "If we treat you as a whole person, they should improve as a side benefit," she says.

The naturopathic physician recommends a diet for Carole that (1) significantly reduces or eliminates foods she is allergic or sensitive to; (2) eliminates unhealthful refined, fatty, and excessively sweet foods; and (3) is high in healthy vegetables, fruits, nonallergenic beans and grains, fiber, and fish. Her doctor carefully explains a 4-day rotation diet chart based on her specific food allergies and known common food sensitivities. This diet will help her select foods and make changing her diet less daunting. They both agree that there is still a lot of work to do together and that it is not easy. "At least I see the tip of the iceberg," Carole says.

The doctor also gives Carole a high-potency, hypoallergenic multivitamin/mineral supplement and natural progesterone cream to apply to her skin for the PMS symptoms. Carole agrees to return in a few days for a series of five acupuncture treatments to help her stop smoking and reduce addictive cravings.

Two weeks later, at the end of the treatments, Carole is down to four cigarettes a day and has stopped drinking alcohol completely. She still drinks one cup of coffee to jump-start herself in the morning but has replaced the other caffeinated drinks with herb teas, water, soda water, and fruit juice. She has only partly changed her diet, but she has eliminated all the foods on her allergy list. She has experienced diarrhea only twice in 2 weeks and significantly less gas.

"The hardest part of the changes came during PMS time," she says. "I wasn't 100 percent sugar free, but this time I knew not to have any sweets in the house or at my desk. The emotional symptoms were greatly diminished. I braced myself for the usual cramps and pain, but they just came and left quickly and were really quite bearable."

Her doctor assures her that the modest positive changes she is experiencing are significant. Real progress toward health may take weeks, months, or even years for deep-seated conditions. "Don't worry if there is a temporary aggravation of symptoms," the doctor says. "Your progression to health should be viewed over the long run, not from one day to the next." Besides learning to take the initiative in effecting change, Carole is learning to view the road to wellness as a process rather than an isolated series of unrelated battles with symptoms.

Nine weeks after her initial evaluation, Carole returns to her naturopathic physician. She has tripped and fallen while carrying an armful of firewood and has pains in her neck and sacrum. After performing an orthopedic exam and taking an x-ray, the doctor concludes that there are no fractures but that there is structural malposition of the bones, swelling, and a mild periosteal bruise. After using ice packs, mild electrical interferential current, and gentle naturopathic manipulation, she instructs Carole to use simple hydrotherapy home treatments of ice packs on her lower back for the next day, then alternating hot and cold packs until the stiffness and pain are reduced. Carole is given two homeopathic medicines—arnica to treat the pain and swelling immediately and symphytum to be used 2 days later to hasten the bone healing.

Two weeks later Carole again sees her naturopathic doctor. By now there is barely any trace of injury. Her digestive symptoms are virtually gone unless she "cheats" for a day or two. "I feel so much better already," she says. "I have more energy, my depression and anxiety are gone. I'm down to one or two cigarettes a day. My last menstrual cycle came and went with only slight symptoms that were totally

continued

BOX 13-4 continued

Case Study

manageable. I feel I have so much more freedom than I've had for years. I am beginning to see that the choices I make everyday affect how I feel."

This is not the end of naturopathic care for Carole. There will be periodic visits with decreasing frequency as she becomes more stabilized, better informed, and more self-reliant in her health care. In time, Carole will return once or twice a year for wellness checkups. But, for now, she is on her way to a life journey of preventively oriented, self-directed natural health care.[1]

REFERENCE

1. Barton, S: Personal communication, adapted from patient case history, January 1998.

RESOURCES

The accrediting agency for naturopathic medical schools and programs in North America is the Council on Naturopathic Medical Education (CNME). The following are accredited schools:

Bastyr University
14500 Juanita Drive, NE
Kenmore, WA 98011
(425) 823-1300
Bastyr Natural Health Clinic: (206) 632-0354

National College of Naturopathic Medicine
049 SW Porter
Portland, OR 97201
(503) 499-4343
Clinic: (503) 255-7355

Southwest College of Naturopathic Medicine and Health Sciences
2140 East Broadway
Tempe, AZ 85282

Canadian College of Naturopathic Medicine
1255 Sheppard Avenue, E
North York, On M2K 1E2
(416) 498-1255

University of Bridgeport College of Natural Medicine
60 Lafayette Street
Bridgeport, CT 06601
(203) 576-4109
This university was granted candidacy status by the CNME on March 31, 2001 at their meeting in Tempe, Arizona.

For further information on accreditation, please contact the CNME at:
P.O. Box 11426
Eugene, OR 97440-3626
(541) 484-6028
www.cnme.org

The American Association of Naturopathic Physicians
8201 Greensboro Drive, Suite 300
McLean, VA 22102
(703) 610-9037
(703) 610-9005 fax
www.naturopathic.org
Founded in 1985, the American Association of Naturopathic Physicians (AANP) is the national professional society representing naturopathic physicians who are licensed or eligible for licensing as primary care providers.

References

1. American Association of Naturopathic Physicians: Definition of naturopathic medicine. AANP Quarterly Newsletter 4(4):22, 1989.
2. National College of Naturopathic Medicine: The profession, philosophy. NCNM Catalog, 1989–91, p 2.
3. Bradley, R: Philosophy of naturopathic medicine. In Pizzorno, J, and Murray, M (eds): A Textbook of Natural Medicine. Bastyr College Publications, Seattle, 1985, p 1.
4. Zeff, J: The process of healing: A unifying theory of natural medicine. Journal of Naturopathic Medicine 7(1):122, 1997.
5. Bradley: Philosophy of naturopathic medicine, p 1.
6. Coulter, H: Divided Legacy: A History of the Schism in Medical Thought (vol 3). Wehawken Book Co., Washington, D.C., 1975, p 8.
7. Kirshfeld, F, and Boyle, W: The Nature Doctors: Pioneers in Naturopathic Medicine. Medicina Biologica, Portland, 1994, p 2.
8. Zeff: The process of healing, p 123.
9. Bradley: Philosophy of naturopathic medicine, p 4.
10. American Association of Naturopathic Physicians: Safety, Effectiveness and Cost-Effectiveness in Naturopathic Medicine. American Association of Naturopathic Physicians, Seattle, 1991, p 5.
11. Bradley: Philosophy of naturopathic medicine, pp 7–9.
12. Ornish, D, et al: Intensive lifestyle changes for reversal of coronary artery disease. JAMA 280(23):2001, 1998.
13. Hudson, T: Consecutive case research of carcinoma in situ of cervix employing local escharotic treatment combined with nutritional therapy. Journal of Naturopathic Medicine 2(1):6, 1991.
14. Frances, D: Crataegus for asthma:case studies. Journal of Naturopathic Medicine 8(2):20, 1998.
15. Standish, L: One year open trial of naturopathic treatment of HIV infection class IV-A in men. Journal of Naturopathic Medicine 3(1):43, 1992.

CHAPTER 14

Homeopathic Medicine

Edward H. Chapman

Edward Chapman, MD, DHt, FAAFP, is board certified in family practice and homeopathy. After completing a 3-year family practice residency, he did a postgraduate fellowship in homeopathy. Since 1983 he has practiced classical homeopathy and family medicine in Newton, Massachusetts.

When Ritalin was first used in 1956 to treat hyperactivity in children, it was hailed as a miracle cure. How could a drug that produced a hyperkinetic, agitated state in most people help modify the same symptoms that accompany attention deficit/hyperactivity disorder?

For proponents of homeopathy, the phenomenon is easy to explain. Homeopathy is a system of therapy based on the observation that a medicine, when administered in very small doses, can cure the same symptoms in an ill person that it produces when given to healthy subjects. Colchicine treats gout when given in pharmaceutical doses, whereas it produces symptoms of gout when given in small doses. Digitalis can produce any arrhythmia it can cure; the differing effects depend on the dose.

Law of Similars

This correlation, known as the "law of similars," was articulated 200 years ago in Germany by Samuel Hahnemann,[1] the founder of homeopathy. The term itself reflects the meaning of the Greek words *omoios,* meaning "the same," and *pathos,* meaning "feeling." The Greek word *allios,* which means "other," is the root of the term *allopathy,* a label that Hahnemann used to describe conventional medical practices that oppose the symptom; for example, using drugs to reduce a fever or cortisone to eliminate a rash.

The homeopathic approach differs from conventional systems of treatment. Conventional medicine acts by such mechanisms as suppressing bodily responses or external disease agents (e.g., an anti-inflammatory or antibiotic); replacing substances that the body is failing to produce (e.g., hormones or insulin); or using small doses of the disease-producing agents to sensitize or desensitize the immune system (e.g., immunization or allergy desensitization). Instead, homeopathy relies on the inherent capacity of an organism to heal itself. The homeopathic medicine initiates the body's return to balance to bring about a healthier state of function using the minimum dose necessary. Homeopaths believe a person's symptoms are clues to workings of the body's homeostatic mechanisms and arise as a result of the whole organism's response to illness.

Homeopathic Treatment

Homeopathic therapy consists of finding a homeopathic medicine that, when given to a healthy person, produces symptoms that are similar to those of the ill person. Hahnemann believed that the medicine creates an artificial disease in the patient that is similar in character to the natural disease. As the body mobilizes its defenses to eliminate the artificial disease, the natural disease, because of its resemblance to the medicinal disease, is also extinguished. This phenomenon can be partially understood by the biological response to immunization or allergy desensitization. In homeopathy a medicinal substance and a disease are related by the similarity of the symptoms they produce.

The homeopathic medicine, or remedy, which stimulates the innate healing capacity of an organism, is person-specific rather than diagnosis-specific. In other words, the remedy given depends on the unique characteristics of the individual and how symptoms are experienced. One size does not fit all.

Once the desired response is initiated, the dose needs to be repeated only when further stimulation is required. Consequently, after a curative response following the dose, the patient may not require additional treatment for months. The dose of homeopathic medicines is so minute that the risk of serious side effects or allergic reactions is minimal. Relative to conventional drugs, the cost of homeopathic medicines is also minimal.

Homeopathy can be helpful in most diseases, but it is especially appropriate to consider as a therapy in a number of situations: when conventional therapy has had no or limited benefit, when the risk of conventional therapies is high (e.g., pregnancy), when side effects limit the usefulness of conventional medications, or when reduction of the dose of allopathic medications in the management of chronic conditions is desirable. Homeopathy also has an important role in the prevention of many common conditions and in the improvement of well-being.

Minimum Dose

Homeopathic medicines are usually manufactured from natural substances—mainly plants, minerals, and substances from animals—by homeopathic pharmaceutical companies according to standards established in *The Homoeopathic Pharmacopoeia of the United States*. A process unique to homeopathy is used. Each remedy is made from a single substance that is repeatedly diluted, mostly using alcohol and water as the solvent. At each dilution, the remedy is mechanically shaken, or succussed. This serial dilution and succussion are repeated until the desired level of dilution, or potency, is reached.

The remedies are then identified by the Latin name for the original substance. Examples of common remedies are belladonna (deadly nightshade), nux vomica (poison nut), calcarea carbonica (oyster shell), aurum metallicum (gold), apis mellifica (honeybee), and crotalus horridus (venom of the rattlesnake).

The two most common potency systems are the centesimal system, with a dilution ratio of 1 part solute to 99 parts solvent, and the decimal system, with a dilution ratio of 1:9. The centesimal potencies are labeled with a *C* and the decimal potencies with either an *X* or a *D*. As each homeopathic potency is produced, it receives a number corresponding to the number of dilutions. For example, the first dilution of a remedy made with the centesimal system is labeled with the name of the medicine followed by the designation "1C." A common potency is 30C. This has been serially diluted and succussed 30 times using a 1:99 ratio with each consecutive dilution.

Potencies 12C and 30X and below are generally considered low potencies and are often given in repeated daily doses. These are generally suitable for use in unsupervised lay self-care. Whereas 30C to 200C are medium potencies, potencies above that considered high. A 1000C potency is labeled "1M." The higher the potency, the less frequently the dose is repeated. (See Box 14–1.)

Because there is not a well-understood mechanism explaining homeopathy, the dilution and succussion process for manufacturing homeopathic medicines is at the center of the debate around its efficacy. Homeopathy's critics say that based on conventional pharmaceutical principles, the medicines are too dilute to be more than placebo. Homeopaths point to the many clinical, in vivo, and in vitro studies, its 200 years of practice, and new basic science research illuminating high-dilution physiology and physics as counterarguments.

The most popular current theory suggesting a mechanism for homeopathy is the "memory of water." This theory proposes that through the process of serial dilution and succussion, "information" contained in the original solute is transferred to the solvent. This information is retained despite further dilutions beyond the point at which molecules of the original substance can be measured. It is then transferred to the organism by the homeopathic medicine. The way this occurs may be explained by recent research[2,3] demonstrating the existence of structures in water called IE crystals. These crystals have been found to act as catalysts in a variety of systems, such as the enhancement of the efficiency of combustion of gasoline[4] and the production of cytokines by white blood cells.[5] IE crystals are only maintained in solutions that have been diluted and then mechanically agitated. The properties of IE crystals meet most of the criteria necessary to explain the observed effects of homeopathic remedies.

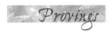

Provings

Homeopaths determine the range of conditions that each homeopathic medicine can heal through toxicological data, information gained in homeopathic drug provings (HDPs), and clinical experience. Pharmacologic and toxicological data, as well as information about the traditional use of medicinal substances in indigenous healing systems, often provide an initial idea of the scope of a homeopathic remedy. Provings test a single substance by administering it in a homeopathic potency, usually the 30C, in a controlled clinical trial to a group of healthy volunteers, or provers. The recorded symptoms the provers developed in response to the substance being proven form the basic symptom picture of that medicine. The full expression of each remedy is completed by adding to it the symptoms that are cured by the homeopathic medicine in clinical cases.

These remedy pictures are living, breathing portraits unique to each medicine, in the same way that each person is unique. They are recorded in reference books called homeopathic "materia medica." Most materia medica place each homeopathic remedy in a separate chapter listed alphabetically, and then in each chapter are found the symptoms associated with that remedy organized according to anatomical structure, such as mind, head, eye, and so forth.

The homeopath seeks to understand the patient's suffering on all levels. Along with the physical signs and symptoms, sensations and disturbances of feeling and thinking are considered. The recognition of symptom clusters in patients that correspond to known pathogenetic patterns of the homeopathic medicines allows for the application of the law of similars.

For instance, the medicine belladonna, the active ingredient of which is atropine, produces signs of cholinergic stimulation: lack of perspiration, flushing and heat of the skin, dilation of the pupils, and visual hallucinations. Provers of belladonna also develop throbbing pains, usually right-sided, which come on suddenly and are associated with agitation. These symptoms and signs are very similar to those that a healthy young child

BOX 14–1
History of Homeopathy

The law of similars—*similia similibus curentur*, or "like cures like,"—was first articulated in 1796 by Samuel Hahnemann, a German physician. He described his observations and discussed this system of healing in the *Organon of the Medical Art*, first published in 1810.[1] The text was printed in six editions over the balance of his career—the last time in 1842, the year before his death.

Hahnemann also discovered that by serially diluting and succussing (vigorously shaking) medicines, one could increase the therapeutic efficacy while limiting the adverse effects of larger doses. Additionally, he developed protocols for testing new medicines on healthy volunteers, whom he called "homeopathic drug provings."

Minute doses of medicines were given in repeated doses to healthy subjects. The symptoms that provers developed were recorded and published between 1825 and 1833 in the six volumes of *Materia Medica Pura*.[2] Through these experiments, he expanded the number of medicinal agents used in the homeopathic treatment of chronic and acute illnesses.

Hahnemann gathered around him a committed group of disciples who assisted and continued his work. Some of these students immigrated to the Americas, where homeopathy flourished throughout the rest of the 19th century.[3]

Hans Graham was the first homeopathic physician to come from Europe to the United States (in 1825). His arrival was soon followed by that of Constantine Hering, who in 1844 helped to found the America Institute of Homeopathy (AIH) to promote the practice of homeopathy by the medical profession. The AIH is the oldest national medical organization, founded 2 years before the American Medical Association, and continues to represent the interests of homeopathic physicians to government and the public.

During the 20th century, many of the original provings of Hahnemann and his disciples were repeated and new substances were also tested. These provings, together with toxicological and clinical observations of the medicines' effects, were compiled in "materia medicas." The most famous of these are *The Encyclopedia of Pure Materia Medica*[4] and *Guiding Symptoms*[5], both of which are used daily by modern homeopaths.

James Tyler Kent authored *Lectures on Homeopathic Philosophy*,[6] *Lectures on Homeopathic Materia Medica*,[7] and *Kent's General Repertory*.[8] *Kent's Repertory*, an index of the symptoms contained in various materia medica, changed the way homeopathy was practiced. Kent's format for indexing the materia medica forms the basis for computerized repertorization systems developed in the last 20 years.

A contentious relationship existed between homeopathic and allopathic physicians during the 19th century. The code of ethics of the American Medical Association, founded 2 years after the AIH in 1846, was designed to prevent medical practitioners from associating with homeopaths:

> No one can be a regular practitioner, or fit associate in consultation, whose practice is based on an exclusive dogma, to the rejection of the accumulated experience of the profession, and of the aids actually furnished by anatomy, physiology, pathology, and organic chemistry.[9]

By 1900, 8 percent of American physicians had incorporated homeopathy into their practices, there were 20 homeopathic medical schools,[10] including Boston University, Hahnemann Medical School, New York Medical, and the University of Michigan. With the changes in medical education catalyzed by the Flexner Report in 1910 and the discovery of antimicrobials, the popularity of homeopathy declined steeply. The homeopathic schools either closed or, to maintain government funding and attract students, converted to the conventional medical paradigm espoused by the authors of the Flexner Report. The Hahnemann Medical School issued its final homeopathic diploma in 1950. By the 1960s, only a handful of medical doctors were practicing homeopathy in the United States. However, the presence of an enthusiastic lay population, self-prescribing over-the-counter (OTC) homeopathic products, kept the American homeopathic pharmaceutical industry alive.

Although the demise of homeopathic medical schools in the United States left a vacuum in homeopathic education and research, homeopathy continued to flourish in Europe, India, Mexico, Argentina, and Brazil. In the educational and political vacuum left in the United States by the decline of the homeopathic medical physicians, the homeopathic community greatly expanded to include other types of health-care professionals. The community of homeopaths now includes naturopathic, osteopathic, and chiropractic physicians; physician assistants; nurse-practitioners; and other regulated

continued

BOX 14–1 continued

History of Homeopathy

health-care professionals. There is also a growing class of homeopaths, called "lay" or "professional" homeopaths, who are trained exclusively in homeopathy and do not have credentials in other health-care professions.

Since the 1970s, there has been a resurgence of the public's interest in homeopathy, prompted by the widespread experience of the limitations of the present medical model: high costs, adverse side effects, lack of a personal relationship with the provider, and ineffectiveness in treating many chronic and acute conditions. Currently an estimated 500 homeopathic medical physicians practice in the United States, and many more use homeopathy on a limited basis.[11] Extrapolation of data reported in January 1993 in the *New England Journal of Medicine*[12] suggested that 2.5 million Americans used homeopathic medicines; of these, about one-third actually visited homeopaths of one type or another in 1990. The 1970s also saw a resurgence of interest by health-care professionals in homeopathy, and since the 1980s sales of homeopathic medicines, 85 percent of them OTC,[13] increased by an average of 20 percent a year.

REFERENCES

1. Hahnemann, S: Organon of the Medical Art (WB O'Reilly, ed). Birdcage Books, Redmond, Wash., 1996.
2. Hahnemann, S: Materia Medica Pura (RE Dudgeon, trans; vols. I and II). Jain Publishing Co., New Delhi, India, 1980.
3. Coulter, HL: Divided Legacy: A History of the Schism in Medical Thought: vol III. Science and Ethics in American Medicine: 1800–1914. McGrath Publishing Co., Washington, D.C., 1973.
4. Allen, TF: The Encyclopedia of Pure Materia Medica, A Record of the Positive Effects of Drugs upon Healthy Human Organism (Indian edition, 12 vols). B. Jain Publishers, New Delhi, India, 1982.
5. Hering, C: The Guiding Symptoms of Our Materia Medica (Indian edition; 10 vols). B. Jain Publishers, New Delhi, India, 1972.
6. Kent, JT: Lectures on Homeopathic Philosophy. Ehrhart & Karl, Chicago, 1929.
7. Kent, JT: Lectures on Homeopathic Materia Medica, ed. 4. Boericke & Tafel, Philadelphia, 1956.
8. Kent, JT: Kent's Repertorium Generale (K von Fimmelsberg, ed). Barthel & Barthel Publishing, Berg, Germany, 1987.
9. Ernst, E, and Kaptchuk, T: Homeopathy revisited. Archives of Internal Medicine 159:2162–2164, 1996.
10. Rothstein, WG: American Physicians in the 19th Century. Johns Hopkins University Press, Baltimore, 1984.
11. Berman, B, et al: Homeopathy and the U.S. primary care physician. British Homeopathic Journal 86:131–138, 1997.
12. Eisenberg et al: Unconventional medicine in the United States. N Engl J Med 328(4):246–353, 1993.
13. Borneman, JP: Homeopathy in the United States and Canada: An analysis of the self-medication market for homeopathic drugs. In Improving the Success of Homeopathy, 23 Jan 97, Royal London Homeopathic Hospital, NHS, 82-89.

might experience with an acute febrile illness or an adult might experience with a cluster headache. Belladonna is frequently prescribed for people with these conditions.

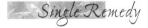 *Single Remedy*

Homeopathic medicine is fundamentally holistic because each organism is seen as responding to an illness as a whole entity, not as separate parts. Therefore, a single remedy is sought for the whole person. One remedy is found that most closely matches, or is similar to, all the symptoms as well as the physical, mental, and emotional characteristics of the patient.

This can be a difficult task even for the trained homeopath, and sometimes people use shortcuts to make it easier. Combination remedies are such a popular shortcut. These combine many remedies that could be helpful for a particular condition into one remedy labeled with that condition. An example would be a remedy labeled "influenza" made up of 6 to 12 individual remedies, where each of the remedies may have the potential of treating one of the different expressions of influenza. This is rarely as effective as giving the correctly matched remedy but is much easier for an untrained person. Combination remedies are generally considered safe to use for acute conditions that are by their nature self-limiting, but most professional homeopaths do not suggest using them for chronic conditions.

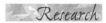 Research

Evidence for the efficacy of homeopathic medicines comes from a number of sources, including epidemiological, clinical, and basic science studies. Eisenberg[6] estimated that 1 percent of Americans used homeopathy in 1991 and that 30 percent of these saw homeopathic providers. Berman surveyed American primary care physicians and found that 13.8 percent refer, 15.9 percent use, and 49 percent want training in homeopathy.[7] According to the homeopathic pharmaceutical industry, sales of homeopathic medicines are increasing by 20 percent a year.[8] A survey of homeopathic use in the Los Angeles area from 1994 to1995 described the population seeking homeopathic services as predominately white, well educated, female, and in fair to good health.[9] Subjects indicated that they were seeking care for more than one medical problem, most of which were chronic and for which they had already attempted conventional treatment. After 4 months of homeopathic treatment, 70 percent reported improvement and 18 percent complete resolution of their complaints; 60 percent had improvement in general health status markers.

Research has demonstrated the activity of serially agitated dilutions (SADs) beyond Avogadro's number[10–23] in a variety of biological systems. Many of the significant experiments are reviewed in three recent publications.[24–26] A meta-analysis of 135 experiments in toxicology found that 80 percent of the experiments showed positive outcomes, with an average 20 percent greater protection effect in SAD-treated animals than placebo-treated ones. For example, mice were pretreated with a SAD derived from the hearts and livers of mice that had died from tularemia, a fatal disease in mice. The treated mice were then exposed to tularemia organisms. Twenty percent of the mice survived. In 1988, *Nature* published a report by Benveniste in which human basophils were shown to degranulate when exposed to antiserum agents IgE at dilutions of $10:120$.[27] The accompanying editorial[28] summarized the incredulity of the scientific community to these findings, which suggest that solutions containing no molecules can affect biological systems.[29–31]

Despite this disbelief, Benventiste's findings have been independently replicated.[32] The principle of restraint that applies is simple: when an unexpected observation requires that a substantial portion of our intellectual heritage should be thrown out, it is prudent to ask whether the observation is correct.[33]

The lack of a plausible mechanism of action for homeopathic medicines underlies the skepticism of modern scientists toward homeopathy. Lo's discovery, arising from research in catalyst chemistry, may contribute to illuminating this gap.[34,35] He discovered that agitated and diluted solutions contain 3 nm IE crystals composed of aggregated water molecules formed in response to the electrostatic forces around individual ions. At dilutions of $10:7$, these aggregates become self-replicating and increasingly stable; at dilutions of $10:16$ the IE crystals may compose almost 4 percent of the solution. Stable over a wide range of pH and temperature, they can be measured using ultraviolet (UV) spectroscopy, electron microscopy, and atomic phase microscopy. The physical characteristics of the aggregates appear to be dependent on the characteristics of the initial solute. It could be surmised that the serially agitated and diluted antiserum in Benveniste's experiments contained IE crystals capable of triggering the cell surface receptors on the basophils, resulting in degranulation. Studies in biological systems to test hypotheses for the action of these structures are in progress.

Research on homeopathy's clinical efficacy has increased in the last decade. High-quality, peer-reviewed, controlled clinical trials have suggested efficacy in diarrhea,[36] asthma,[37] seasonal rhinitis,[38] mild head trauma,[39] otitis media,[40,41] fibrositis,[42] migraine,[43] and other conditions. Three meta-analyses of a number of research studies[44-46] of homeopathic clinical trials have similarly concluded that the activity of homeopathic potencies cannot be explained by placebo; but that the lack of large-scale, independently replicated trials limits the conclusions that can be inferred from single studies. Two attempts to replicate the trial in migraine have failed to find effects for homeopathy.[47,48]

The creation of the Office of Alternative Medicine (OAM) at the National Institutes of Health in 1992 marked the first time federal funding became available for research into any alternative therapies. To date, the only federally funded clinical trial in homeopathy was in mild traumatic brain injury.[49] The OAM's current budget of $12 million is insufficient to fund large controlled trials. The OAM has provided an invaluable service by legitimizing the links between academic institutions and alternative medicine providers. As a consequence, a number of high-quality research efforts are underway in the United States.

Clinical Example

Mild traumatic brain injury (MTBI) is a traumatically induced condition that affects about a million people a year in the United States. Five to fifteen percent of them have persistent physical, emotional, or cognitive deficits that persist beyond 3 months; spontaneous recovery after 6 months is unusual. There is no pharmacologic treatment that affects the breadth of the disorder. Rather, clinicians must utilize rehabilitation techniques to develop coping strategies together with polypharmacy to address the multiple complaints. The positive effects of medications used for pain, vertigo, anxiety, or depression are frequently limited by side effects that further impair cognitive functioning.

The outcome of a study of the homeopathic treatment of MTBI documented statistically significant improvements in subjects' symptoms and functioning in life situations.[50] No significant side effects of homeopathic medicines were noted. Larger-scale, independently replicated studies are needed to confirm the findings of this pilot study. The following case of a subject in the treatment group of this study is presented to exemplify the homeopathic prescribing process.

A CASE OF MTBI

A 32-year-old woman, Rose, entered the study 2½ years after suffering a head-on automobile accident in which she lost consciousness for several minutes and fractured her knees, cervical spine, clavicle, shoulder, and ribs, resulting in a 4-week hospitalization. Her intelligence was affected and she lost many skills, preventing her from continuing gainful employment.

Prior to the accident, she was employed in desktop publishing. After her MTBI, she could not remember how to turn on the computer. Her math skills were severely affected; she was unable to conceptualize 3 inches and no longer knew the multiplication tables. When she was writing, her hand would tremble. Her concentration and short-term memory were poor. She could not think at the same time that she spoke.

Nine months after her accident, she had a psychiatric admission. She was at an auction and suddenly became catatonic. She was not frightened, just blank, like a zombie. For 3 months afterwards, she needed a baby-sitter. After a second accident, she experienced flashbacks of the original accident, accompanied by panic attacks, and was again hospitalized. This prompted her husband to call a meeting of her nine doctors and arrange for her transfer to a regional inpatient pain treatment center.

She slept 19 hours a day for a year after the accident. The sleepiness, imbalance, and tremor she felt were caused by medication, including amitriptyline, Xanax, Klonopin, Prozac, and Stadol nasal spray prescribed to manage problems with mood and pain. She was weaned from these medications at the inpatient pain treatment center. At enrollment she was taking no medications for MTBI but was on oral contraceptives and urinary tract infection prophylaxis with Bactrim and Nitrofurantoin, as well as vitamins.

She feared driving in a car. She had frightening dreams. She feared taking drugs. She was startled by sudden noise. She felt chillier and had night sweats. Her sex drive disappeared. She experienced left-sided headaches secondary to neck injury. Moving her eyes caused pain. Her head felt as though it would explode, made worse by excitement, stress, stooping (she blacks out and can hear rushing in neck), noise, light, and the odor of perfumes and smoke as well as paint fumes, but made better by relaxation and quiet.

She had back pain; her legs got numb while sitting. The sound of a voice irritated her. She experienced a driven feeling—things must be done now. She felt impatient when things got out of order. Everything had to be on time. Prior to the accident, she had been happy-go-lucky and friendly. She didn't like to spoil others' fun, so didn't say a lot about her symptoms. Only close friends knew.

Assessment. Rose is a woman who sustained a MTBI. She is in an oversensitive state that appeared after being overmedicated. Her headaches and mental state are made worse by stimulation of all kinds. She is impatient, intolerant, and chillier than usual.

The process of a homeopathic prescription involves translating the patient's expressions of disease into language that can be used to identify the appropriate homeopathic remedy. Two primary resources are utilized: (1) the materia medica, listing the medicines and their respective characteristics, and (2) the repertory,[51] indexing the symptoms, or rubrics, and organized anatomically. Each rubric is associated with a list of homeopathic medicines that have been linked with that symptom. The materia medica and repertory both contain approximately the same information but organized in a complementary manner. A repertorization allows the homeopath to tabulate the patient's symptoms and identify which remedies are best associated with these symptoms and might be appropriate for the specific patient. The details of the remedies are then studied in the materia medica, and a prescription is made.

The following rubrics were chosen to represent her symptoms (numbers in parentheses indicate the number of remedies in the rubric):

MIND; IMPATIENCE (138)
MIND; HURRY, haste; tendency (138)
MIND; STARING, thoughtless (17)
MIND; MEMORY; weakness, loss of; mental exertion; from (14)
MIND; MEMORY; weakness, loss of; words, for (64)
MIND; MISTAKES, makes; calculating, in (21)
MIND; MEMORY; weakness, loss of; say, for what he is about to (41)
HEAD PAIN; GENERAL; injuries, after mechanical (24)
HEAD PAIN; GENERAL; noise, from (98)
HEAD PAIN; GENERAL; excitement of the emotions, after (58)
HEAD PAIN; GENERAL; odors; strong, from (22)
HEAD PAIN; GENERAL; stooping; from (140)
HEAD PAIN; LOCALIZATION; sides; left (197)

BLADDER; INFLAMMATION; chronic (53)
GENERALITIES; MEDICAMENTS, allopathic medicine; oversensitive to (18)
EXTREMITIES; NUMBNESS, insensibility; lower limbs; sitting; while (22)
GENERALITIES; INJURIES, blows, falls and bruises; concussion; actual or tendency (61)

When these symptoms are graphed against the remedies included under each rubric, the graph shown in Figure 14–1 is generated.

The study of the materia medica leads to the prescription of the most similar remedy for the case. One must match not only specific symptoms but also the characteristic state that is represented by these symptoms. The materia medica description of the remedy nux vomica has a marked similarity to the essence of the case presented.[52]

Nux Vomica

Nux vomica is frequently the first remedy indicated for patients with a history of using many medicines and/or stimulants. It helps to re-establish equilibrium and counteracts the chronic effects of the drug use. Nux vomica is pre-eminently the remedy for many of the conditions incident to modern life.

FIGURE 14-1

A "repertorization" allows the homeopathic physician to tabulate the patient's symptoms and identify which remedies are best associated with these symptoms and would be most appropriate for the individual patient.

	Sulph.	Nux-v.	Puls.	Nat-m.	Sil.	Calc.	Bell.	Lyc.	Lach.
Total	29	28	23	22	21	20	20	19	19
Rubrics	14	13	12	11	12	12	9	14	11
Family									
MIND; IMPATIENCE (138)	3	3	2	2	3	2	1	2	2
MIND; HURRY, haste; tendency (138)	3	2	2	3	3	1	2	1	2
MIND; STARING, thoughtless (17)			2						
MIND; MEMORY; weakness, loss of; mental exertion; from (14)	3	3	1	2	2	2			2
MIND; MEMORY; weakness, loss of; words, for (64)	2	2	1	2	1	1		2	2
MIND; MISTAKES, makes; calculating, in (21)		2				1		2	1
MIND; MEMORY; weakness, loss of; say, for what he is about to (41)	2			2				1	
HEAD PAIN; GENERAL; injuries, after mechanical (24)	1		1	2		1	2		1
HEAD PAIN; GENERAL; noise, from (98)		2		1	2	3	4	1	2
HEAD PAIN; GENERAL; excitement of the emotions, after (58)	1	3	3	3	1	2	2	2	2
HEAD PAIN; GENERAL; odors; strong, from (22)	2	1			2		2	2	
HEAD PAIN; GENERAL; stooping; from (140)	3	2	3	2	2	2	3	1	1
HEAD PAIN; LOCALIZATION: Sides; left (197)	2	2	1	1	1	2	2	1	2
BLADDER; INFLAMMATION; chronic (53)	2		2					1	
NUMBNESS, insensibility; Lower Limbs; sitting; while (22)	1	1			1	1		1	
INJURIES, blows, falls and bruises; concussion; actual or tendency (61)	1	2	2	2	2	2	2	1	2
MEDICAMENTS, allopathic medicine; oversensitive to (18)	3	3	3		1			1	

Typical patients who need nux vomica are rather thin, spare, quick, active, nervous, and irritable. They do a good deal of mental work and have mental strains that lead to use of stimulants, coffee, wine—possibly in excess—and rich and stimulating food; a thick head, dyspepsia, and an irritable temper are the next day's inheritance. These conditions produce an irritable nervous system, hypersensitive and overimpressionable, which nux vomica will do much to soothe and calm. These patients may also have convulsions and periods of unconsciousness; they are aggravated by touch and movement; and they are easily chilled, often avoiding fresh air. Nux vomica patients always seems to be out of tune—with inharmonious spasmodic action; a tense contracted feeling; bruised soreness of the abdomen, brain, and so forth; contractive pains throughout the body; and a generally bruised feeling in the morning in bed. They may have great debility and oversensitiveness of all the senses—with everything making too strong an impression, with stitches and jerks throughout the whole body, and with trembling all over, although mostly in the hands, especially in the morning and among those who drink too much.

Plan. The similarity of this portrait to the patient's case, together with the matching of most of the specific symptoms displayed in Figure 14–1, led to the prescription of nux vomica 200C/day for 7 days.

One-month follow-up. The improvement was fairly sudden. Rose felt better, and her mind was working again; she stated she could remember things more. She felt ready to try to work at a computer and had bought one 2 weeks earlier. She could read manuals and follow directions. Her husband commented that she was sharper across the board. She had not tried to do math and still had difficulty conceptualizing 3 inches.

Her general energy level was changed; she could go all day long, from 8 AM to 3:30 PM nonstop, on the computer. She was tired by evening and went to bed early. Her headaches were better, coming on after concentrating for 2 days or excitement. Back pain had gotten worse after the remedy, peaking the same week she took it, but had gradually improved since. When asked about her irritability, she replied that she was in a better mood and felt more useful, but the driven feeling was still there. She suffered from sleeplessness. Her sexual desire remained the same. Doing two things a once was still hard. Chilliness was still there. Her ability to initiate activity was the same.

Assessment. She rated her improvements in three areas (on a scale of 10 to 0, poor to good) as (1) cognitive: from 10 to 4 and continuing to improve; (2) physical: from 10 to 8, continuing to have back pain; and (3) emotional: from 10 to 0. She said her sense of usefulness had returned. There was a clear and dramatic improvement in her state.

Plan. Do nothing. Homeopathic medicines act as catalysts and do not need repetition unless the remedy reaction ceases. Rose was asked to call if she relapsed or stopped improving.

Two-month follow-up. She had a mild relapse of her symptoms 2 weeks after the visit and repeated the nux vomica 200C in water for 3 days, after which she continued to improve.

Three-month follow-up. She had to repeat the nux vomica in water several times, with minimal improvement. Her energy level was lower and she had fewer useful hours in the day. She was working 3 days a week for 5 to 6 hours a day. Memory remained an issue; she could not remember to take her oral contraceptive or antibiotic. She had an unpleasant dream of a friend having a heart attack, and she didn't know what to do;

someone else was drowning. She had drenching night sweats at 1 or 2 AM. She felt hot, especially her chest and thighs, and radiated heat when asleep. She would leave the window open. Her moods were more stable; she felt less cranky, agitated, and frustrated. She was craving fat, pizza, hot spices, and creamy foods.

Assessment. She was better but had reached the maximum benefit from the 200C potency of nux vomica. The driven feeling and dreams of fatal accidents are characteristic of nux vomica. In routine circumstances the potency would be increased to nux vomica 1000C (1M); but in the study protocol only the 200C potency was available. Some fundamental shifts in her state had begun to appear: body warmth, desire for spices, and an increase of her night sweats. The warmer body temperature was a return of a state normal for her prior to the accident.

Plan. In the absence of a higher potency of nux vomica, she was given the complementary remedy sulphur 200C/day for 7 days.

Four-month follow-up. She felt excellent and was back at work, on her own schedule, building up slowly, now averaging 20 hours per week. After taking the second remedy, she developed intense headaches; she repeated nux vomica 200C in water and then gradually improved. In general she felt great. She had to go to bed by 9:30 PM, and usually awoke on weekdays at 6:30 AM with an alarm and on weekends at 8 AM. She was still waking at around 1 or 2 AM with night sweats. She still had nightmares. Her bladder was stable, and she planned to speak her primary care doctor the next week about going off antibiotics. The disks in her back felt swollen in wet weather. A bad cold and possible pneumonia resolved; she used echinacea. Her short-term memory was still limited.

Assessment. She was better. She had an initial aggravation by the sulphur, during which time she took nux vomica. It was unclear whether the subsequent improvement was due to repeating the nux vomica.

Plan. She was terminated from the study after the prescribed 4-month treatment period and referred to a local homeopathic physician for follow-up. She will need a higher potency of nux vomica and then possibly sulphur, if indicated, but starting with a lower potency. Herbal support for her urinary tract infection might allow her to discontinue the antibiotics, which could be interfering with the homeopathic medicine.

This case illustrates the classical homeopathic method, which matches the symptoms of homeopathic medicines collected from provings and cured clinical cases to the total symptom picture of the sick person. The relevant symptoms relate to the mental, emotional, physical, and general symptoms of the person. The medical diagnosis is secondary in importance to the actual symptoms, which represent clues to the individuality of the person.

The process of case taking, repertorization, and materia medica study leads to the prescription of a single remedy that acts as a catalyst to stimulate a curative response, bringing about healing at all levels in the organism. Along with the homeopath's observation of changes in symptoms and signs, judgments about improvement include how the patient feels as a whole and functions according to his or her own individual standards.

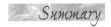

Summary

Homeopathy has been adapted for use across the spectrum of medical care, from medical and veterinary professionals to consumers in their own self-care. Despite its growing popularity and accumulating clinical evidence for its efficacy, homeopathic medicine engenders more skepticism among scientific minds than most other alternative/complementary therapies. Homeopathy's basic principles—the law of similars and the minimum dose—are radical concepts for the conventional scientific mind to accept, but the absence of a plausible mechanism of action is the source of the major controversy limiting the acceptance of homeopathy.

Advances in the understanding of cellular physiology and of water and catalyst chemistry promise to shed light on mechanisms by which homeopathic medicines affect biological systems and add scientific credibility to observed clinical outcomes.

Homeopathy offers a vehicle for a transforming medical practice grounded in the biomolecular model,[53] which identifies and treats lesions, disease agents, and pathology with surgery and bioengineered molecules, to a complexity model,[54] which emphasizes homeostasis, autoregulation, host responses, information, communication, and function.

The biomolecular model assumes we can find the cause of a disease and fix it as if it existed in isolation from the whole organism and the environment in which that organism lives. The model works well in surgically amenable conditions, for acute infectious diseases, and for medical emergencies treated in the intensive care unit. In that world the randomized, placebo-controlled clinical trial (RCT) is the gold standard for determining efficacy of a treatment. Today, however, health practitioners are being forced to consider other models because of (1) the limitation of this approach in dealing with chronic disease, (2) the issue of the clinical significance of the effects measured by RCTs, and (3) the economic burden placed on our society by a medical-industrial complex built on these assumptions.

The evolving paradigm of evidence-based medicine is taking root.[55] This approach recognizes that we have incomplete knowledge of most medical conditions and must do our best to treat them within our current limits. Beginning with a clinical problem, the physician must research databases for clinical information, appraise evidence for validity and usefulness, and then implement a treatment plan into daily practice. It is quite reasonable to use an evidence-based approach that incorporates homeopathy and other alternative modalities in clinical situations when there is no effective allopathic treatment, when conventional treatment is too risky, when side effects limit drug use, when there is a need to reduce the economic and personal burden of conventional therapies, or when prevention of chronic disease is paramount.

Homeopathy is not magic; in the hands of a trained professional it is an effective method, applied using time-tested principles and medicines produced by standardized techniques. Despite 200 years of experience, homeopathy is in its infancy. The revival of homeopathy since the 1970s is being fostered by computers, which have made the search of the homeopathic database into a rapid and flexible process. This development has made homeopathy accessible to contemporary medical practice. It can be used by homeopathic specialists in the treatment of chronic diseases, by primary care practitioners as a complement to the medical management of common acute and chronic illness, and by consumers in self-care. Homeopathy offers a safe, effective, low-cost alternative that is welcome in the current environment of scarce health-care resources.

Homeopathy's growing popularity among consumers reflects their dissatisfaction with the efficiency-based, impersonal, and technologically dependent practices of the dominant medical paradigm. People who seek to be seen and understood as individuals, to take responsibility for their own health through self-care, and to have an active relationship with their health-care provider will be attracted to homeopathy. A combination of consumer demand and a mosaic of evidence,[56] based on clinical outcomes and cost-efficacy studies, will gradually increase the inclusion of homeopathy into mainstream medicine.

RESOURCES

American Homeopathic Pharmaceutical Association
Box 174
Newtown, PA 19073
(610) 325-7464
Information on manufacturing and distribution of homeopathic medicines.

Council for Homeopathic Education
801 N. Fairfax St., Suite 306
Alexandria, VA 22314
Phone: (703) 548-7790
Fax: (703) 548-7792
Accreditation of homeopathic education programs.

Homeopathic Educational Services
2124 Kittredge St.
Berkeley, CA 94794
(510) 649-0294

Minimum Price Homeopathic Books
P.O. Box 2187
Blaine, WA 98231
(800) 663-8272

National Center for Homeopathy
801 N. Fairfax St., Suite 306
Alexandria, VA 22314
Phone: (703) 548-7790
Fax: (703) 548-7792
Information on homeopathy.

REFERENCES

1. Hahnemann, S: Organon of the Medical Art (WB O'Reilly, ed). Birdcage Books, Redmond, Wash., 1996.
2. Lo, SY: Anomalous state of ice. Modern Physics Letters B 10(19):909–910, 1996.
3. Lo, SY: Physical properties of water with IE structures. Modern Physics Letters B 10(19):921–930, 1996.
4. Bonavida, B: Induction and regulation of human peripheral blood TH1-TH2 derived cytokines by IE water preparations and synergy with mitogens. Proceeding of the First International Symposium of the Physical, Chemical and Biological Properties of IE Clusters, 1997, 4–6. *http://www.atcg.com/randd/workshop.html* (accessed April 29, 1998).
5. Sinitsyn, AP: Effect of IE solutions on enzymes and microbial cells. Proceedings of the First International Symposium of the Physical, Chemical and Biological Properties of IE Clusters, 1997, 6–7. *http://www.atcg.com/randd/workshop.html* (accessed April 29, 1998).
6. Eisenberg, DM, et al: Unconventional medicine in the United States. N Engl J Med 328(4):246–252, 1993.
7. Berman, B, et al: Homeopathy and the U.S. primary care physician. British Homeopathic Journal 86:131–138, 1997.

8. Borneman, JP: Homeopathy in the United States and Canada: An analysis of the self-medication market for homeopathic drugs. In Improving the Success of Homeopathy, 23 Jan 97, Royal London Homeopathic Hospital, NHS; 82-89.

9. Goldstein, MS, and Glick D: Use of and satisfaction with homeopathy in a patient population. Alternative Therapies 4(2):60–65, 1998.

10. Kent, JT: Lectures on Homeopathic Philosophy. Ehrhart & Karl, Chicago, 1929.

11. Kent, JT: Lectures on Homeopathic Materia Medica, ed. 4. Boericke & Tafel, Philadelphia, 1956.

12. Kent, JT: Kent's Repertorium Generale (K Fimmelsberg, ed). Barthel & Barthel Publishing, Berg, Germany, 1987.

13. Ernst, E, and Kaptchuk T: Homeopathy revisited. Arch Intern Med 159:2162–2164, 1996.

14. Rothstein, WG: American Physicians in the 19th Century. Johns Hopkins University Press, Baltimore, 1985.

15. Berman et al: Homeopathy and the US primary care physician.

16. Eisenberg et al: Unconventional medicine in the United States.

17. Borneman: Homeopathy in the United States and Canada.

18. Lo: Anomalous state of ice.

19. Lo: Physical properties of water with IE structures.

20. Bonavida: Induction and regulation of human peripheral blood.

21. Sinitsyn: Effect of IE solutions on enzymes and microbial cells.

22. Davenas, E, Beauvais, F, and Amara, J: Human basophil degranulation triggered by very dilute antiserum against IgE. Nature 333:816–818, 1988.

23. Bellavite, P, and Signorini, A: Homeopathy—A Frontier in Medical Science (A Steele, trans). North Atlantic Books, Berkeley, 1995.

24. Davenas, Beauvais, and Amara: Human basophil degranulation.

25. Bellavite and Signorini: Homeopathy—A Frontier of Meical Science.

26. Endler, PC, and Schulte, J: Ultra High Dilution Physiology and Physics. Kluwer Academic Publishers, Boston, 1994.

27. Bastide, M: Signals and Images. Kluwer Academic Publishers, Boston, 1997.

28. When to believe the unbelievable [editorial]. Nature 333:787, 1988.

29. Davenas, Beauvais, and Amara: Human basophil degranulation.

30. Bellavite and Signorini: Homeopathy—A Frontier in Medical Science.

31. Endler and Schulte: Ultra High Dilution Physiology and Physics.

32. Belon, P, et.al: Inhibition of human basophil degranulation by successive histamine dilutions. Inflamm Res 48:17–18, 1999.

33. When to believe the unbelievable.

34. Lo: Anomalous state of ice.

35. Lo: Physical properties of water with IE structures.

36. Jacobs, J, et al: Treatment of acute diarrhea with homeopathic medicine: A randomized clinical trial in Nicaragua. Pediatrics 93(5):719–25, 1994.

37. Reilly, DT, et al: Is evidence for homeopathy reproducible? A controlled trial of allergic asthma. Lancet 344(8937):161–166, 1995.

38. Taylor, MA, et al: Randomized controlled trial of homeopathy versus placebo in perennial allergic rhinitis with overview of four trial series. BMJ 321:19–26, 2000.

39. Chapman, E, et al: The homeopathic treatment of mild traumatic brain injury. Manuscript submitted for publication.

40. Jacobs, J: Homeopathic treatment of acute otitis media in children—a randomized placebo-controlled trial. Manuscript submitted for publication.

41. Friese, KH, et al: The homeopathic treatment of otitis media in children—comparisons with conventional therapy. Int J Clin Pharmacol Ther 35(7):296–301, 1997.

42. Fisher, P, et al: Effect of homeopathic treatment on fibrositis. BMJ 299:365–366, 1989.

43. Brigo, B, and Serpelloni, G: Homeopathic treatment of migraines: A randomized double-blind controlled study of sixty cases. The Berlin Journal on Research in Homeopathy 1:98–105, 1991.

44. Kleijnen, J, et al: Clinical trials in homeopathy. BMJ 302:316–23, 1991.

45. Linde, K, et al: Are the clinical effects of homeopathy placebo effects? A meta-analysis of placebo controlled trials. Lancet 350:834–843, 1997.

46. Boissel, JP, et al: Overview of data from homeopathic medicine trials: Report on the efficacy of homeopathic interventions over no treatment of placebo. In Report of the Homeopathic Medicine Research Group. European Commission, Brussels, 1996.

47. Walach, H, et al: Classical homeopathic treatment of chronic headaches. Cephalgia 17:119–126, 1997.

48. Whitmarsh, THE: Double-blind randomized placebo-controlled study of the homeopathic prophylaxis of migraine. Cephalgia 17:600–604, 1997.

49. Chapman et al: The homeopathic treatment of mild traumatic brain injury.

50. Ibid.

51. Warkentin, DK, and van Zandvoort R: The Complete Repertory. MacRepertory, Kent Homeopathic Associates, 710 Mission Ave., San Rafael, CA, 94901. (415) 457-0678.

52. Vermeulen, F: Concordant Materia Medica, ed. 2. Emryss bv Publishers, Haarlem, The Netherlands, 1997, p 1216.

53. Bellavite and Signorini: Homeopathy—A Frontier in Medical Science.

54. Ibid.

55. Geyman, JP: Evidence-based medicine in primary care: An overview. Journal American Board of Family Practice 2(1):46–56, 1998.

56. Reilly, D: The evidence profile for homeopathy—creating the verification mosaic. In Improving the Success of Homeopathy, 23 Jan 97, Royal London Homeopathic Hospital, NHS, 63-68.

BIBLIOGRAPHY

Bellavite, P, and Signorini, A: Homeopathy—A Frontier in Medical Science (A Steele, trans). North Atlantic Books, Berkeley, 1995.

Castro, M: The Complete Book of Homeopathy. St. Martin's Press, New York, 1990.

Jonas, W, and Jacobs J: Healing with Homeopathy: The Way to Promote Recovery and Restore Health.. Warner Books, New York, 1996.

Ullman, D: Discovering Homeopathy: Medicine for the 21st Century. North Atlantic Books, Berkeley, 1991.

CHAPTER 15

Anthroposophic Medicine

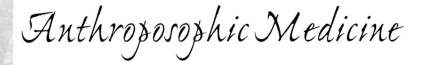

Alicia Landman-Reiner

Alicia Landman-Reiner, MD, is board certified in both family and anthroposophic medicine. After receiving her MD degree in 1982, she became one of the few medical physicians in the United States who also practiced in an integrative way. Landman-Reiner currently has a solo practice in anthroposophic and integrative medicine in Northhamptom, Massachusetts.

A 29-year-old man visits his doctor, an MD, because of a cough and fever. The doctor takes the patient's temperature, pulse, and blood pressure and then orders blood work. The blood cell count indicates infection; a microscope reading of the man's sputum, which defines the number and kind of bacteria and immune cells, indicates pneumonia.

Like most conventional MDs, the doctor diagnoses the patient's condition based on quantitative and microscopic findings. Although the doctor may be sympathetic as a person, he or she does not rely on emotions or artistic judgment to make the diagnosis, which is a purely objective, logical process.

The anthroposophic physician, on the other hand, listens carefully to the patient's experience. "Doctor, I'm cold and thirsty. This wet cough is heavy in my chest. I'm so tired of this thing; it's giving me the blues." The doctor observes the patient for physical clues as well: he is sitting slightly slumped on the examining table, touching his chest with each loose, rattling cough; his skin is sallow and moist, the hands and feet slightly cool. The doctor uses artistic and emotional capacities, not only logical thinking, to achieve a picturelike description of the presenting symptoms, concluding, "This patient is too watery." Therapy will try to reduce wateriness in the respiratory system, where it is excessive.

Although this picture of the patient's "watery quality" has no underlying biochemical correlate, anthroposophic medicine views it as a philosophically valid way to formulate the patient's problem.

What is anthroposophy? It is a system of healing based on the belief that the human being is much more than a physical body. It encompasses life-essence, soul, and spirit, as well as the physical organism. Anthroposophic doctors consider these spiritual aspects of a person when diagnosing and treating disease as much as they do the physical aspects.

The word *anthroposophic* is derived from the Greek words *anthropo,* meaning "human," and *sophos,* meaning "wisdom." Over the last 75 years this new wisdom about the human being has been developed into a comprehensive medical and therapeutic approach that is practiced by physicians, along with nurses and other therapists, in outpatient and inpatient settings around the world. (See Box 15–1.)

BOX 15–1

The Origin of Anthroposophic Medicine

Rudolf Steiner (1861–1925), an Austrian-born scientist and philosopher, sought to unite the ideals of modern scientific training with millennia-old wisdom traditions based on meditative practice. This marriage he called "anthroposophy."

Western medicine is built on materialism, the viewpoint that reality is made up only of sense-perceptible matter. Steiner argued that many ancient peoples, however, had direct experience with other, nonmaterial, levels of reality. Ancient Chinese and Indian healers actually experienced life-essence as a reality. They called it "chi" and "prana" and built medical systems mapping these energies and working with them. Trained shamans of Native-American traditions perceived soul activity and the movement of spirit in their patients. Steiner argued that these faculties are latent in every modern person as well and can be reawakened.[1]

Schooled in mathematics, physics, and chemistry, Steiner wrote a doctoral thesis in philosophy. Ever since his childhood, he had experienced a hidden spiritual dimension in the world, a capacity he had nurtured and disciplined but kept separate from his outer life. His career as a writer and teacher in the intellectual centers of Weimar and Berlin took a decisive turn when, at the age of 39, he began to speak openly of his spiritual insights and present his synthesis of Western and Eastern spiritual traditions.[2]

He described three higher levels of reality: life-essence, soul, and spirit.[3] His aim was to outline a method for retraining the eyes and ears to directly know the life body, the soul, and the spirit. He emphasized that such teachings have existed throughout human history and that his contribution was to present those teachings in a form suitable to the scientifically trained mind.[4-6]

The spiritual content was shocking to his mainstream audiences. His new followers, however, were men and women who felt burdened and stifled by the late-19th-century materialism that gripped their diverse fields and institutions. They urgently sought "to introduce into life the impulses from the world of the spirit,"[7] and they found the means through Steiner's anthroposophy.

Steiner and his coworkers founded numerous projects: Waldorf education, now the largest independent school movement in the world; biodynamic agriculture, one of the earliest organic agricultural methods, practiced today worldwide; and other initiatives in the arts, religion, and science. The Goetheanum, in Switzerland, today the world center for anthroposophy, was built during World War I by coworkers from many nations. Steiner himself wrote and lectured prolifically, producing some 30 books and 6000 lectures.

In 1920, Steiner was approached by a circle of physicians seeking to expand the boundaries of medicine in such a way as to include the soul and the spirit in issues of illness and healing. Collaborating with Ita Wegman, a Dutch physician, Steiner helped them develop a new medical approach. They founded a hospital, an outpatient clinic, and a pharmaceutical company which are still active today. Wegman wrote: "From time immemorial . . . the attainment of spiritual knowledge was brought into connection with the healing of the sick. We had no thought . . . of underrating the scientific medicine of our time. We recognized it fully. Our aim was to supplement the science already in existence by the illumination that can flow from a true knowledge of the spirit, towards a living grasp of the processes of illness and of healing."[8] A new medical movement had begun.

Currently anthroposophic medicine is a widely known complementary medical approach in Europe and is becoming familiar in North America. There are more than 1000 anthroposophically trained medical doctors, mostly in Germany, Switzerland, Holland, and Sweden; another 16,000 prescribe some anthroposophic remedies.[9] Individual and group practices exist all over the world, including the Middle East, Africa, and North and South America. About 20 hospitals in Europe combine anthroposophic and standard medical approaches; one of these specializes in cancer care and one in psychiatry. Several pharmaceutical companies, notably Wala and Weleda (with branches in 36 countries), produce and distribute herbal, mineral, and homeopathically prepared remedies of high quality.[10,11]

continued

BOX 15–1 continued

The Origin of Anthroposophic Medicine

All anthroposophic doctors must first acquire standard medical training and licensure. Only in Germany, at the University of Witten, does a medical college integrate standard and anthroposophic training. The Lukas Klinik in Switzerland offers medical courses in English, Spanish, and German, and the North American anthroposophic physicians' organization sponsors courses and conferences.[12] The American College of Anthroposophically Extended Medicine certifies trained doctors.[13] Training in anthroposophic approaches to nursing and to massage, art, and movement therapies is also available in the United States.

REFERENCES

1. Steiner, R: Knowledge of the Higher Worlds and Its Attainment. Anthroposophic Press, Hudson, N.Y., 1947.
2. Steiner, R: Chapters in the Course of My Life. Anthroposophic Press, Hudson, N.Y., 1999.
3. Steiner, R, and Wegman, I: Fundamentals of Therapy. Rudolf Steiner Press, London, 1983. (Original work published 1925)
4. Steiner: Knowledge of the Higher Worlds and Its Attainment.
5. Steiner, R: Philosophy of Freedom. Rudolf Steiner Press, London, 1964.
6. Steiner and Wegman: Fundamentals of Therapy.
7. Steiner, R: The Course of My Life. Anthroposophic Press, New York, 1951, p 300.
8. Steiner and Wegman: Fundamentals of Therapy, p vii.
9. Murphy, F: Personal communications with author. Waleda, Congers, N.Y., 18 June 2001.
10. Wala Therapeutic Preparations, ed. 4. Wala-Heilmittel GMBH, Eckwaelden, Germany, 1981.
11. Weleda Medicine List, ed. 15. Weleda, Congers, N.Y., 1995.
12. See Physicians Association for Anthroposophical Medicine (PAAM) in the "Resources" section for further information.
13. Board of the American College of Anthroposophically-Extended Medicine, 241 Hungry Hollow Road, Chestnut Ridge, NY 10977.

Three-Part Physiology

While standard medicine views health as merely the absence of disease and disease as the breakdown of some part of the great machine, the human body, anthroposophic medicine views health and illness as more active processes. Health is a state of dynamic balance between opposing principles within the human being. The organism is always mediating between extremes, creating and re-creating balance.

How is the human body created? Rudolf Steiner, the founder of anthroposophy, asserted that the human body emerges from the fundamental polarity of heaven and earth. He believed that the body is created by cosmic forces, on the one hand, "propelling the organs out of the spiritual-etheric world, and on the other hand, earthly forces, building up the body, assembling and consolidating it."[1–4] Steiner depicted the human being dynamically set between earth and heaven.

Anthroposophy views the human body as having three distinct parts: two opposing systems, with a third system actively mediating between them. The first pole is termed the "nerve-sense system." It is centered in the head, containing the brain and the sense organs, namely, the eyes, ears, and organs of smell and taste. The opposing pole, centered in the abdominal organs and the reproductive system and including the limbs, is termed the "metabolic-limb system." These two systems oppose each other on several levels. Anatomically, the head sits at the opposite end of the body from the metabolic digestive organs and limbs. Observing the skeleton, we see that the bones of the head (the nerve-sense system) are rounded and contain the organs within them. The limbs and body, on the other hand, have bones inside, with the organs arranged around them.

These systems also differ functionally. The nerve-sense system is designed to take in impressions, the intangible, and integrate them. The metabolic-limb system, on the other hand, takes in substance—the food we eat—and integrates it into the body. This system enables the body to be active in the world.

In addition, the nerve-sense system, especially the brain, functions as the seat of consciousness—of thinking and sensing. In contrast, the metabolic-limb system, in the digestive organs, functions unconsciously. It has tremendous vitality. In the intestines, for example, millions of new cells are produced every day: there is burgeoning life. The liver, an essential metabolic organ, has so much vitality that it can function with only 10 percent of its capacity. There is also continuous movement in the intestinal tract. In contrast, the organs of the nerve-sense system are much less full of life. Whereas the cells of the intestine are constantly being renewed, nerve tissues are fully formed early in life, with minimal capacity for regeneration. The sense organs are almost devoid of life; for example, the eye is like a crystal, precisely so that it can receive and transmit messages without distorting them.

In sum, the nerve-sense system is centered in the head, with less vitality and more consciousness, whereas the metabolic-limb system is centered in the body, with great vitality and little consciousness.

We would be constantly ill if we did not have in our bodies a third system, whose activity mediates between the two extremes. This system is physically situated between the nerve-sense system and metabolic-limb system—in the chest, between the head and the abdomen. Because its organs are the heart and lungs, whose functions are heartbeat and rhythmical breathing, it is called the rhythmic system.[5]

Each breath and impulse of the circulation move between two polarities: inhaling toward the nerve-sense system and exhaling toward the metabolic-limb system. As the heart contracts in systole, we become subtly more awake, more in our nervous system; as

FIGURE 15–1   Polarity of Nerve-Sense System and Metabolic-Limb System

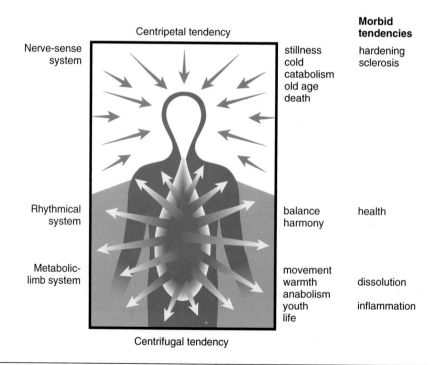

Reprinted with permission from Weleda AG, Arlesheim (Switzerland) and Schwäbisch Gmund (Federal Republic of Germany).

it expands in diastole, we become subtly more relaxed, less conscious, therefore more metabolic. This back-and-forth activity of breathing and heartbeat, which accompanies every moment of our lives, physically expresses the mediating role of the rhythmic system.[6]

Anthroposophic medicine is not alone in recognizing breathing as the key to healing: this is known by many healing traditions. Yogic breathing exercises are one example. In Chinese medicine, the organs of breathing and respiration are seen as regulating living energy for the whole body.[7] In the Greek language, "breath" and "spirit" are called by one word, *pneuma*. From the Latin, we have derived both *spirit* and *inspire,* or *breathe.* The linguistic connection of *breath* and *spirit* points to the centrality of breath to our wholeness, which is to say, our healing.

From the anthroposophic medical viewpoint, the threefold organism is continually healing itself, continually and actively moving toward wholeness. This is seen graphically in the threefold picture of nerve- sense, metabolic-limb, and rhythmic systems. (See Fig. 15–1.)

Imbalance Leads to Illness

As just described, the two polar aspects of our organism oppose each other. The rhythmic system mediates and much of the time is able to restore balance. However, when a physiological imbalance becomes fixed, illness results. Therefore, many illnesses can be understood as being the result of a chronic dominance of the nerve-sense system or the metabolic-limb system that cannot be resolved by the intrinsic activities of breathing and circulation.[8]

Exaggerated dominance of the nerve-sense system leads to what anthroposophic medicine calls "sclerotic illnesses." In these conditions the whole organism, not just the nerve-sense system, becomes devitalized. These include illnesses in which movement is diminished or frozen (e.g., arthritis or asthma), conditions characterized by low energy (e.g., chronic fatigue or mononucleosis), and conditions in which hardened mineral deposits appear (e.g., gout or kidney stones). These illnesses tend to be chronic. Typical diseases of the elderly fall into this category (e.g., arthritis, hardening of the arteries, and cancer).

Exaggeration of the metabolic-limb system, on the other hand, leads to inflammatory illnesses, ones in which we become too warm, too sleepy, too full of life. Our metabolism is very active, but we are less alert. This metabolic activity includes aspects of what Western medicine describes as immune activity. Examples of inflammatory illnesses include strep throat, pneumonia, and acne. These types of illnesses often afflict children.[9]

A Fourfold Spiritual Anatomy

The anthroposophically trained physician also bases his or her diagnosis on four levels of reality described by Steiner, which are organized in the human being as separate but interrelated "bodies." The first level, our physical body, is what we ordinarily perceive. It gives us materiality and structure. It is permeated by and formed by physical forces, such as gravity.

The second level, the "life" or "etheric" body, is not based on physical and chemical forces; rather, it "rests on a quite different foundation: in effect the physical substances, as they pour into the etheric realm, divest themselves . . . of their physical forces."[10] The etheric body is the source of growth and regeneration, of the inexhaustible vitality that is typical of the plant world. It is especially strong in the young child. The etheric body is closely associated with fluids in our organism: it has an affinity for the flowing, the mutable, all that is watery.

The third level, the soul body, Steiner termed the "astral" body. This level of organization underlies movement and dynamic processes, such as nerve conduction, glandular secretion, and breathing. Closely connected with our emotions, the astral body has an affinity for air, changing its configuration with every breath.

The fourth level is the ego, the most purely spiritual level, whose nature is farthest of all from the ordinary physical. This ego enables us to express ourselves as individuals, to view ourselves as an "I." Our unique human individuality manifests itself via the ego through our body's warmth.[11] As our body temperature increases in fever, our ego-presence intensifies within our metabolism; this is part of the process of "fighting off" an illness and reestablishing our integrity. Each of these four levels functions in our organism as a whole and in distinct ways within each of our organs. If one or several of the bodies do not function harmoniously with the others, illness results.[12]

In diagnosing illness, the anthroposophic physician views the patient in terms of the fourfold bodies and the threefold realms of function described earlier. He or she might ask: (1) How is an individual configured, in terms of the physical body, etheric body, astral body, and ego. (2) How is each of these four members active in the nerve-sense, rhythmic, and metabolic-limb systems? All these factors—as well as others—must be taken into account to come to a diagnosis.

The following are examples of the fourfold and threefold principles in illness:[13]

- The physical body acts too independently in the reproductive system (a part of the metabolic-limb system), resulting in a fibroid tumor—a benign growth—in the uterus.
- The etheric body is overactive, overwhelming the nerve-sense system in the region of the head, resulting in a cold with watery nasal discharge, sore throat, and headache.
- The astral body acts too strongly in the nerve-sense system; after some years of more subtle symptoms, there is an asthma attack.
- The ego works too weakly in the digestive system, reflected in sugar cravings with shakiness and feelings of faintness.

These concepts, however, are valuable only when used in a flexible way. The art of anthroposophic diagnosis lies in acquiring knowledge of the human organism while remaining open to what is unique in each patient.[14]

Anthroposophic Medicines and Other Therapies

A wide range of therapies, which are prepared from a variety of minerals, plants, and animal sources, are used in anthroposophic medicine. Great care goes into obtaining ingredients of high quality, picked in the wild or grown without pesticides (when possible) and harvested in a season and at a time of day specific to each remedy. (See Fig. 15–2.) Attention is paid even to the inner mood of those preparing the remedies, because thoughts and feelings are forces that affect the material world and could have an impact on the quality of the remedy.

There are similarities between anthroposophy and homeopathy. Many of the early anthroposophic physicians were homeopaths, and homeopathy and anthroposophic medicine have much in common. Both approaches strive to understand the use of dilute substances in a rational way.[15] Eighty-five percent of remedies are diluted homeopathically; the rest are prepared at full strength. Processes unique to anthroposophic medicine, such as rhythmically heating, cooling, and exposing the remedies to light and dark, may also be used to enhance certain qualities.[16–19] (See Fig. 15–3)

FIGURE 15–2   Plant Remedies

Ingredients for anthroposophic remedies are picked in the wild or grown without pesticides whenever possible.

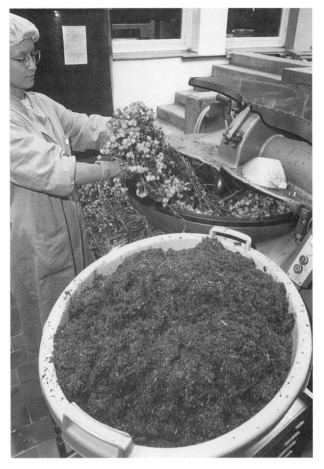

Reprinted with permission from Weleda AG, Arlesheim (Switzerland) and Schwäbisch Gmund (Federal Republic of Germany).

The anthroposophic physician seeks to match the specific arrangement of forces in the remedy with the imbalanced forces in the person who is ill. A prime example is the threefold plant. Three aspects of plant anatomy—root, flower, and leaf—correspond to the threefold human being, but inverted so that the root corresponds to the nerve-sense system, the stem and leaves to the rhythmic system, and the flower to the metabolic system.[20] (See Fig. 15–4.)

The root is typically used to treat problems of the nerve-sense system. Examples of this include using lovage root to treat ear infections and chamomile root to treat digestive problems caused by the improper working of the nerve-sense system, such as irritable bowel syndrome. Leaves and stems are preferred for problems seen in the rhythmic system. Examples include using cactus stem to treat certain cardiac problems and a mixture of fern and willow leaves to harmonize rhythmic activity in the digestion, such as in constipation. Flowers are used to treat the metabolic-limb system. For example, elder flowers may be used to strengthen the metabolism in a sclerosing condition such as arthritis.[21]

FIGURE 15–3

Anthroposophic remedies are often rhythmically heated, cooled, and exposed to light and dark to enhance certain qualities.

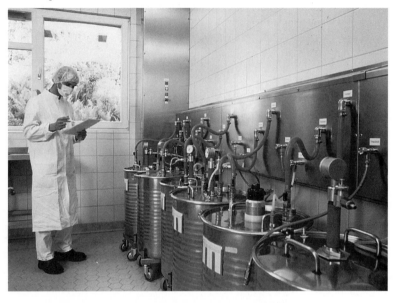

Photo courtesy of WALA-Heilmittel GmbH. Reprinted with permission.

FIGURE 15–4   Plant Remedies and Threefold Human Being

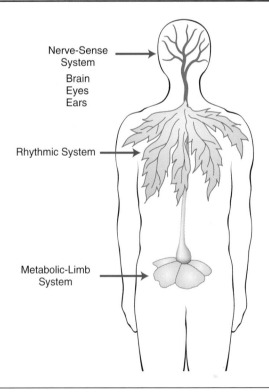

Nerve-Sense
System
Brain
Eyes
Ears

Rhythmic System

Metabolic-Limb
System

Photo courtesy of WALA-Heilmittel GmbH. Reprinted with permission.

Rudolf Steiner asked us to consider the proposition that "the substance appearing in the outer world to our senses is nothing more than a process come to rest."[22] Anthroposophy strives to utilize natural substances in a way that does not merely reduce them to their chemical components. The goal is to read and understand how the substance appears in nature—whether in mineral form, in a plant, or in an animal—and to apply its gesture to a pathological process in the human organism.

An example is the medicinal use of calcium carbonate from oyster shell. The oyster's metabolic aspect (its soft body) and its mineral, devitalized aspect (the oyster shell) are anatomically separated. The two realms are polarized. Oyster shell is used in anthroposophic medicine, after appropriate pharmaceutical processes, to treat an illness in which the nerve-sense and metabolic aspects of the human being are too close together and need to be separated.[23] An example is a child with chronically enlarged tonsils; that is, there is too much metabolic activity in the child's nerve-sense system. Calcium carbonate, from oyster shell, might be an appropriate therapy. In this way, the gesture made by the substance in nature acts as a model for the organism to follow.

Many other therapies, not just medications, are used today in anthroposophic medicine. A gentle massage technique, called rhythmical massage, is taught and practiced in the United States and Germany. Therapeutic baths may be prescribed. Art therapies of great variety—using painting, sculpture, music, and recitation—are offered to medically ill patients in the anthroposophic hospitals of Europe, whereas in standard medicine such therapies are usually reserved for treating mental health problems.[24–26]

Eurythmy is a form of healing movement in which highly trained practitioners teach the patient movements corresponding to the sounds of language, the vowels and consonants. These exercises stimulate forces that resound deep within the patient. Eurythmy exercises can work in a highly potent way to mobilize inner healing forces, sometimes in tenacious chronic disease.[27]

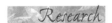

Research

In the earlier years of anthroposophic medicine, most published research was of a descriptive nature, such as individual case descriptions, notably in 60 years of the German medical journal *Merkurstab*.[28] During the past quarter-century, collaboration between anthroposophically trained scientists and conventional researchers has resulted in some 500 papers by Hildebrandt and associates at the University of Marburg, in Germany, extensively exploring biorhythms in human physiology.[29]

Von Lauer and Henn[30] have researched physiological rhythms in cancer patients; they suggest that circadian temperature curves are disturbed in cancer and have explored temperature curves as an index of therapeutic efficacy. Alm and colleagues[31] reported on 675 children's allergic illness in the *Lancet*. They found that Swedish children raised according to an "anthroposophic lifestyle"—diet and use of anthroposophic medicine, with avoidance of antibiotics and some vaccines—had fewer allergies and were less likely to have asthma. Research projects currently in progress include an international study of anthroposophic and homeopathic treatment for colds and two studies of the anthroposophic approach to attention deficit disorder in children.[32–34]

Substantial research has focused on the use of extract of the European mistletoe (viscum album) in cancer therapy. Mistletoe therapy is now a widely used complementary treatment for cancer in Europe.[35] Iscador (the most studied mistletoe preparation) has been found to be cytostatic or cytotoxic (stopping the growth of, or killing, cancer cells) and immunomodulatory. In this, mistletoe appears to assist the body in eliminating tumor cells via the immune system. Components of Iscador extract, including viscotoxins and mistletoe lectins, have been extensively studied. In white blood cells exposed to mistletoe lectins, positive effects were measured on the activity of natural killer cells (cells that are active in the immune response to cancer) and on cytokines (mediator proteins of the immune system).[36,37]

Some 50 studies and clinical series report survival advantage and/or improvement of quality of life in cancer patients treated with mistletoe. Some of these studies, however, are of poor quality. Few studies are randomized.[38] A critical examination of 36 clinical trials of mistletoe treatment found nine studies supporting the life-extending effect of mistletoe.[39] The treatment, administered by physicians, is generally well tolerated and safe.[40] Mistletoe is used in anthroposophic hospitals, along with a spectrum of other remedies, therapies, and counseling. Patients receiving this comprehensive cancer care treatment report such benefits as improved quality of life, reduced pain, and improvements in mood and overall coping.[41] Mistletoe therapy should be seen as one element of a coordinated approach to the whole patient with cancer. Much more research is needed, and significant funding is required for trials meeting the highest methodological standards.

Anthroposophic researchers have also considered issues of method and design. How can controlled clinical trials be adapted to highly individualized therapy regimens? How can qualitative thinking be incorporated into research methods developed around the quantitative? In other words, how can research be adapted to the subtle, living, complex activity of anthroposophic therapy?[44,45] Ongoing presentation of research results and issues takes place in the journals *Merkurstab* and the *Journal for Anthroposophic Medicine.*[46]

Summary

The practice of anthroposophic medicine is meant to be integrated into a standard medical approach. The anthroposophic doctor performs standard medical tests for diagnosis and interacts with other medical professionals, as needed, regarding the patient's course. There are circumstances in which standard Western medicine is the most appropriate therapy, such as treatment of traumatic injuries or organ failure, where high-technology support is life saving. In European anthroposophic hospitals, such treatment is combined with complementary therapy in a way that offers the best of all care. In the United States, an anthroposophic doctor fully incorporates conventional modalities when the patient needs them.

Anthroposophic medicine does not view illness as failure on the patient's part, nor is perfect health necessarily the goal. Illness is part of the human condition and may even become a turning point in the patient's course of life. Rudolf Steiner, in a lecture to young doctors and medical students, counseled them to develop and maintain a strong "will to heal"—that is, not to abandon hope for healing, no matter how desperate the illness—yet nevertheless to respect and accept the patient's unique path, of which the illness is a part.[47]

The anthroposophic physician or therapist is also on a path of inner development. In the anthroposophic view, if the doctor's or therapist's personal attributes do not contribute to healing, then neither knowledge of threefold physiology and fourfold spiritual anatomy, nor mastery of the complex language of minerals, plants, and animals, will bear fruit. The first step on the anthroposophic path, and one to which the doctor and therapist are encouraged to return again and again, is deep reverence for all that manifests in nature and in each human being who seeks healing.[48] (See Box 15–2.)

BOX 15–2

Clinical Example

A 4-year-old girl was brought to this author's anthroposophic medical practice because of recurrent ear infections since the age of 18 months. She had had four episodes of middle ear infection the prior winter. Her parents had tried treating her with dietary changes and some home remedies, without apparent improvement. Otherwise she was generally healthy but a picky eater, and she occasionally wet her bed. There was a family history of hay fever.

A fair, slender, active child, she interacted readily with the examiner. Her voice was high pitched, even "squeaky." She appeared tired, with dark circles under the eyes. Lab results showed a mild anemia.

This was a child with a strong nerve-sense system and a relatively weaker metabolic-limb system, as shown by her slender build, ready interaction, and fatigue. The bed wetting, food selectivity, and anemia all pointed to a weakness in metabolism, especially in the kidney area. In reaction to that weakness, there were recurrent inflammations in the nerve-sense system—that is, the ears, which have a certain relationship to the kidneys. The ear infections were a symptom of her body's efforts to balance the more fundamental problem. Some of her symptoms were "allergic," which anthroposophy sees as a "cry for help" of a weakened system or organ. The high-pitched voice pointed to deficient iron forces.

The doctor first prescribed homeopathic (highly dilute) silver to give an impulse to the etheric body, then oyster shell and oak bark to support the healthy working of the etheric body in her metabolism. A remedy from nettle *(Urtica dioica),* cultivated by a process that enhanced its iron forces, was given to strengthen the kidney forces in the metabolic system. Root of lovage *(Levisticum officinale),* chosen because the problem occurred in the nerve-sense system, was used to tame the excessive etheric fluid activity in the ear.

The doctor also advised a low-allergen diet to lighten the metabolic work, as well as increased naps, an earlier bedtime, and warmer clothes to strengthen her metabolic forces and support healing. The doctor told the parents to allow their daughter to play actively and imaginatively, especially outdoors, but to have her avoid excessive intellectual activity until her health improved because this would further burden her nerve-sense system.

The patient subsequently had several colds with fevers. There were no further middle ear infections. Six months after starting treatment, she had one outer ear infection. This more superficial problem signaled that her organism was working more harmoniously. Over 5 years of follow-up there were no further middle ear infections.

RESOURCES

Anthroposophic Press
P.O. Box 960
Herndon, VA 20172-0960
(800) 856-8664
anthropres@aol.com

Anthroposophical Society in America
1923 Geddes Ave.
Ann Arbor, MI 48104
Phone: (734) 662-9355
www.anthroposophy.org

Artemisia—Association for the Anthroposophical Renewal of Healing
1923 Geddes Ave.
Ann Arbor, MI 48104
Phone: (734) 761-5172
www.artemesia.net

This organization has information on professional training and conferences on nursing, therapeutic massage, art therapy, therapeutic eurythmy, and other topics.
Inquiries regarding conferences, newsletters, and publications are welcome from all those interested in learning more about the anthroposophic therapeutic approach.

Lilipoh
P.O. Box 649
Nyack, NY 10960
Phone: (914) 268-2627
A journal dedicated to natural medicine.

Physicians Association for Anthroposophical Medicine (PAAM)
1923 Geddes Ave.
Ann Arbor, MI 48104
Phone: (734) 930-9463
www.paam.net
PAAM has information, a newsletter, and membership options for interested physicians or physicians-in-training. The organization also sponsors conferences and trainings. In addition, PAAM has information for patients seeking anthroposophically trained doctors.

Rudolf Steiner Library
RD 2, Box 215
Ghent, NY 12075
Phone: (518) 672-7590
The library has 8000 volumes available by mail.

REFERENCES

1. Steiner, R: Curative Eurythmy. Rudolf Steiner Press, London, 1983. (Original work published 1921–1922)
2. Steiner, R: Spiritual Science and Medicine. Rudolf Steiner Press, London, 1975. (Original work published 1920)
3. Steiner, R: Course for Young Doctors. Mercury Press, New York, 1994. (Original work published 1924)
4. Steiner, R: Polarities in Health, Illness and Therapy. Mercury Press, Spring Valley, N.Y., 1987. (Original work published 1923)
5. Ibid.
6. Ibid.
7. Kaptchuk, TJ: The Web That Has No Weaver. Congdon & Weed, New York, 1983.
8. Steiner: Polarities in Health, Illness and Therapy.
9. Bott, V: Anthroposophical Medicine. Rudolf Steiner Press, London 1978, p 48.
10. Steiner, R, and Wegman, I: Fundamentals of Therapy. Rudolf Steiner Press, London, 1983. (Original work published 1925)
11. Steiner, R: The Bridge between Universal Spirituality and the Physical Constitution of Man. Anthroposophic Press, Hudson, N.Y., 1983. (Original work published 1920)
12. Steiner and Wegman: Fundamentals of Therapy.
13. Author's own clinical examples.
14. Steiner, R: An Outline of Occult Science. Anthroposophic Press, Hudson, N.Y., 1972. (Original work published 1909)
15. Scharff, PW: What Is Anthroposophical Medicine? Weleda, Inc., Congers, N.Y., 1980.
16. Ibid.
17. Wala Therapeutic Preparations, ed. 4. Wala-Heilmittel GMBH, Eckwaelden, Germany, 1981
18. Weleda Medicine List, ed. 15. Weleda, Inc, Congers, N.Y., 1995.
19. Scharff, PW: Anthroposophically extended medicine. ANTHA Newsletter 1, 1994, p 1.

20. Steiner: Polarities in Health, Illness, and Therapy.

21. Steiner, R: Anthroposophical Spiritual Science and Medical Therapy. Mercury Press, Spring Valley, N.Y., 1991. (Original work published 1921)

22. Ibid.

23. Ibid.

24. Hauschka, M: Rhythmical Massage. Rudolf Steiner Press, London, 1979.

25. Schmidt, G: The Oil-Forming Process. Mercury Press, Spring Valley, N.Y., 1978.

26. Husemann, G: The Artistic Approach to Therapies. Mercury Press, Spring Valley, N.Y., 1994.

27. Ibid.

28. Merkurstab, Gesellschaft Anthroposophischer Aertzte in Deutschland, Stuttgart, Germany.

29. Hildebrandt, G, and Bandt-Reges, I: Chronobiologie in der Naturheilkunde: Grundlagen der Circaseptanperiodik Karl F Haug Verlag, Heidelberg 1992; Hildebrandt, G, and Hansel, H (eds): Biological Adaptation: International Symposium. Thieme-Stratton, Stuttgart and New York, 1982. (These are two examples of this author's many publications.)

30. Von Lauer, A, and Henn, S: Alternative medicine: Expanding medical horizons (report to the NIH). Office of Alternative Medicine Workshop on Alternative Medicine, Chantilly, Va., 1992.

31. Alm, JS, et al: Atopy in children of families with an anthroposophic lifestyle. Lancet 353:1485–1488,1999.

32. Bristol, E: Personal communications with author, Anthroposophical Society.

33. Payne, K, and Rivers, B: A Creative Way to Understand and Help Children with Difficult Behavior (Waldorf attention-related disorders research project, study in process 2000–2001).

34. Personal communication, Kim Payne, regarding ongoing study at University of Bern on eurythmy therapy in attention deficit disorder.

35. Kienle, GS: The story behind mistletoe: A European remedy from anthroposophical medicine. Alternative Therapies 5:6, 1999.

36. Office of Technology Assessment: Unconventional Cancer Treatments. U.S. Government Printing Office, Washington, D.C., 1990 (reprinted 1993).

37. Hajto,T, et al: Increased secretion of tumor necrosis factor alpha, interleukin 1, and interleukin 6 by human mononuclear cells exposed to B-galactoside-specific lectin from clinically applied mistletoe extract. Cancer Res 50:3322–3326, 1990.

38. Kienle: The story behind mistletoe.

39. Anthroposophical medicine (report prepared for the Ministry of Science and Technology of the Federal Government of Germany, Bonn, 1992). In Cancer, Anthroposophically-Extended Viewpoints on Its Treatment. Fellowship Community Associates, Chestnut Ridge, N.Y., 1994.

40. Gorter, RW, et al: Tolerability of an extract of European mistletoe among immunocompromised and healthy individuals. Alternative Therapies 5:6, 1999.

41. Kienle: The story behind mistletoe.

42. Gorter, R, and Linder, M: Prospektive, longitudinale, dosiseskalierende, randomisierte phase l/ll Studie mit Iscador. Forschende Komplementarmedizin 3:4, 1996; and personal communication.

43. Ibid.

44. Kienle: The story behind mistletoe.

45. Anthroposophical medicine.

46. Journal for Anthroposophical Medicine, published by Physicians' Association for Anthroposophical Medicine, 1923 Geddes Ave., Ann Arbor, MI 48104.

47. Steiner: Course for Young Doctors.

48. Steiner, R. Knowledge of the Higher Worlds and Its Attainment. Anthroposophic Press, New York, 1947.

CHAPTER 16

Osteopathy

Jayne Alexander and Andrew Goldman

Jayne Alexander, DO, maintains a private practice in Bridgewater, Massachusetts.
Andrew Goldman, DO, a board member of the Sutherland Cranial Teaching
Foundation, maintains a private practice in Sharon, Connecticut.

Osteopathy is a dynamic system of holistic health care that has been in existence for more than a century. A philosophy, an art, and a science, osteopathy emphasizes the importance of the neuromusculoskeletal system in the diagnosis and treatment of many illnesses. Because doctors of osteopathy (DOs) are accorded unlimited licensure and full medical and surgical practice privileges, they are frequently considered mainstream practitioners. The majority of osteopaths engage in some form of primary care, such as general or family practice, internal medicine, gynecology, obstetrics, or pediatrics. Many pursue specialties in psychiatry, radiology, anesthesiology, cardiology, or surgery.

Although allopathic medicine has not provided a context for the unique message of osteopathy, the profession has flourished because of the unmitigated enthusiasm and ardent support of the patients whom it has served.

Fundamental to osteopathy, in all its aspects, is a profound respect for nature and nature's laws. Dr. Andrew Taylor Still,[1] the founder of osteopathy, wrote, "An osteopath is taught that Nature is to be trusted to the end." Inherent in that respect for nature is the belief that *health* is the natural state of living beings. Aberrations from health are indicative of an interference with nature's design.

Osteopathy emphasizes the following four principles:

1. The human being is a dynamic unit of function.
2. The body possesses self-regulatory mechanisms that are self-healing in nature.
3. Structure and function are interrelated at all levels.
4. Rational treatment is based on the previous principles.[2]

Dynamic Unit of Function

Osteopathic philosophy holds that the human being, in all its dimensions, functions as a dynamic whole. It recognizes the importance of the physical, mental, and spiritual attributes of each being and honors the whole person. At the same time, it acknowledges that distinctions such as "body," "mind," and "spirit" are functionally artificial. Although these distinctions may facilitate speaking and stimulate thinking, all aspects of the being are, of necessity, interrelated, interdependent, and integrated, for the human being manifests as a multidimensional whole.

Still,[3] the founder of osteopathy, said, "I find in man a miniature universe. I find matter, motion, and mind." He elaborated: "The three [matter, motion, and mind], when united in full action, are able to exhibit the thing desired—complete."[4] (See Box 16–1.)

Self-Regulation and Self-Healing

Throughout nature, living systems demonstrate self-regulatory and self-healing mechanisms. In humans, self-regulation is manifest in such processes as the phenomenon of growth from fetus to adult, the ability of the body to maintain a constant internal temperature regardless of external conditions, the cyclic nature of menstruation, and the elegantly orchestrated feedback mechanisms of the endocrine system and the autonomic and central nervous systems. Self-healing is clearly exemplified by the body's ability to recover from a cold or viral infection, to mend a broken bone, and to form a clot at the site of a cut. All healing, however, is ultimately "self-healing." Physician, shaman, minister, and therapist may perform various functions to *assist* in the healing of the patient, but the actual capacity to heal resides within the patient.

Still said, "I have never failed to find all remedies in plain view on the front shelves and in the store house of the Infinite—the human body." He also commented, "Every living organism has within it the power to manufacture and prepare all chemicals and forces needed to build and rebuild itself."[5] Considering the vast array of neurotransmitters, immune system modulators, and other biochemical entities that have been discovered in recent years, Still[6] was indeed prescient in his 1897 statement: "Man should study and use the drugs compounded in his own body."

William Garner Sutherland, a graduate of the American School of Osteopathy, made a significant contribution to osteopathy and to the well-being of humanity through his discovery of the self-regulatory mechanism that he named the "primary respiratory mechanism" (PRM). Sutherland observed that the bones of the living human cranium are designed for motion and move in an organized fashion relative to each other. Moreover, he observed that motion at the cranial sutures occurs in response to and in concert with an involuntary, inherent, rhythmic motion within the central nervous system.[7] Osteopathic attunement to this mechanism has enabled those members of the profession who have pursued Sutherland's teaching in depth to be of service to a wide population of patients, from the newborn infant to the adult, through the diagnosis and treatment of restrictions of motion within this mechanism.

Interrelatedness of Structure and Function

The osteopath thinks in terms of the effect that structure has on function and vice versa. Changes in structure, whether visceral, somatic or psychic, macroscopic or microscopic, peripheral or deep, ultimately affect function. Still[8] said, "Osteopathy deals with the body as a perfect machine, which if kept in proper adjustment, nourished and cared for, will run smoothly into ripe and useful old age. . . . When every part of the machine is properly adjusted and in perfect harmony, health will hold dominion over the human organism by laws as natural and immutable as the laws of gravity." More pointedly, he said, "In the year 1874 I proclaimed that a disturbed artery marked the beginning to an hour and a minute when disease began to sow its seeds of destruction in the human body. . . . The rule of the artery is absolute, universal, and it must be unobstructed, or disease will result."[9]

Aberrations in structure and function—that is, anatomy and physiology—have a cause, and the aberrations themselves are the effects. Dr. Still[10] stated, "We say disease when we

BOX 16–1

A History

Osteopathy came into existence against the backdrop of post–Civil War Kansas. Andrew Taylor Still, a frontier physician, farmer, inventor, and legislator, returned home from the war in 1864 deeply affected and frustrated by the relative failure that he and his medical colleagues had experienced in caring for the sick and wounded soldiers. The medicinal agents employed by physicians during the war were toxic and often addictive. Surgeries were grueling and were often followed by infection and death. Then, soon after he returned home, three of his children contracted spinal meningitis; despite the efforts of Still and his colleagues, all three children died. A few weeks later, his 1-year-old daughter died of pneumonia. Following this devastating series of events, he wrote, "Not until my heart had been torn and lacerated with grief and affliction could I fully realize the inefficacy of drugs."[1]

These profound demonstrations of the inadequacy of medicine as it was being practiced led Still to question the nature of medical practice, the physiological soundness of the human species, and, in fact, the nature of God. Of that time in his life, he wrote, "I proposed to myself the serious questions, 'In sickness, has God left man in a world of guessing? Guess what is the matter, what to give, and guess the result?' . . . I decided that God was not a guessing God, but a God of truth. . . . So wise a God had certainly placed the remedy within the material house in which the spirit of life dwells."[2] With the burgeoning conviction that the human body had within it the elements essential to its own health, Still embarked on a period of deep study and contemplation.

Still's focused intention and deep inquiry culminated at 10 AM on June 22, 1874, in a moment of illumination. On that date, the concept, which he named "osteopathy," became clear to him. In a lecture he gave on his 69th birthday, Still said of that experience, "Who discovered Osteopathy? Twenty-four years ago, the 22nd day of June, at ten o'clock, I saw a small light in the horizon of truth. It was put into my hand, as I understood, by the God of nature."[3] He also stated, "I do not claim to be the author of this science of Osteopathy. No human hand framed its laws; I ask no greater honor than to have discovered it."[4]

As is often the case with radical innovators and paradigm shifters, Andrew Taylor Still was derided and accused of heresy. He wrote that people avoided him on the street because he said that he "did not believe God was a whisky and opium-drug doctor."[5] He was shunned by former associates and was prohibited from explaining the concept of osteopathy at Baker University in Baldwin, Kansas, an institution to which he had donated hundreds of acres of land and which he had physically helped to build.[6]

Still subsequently left Kansas and traveled throughout Missouri as an itinerant physician, applying his concept to the patients he treated. Application of the concept of osteopathy met with great success, and, as word of its benefits spread, Still became unable to single-handedly attend to the great number of patients who sought his help. Therefore, in 1892, in Kirksville, Missouri, Still founded the American School of Osteopathy, later renamed the Kirksville College of Osteopathic Medicine. A revised charter for the school issued under Missouri law in 1894 states:

> The object of this corporation is to establish a College of Osteopathy, the design of which is to improve our present system of surgery, obstetrics and treatment of disease generally, and place the same on a more rational and scientific basis, and to impart information to the medical profession, and to grant and confer such honors and degrees as are usually granted and conferred by reputable medical colleges.[7]

Although, according to the charter, an MD degree could have been awarded to the school's graduates, Still wanted his students to receive a degree that would distinguish them from traditionally trained MDs. He chose to award his graduates with the degree DO.

The first class of students—5 women and 16 men—entered the American School of Osteopathy in 1892. Before commencing study, one of those women, Mrs. Jenette Bolles, asked Still if women could learn to practice osteopathy. He responded that a woman could learn to do anything a man could do.[8] Women were welcomed into the profession, and the 1901–1902 catalog of the American School of Osteopathy stated, "Women are admitted on the same terms as men. It is a policy of the school that there shall be no distinction as to sex. All have the same opportunities and the same requirements."[9]

continued

BOX 16–1 continued

A History

Professional recognition and legal provision for the practice of osteopathy were forthcoming, with the Vermont state legislature in 1896 being the first to grant licensure for the practice of osteopathy. Other states rapidly followed suit, despite opposition from the medical establishment.

REFERENCES

1. Still, AT: Autobiography of A. T. Still. Author, Kirksville, Mo., 1908, p 87.
2. Ibid, p 88.
3. Ibid, p 339.
4. Ibid, p 302.
5. Ibid, p 107.
6. Ibid, p 97.
7. Quoted in Booth, ER: History of Osteopathy and Twentieth-Century Medical Practice, ed. 2. Caxton Press, Cincinnati, Ohio, 1924, pp 79–80.
8. Walter, GW: Women and Osteopathic Medicine: Historical Perspectives. Kirksville College of Osteopathic Medicine, Kirksville, Mo., 1994.
9. College catalog, 1901–1902, American School of Osteopathy, Kirksville, Mo.

should say effect; for disease is the effect of change in the parts of the physical body. Disease in an abnormal body is just as natural as is health when all parts are in place."

Rational Treatment

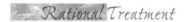

The osteopathic approach both to the understanding of health and to the designing and rendering of treatment is based on inclusionary thinking that appreciates the dynamic, multidimensional, self-regulatory, and self-healing nature of the human being. It requires that the physician have a thorough knowledge of anatomy, physiology, and chemistry and be able to reason from that knowledge. It directs the physician to discover and eliminate the *cause* of disease rather than "dally with effects," or symptoms.[11]

A thread that is present throughout all of osteopathy and that unifies these principles in the rendering of treatment is that of respect—respect for the body's inherent wisdom and the manifestation of nature's laws, and respect for the health that is present and dynamically operative within the patient. Sutherland and Wales[12] stated, "The goal with your patients is to find the way to healthy function within the mechanism that they bring to you."

CASE STUDY

Ruby

Ruby, a 16-year-old dancer, returned home from a week-long modern dance program during which she had been dropped on the top of her head during a routine. She was fatigued and complaining of a one-sided frontal headache. Within 48 hours of arriving home, she developed a fever. During the night, her fever exceeded 104°, and Ruby's mother took her to the local emergency room. There, lab work was run, and she showed an elevated white blood cell count, indicative of infection. She was hydrated with intravenous fluids, and was administered acetaminophen and an intravenous antibiotic. Within 2 hours, her temperature normalized. The source of her symptoms was not identified, and she was sent home with the diagnosis of nonspecific viral syndrome. She was told to rest and to use acetaminophen or ibuprofen if her temperature rose again.

Twenty-four hours later, Ruby was still requiring medication to control her fever. Her headache persisted, and she was noting clear fluid draining continuously from one side of her nose. She was taken to the office of her pediatrician, Dr. Hart, an osteopath. Dr. Hart took a thorough history from Ruby, reviewed the lab results from the previous day's emergency room visit, and conducted a thorough physical exam. Although Ruby's neurological examination result was normal, her symptoms, in conjunction with her history of being dropped on her head, led Dr. Hart to consider the possibility of a skull fracture or bleeding in the head. She called a neurosurgeon to discuss the case, and he concurred with her thought that a computed tomography (CT) scan of the head should be performed promptly.

Dr. Hart wrote orders for updated blood work and for a CT scan of the head and sent Ruby to the hospital to have the tests performed. The white blood count continued to be elevated. However, the CT scan offered an explanation: it showed a full-blown left-sided sinusitis. The hospital's physician wrote Ruby a prescription for one 14-day course of antibiotics and told her that she might actually require up to 6 weeks of antibiotics to eradicate the infection.

The next day Ruby's mother contacted Dr. Hart, who was satisfied that an acute sinus infection accounted for Ruby's elevated temperature, elevated white blood cell count, and unilateral headache. But why, she asked, employing osteopathic thinking, should a unilateral sinus infection occur in this otherwise healthy 16-year-old? Treating the bacterial infection with antibiotics might eliminate the symptom, she reasoned, but if the cause was not found and eliminated, the infection could persist or recur. Dr. Hart wondered whether the force involved in Ruby's landing on her head had impaired lymphatic drainage from the head or had altered the function of the mechanism that enables the sinuses to drain properly.

Determined to seek out and eliminate the cause of Ruby's sinusitis, Dr. Hart referred Ruby to Dr. Taylor, an osteopath who was particularly proficient in osteopathic manipulative medicine—that is, the diagnosis and manual treatment of structural abnormalities that can lead to impaired physiology. Dr. Hart explained to Ruby's mother that although she herself had learned these methods of diagnosis and treatment in school, she, regrettably, had not used these skills sufficiently to be comfortable in applying them.

When Ruby arrived in Dr. Taylor's office, she was observed as she sat, stood, and walked. A history was taken. Then, Dr. Taylor, with her hands placed lightly on Ruby, gathered information regarding the motion and position of various structures in Ruby's body. She determined that Ruby's craniovertebral (head-neck) junction and cervical spine (neck) were mechanically strained, potentially interfering with lymphatic drainage from the head and altering nerve input to the lining of the sinuses. Additionally, she noted that the motion in the cranium, including the bones that house the sinuses, was restricted, potentially interfering with sinus drainage. Using her hands in a precise and subtle manner, Dr. Taylor relieved the strain pattern and restored normal position and motion to the neck and head.

Ruby was asymptomatic the next day. She completed the 14-day course of antibiotics as directed, and a follow-up sinus x-ray showed complete resolution. There was no relapse or recurrence. Eliminating the probable cause of or predisposing factor to her infection potentially saved Ruby from the need for additional antibiotics and a prolonged convalescence.

Osteopathic Manipulation

Osteopathic manipulative medicine, a method of manual diagnosis and treatment unique to osteopathy, is often incorporated into primary and specialty care practices and is sometimes practiced as a specialty unto itself. Using their hands diagnostically, osteopaths are able to perceive and diagnose many joint dysfunctions—or ligamentous articular strains—that are not perceptible on x-rays or other imaging studies. They can feel in strained or sprained tissues the vectors of force responsible for injury. Those trained in osteopathy in the cranial field can perceive dysfunction within the primary respiratory mechanism, or "craniosacral mechanism," as Rollin Becker[13] sometimes called it. Using their trained hands to render treatment, osteopaths can undertake, among other things, to normalize joint mechanisms, eliminate strains, and facilitate the function of the primary respiratory mechanism.

Although not all osteopaths—whether because of time constraints or personal preference—apply the principles of osteopathic manipulative medicine in their practices, those who do develop and utilize this aspect of osteopathy possess a valuable means of detecting and eliminating the source of many physical dysfunctions. Osteopathic pediatricians, neurologists, neonatologists, and cardiologists augment their diagnostic ability and facilitate healthy function when they employ this skill. Those osteopaths who practice osteopathic manipulative medicine as a specialty unto itself treat patients who present with a wide variety of issues.

Typical case scenarios presenting to such a practice would include a newborn who has undergone a prolonged or traumatic delivery and is experiencing regurgitation and having difficulty sucking; a pregnant women with low back pain and fluid retention; a child with a spastic disorder or developmental delay; a car accident victim with whiplash; a dental patient undergoing orthodontia or having recently had a tooth extraction; a child or teenager with scoliosis; a migraine headache sufferer; and a young mother with postpartum depression.

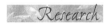

Research

Still saw research as primary to osteopathy. He said: "Osteopathy is a science. Its use is in the healing of the afflicted. It is a philosophy which embraces surgery, obstetrics, and general practice. An osteopath must be a man of reason and prove his talk by his work. He has no use for theories unless they are demonstrated."

Traditionally, osteopathic medicine has viewed the human body as a unit. For this reason, modern research techniques, which demand separation of the whole into its parts in order to allow for carefully controlled experimentation, have inherent limitations. We humans are more than our component parts. We are an integrated whole, our parts inseparable. The osteopathic physician is constantly aware of this when interacting with a patient. Too often in modern medicine, fragmented information is used in an overspecialized approach to patient care.

The osteopathic profession has begun to realize the need for a paradigm shift in our scientific inquiry. I. M. Korr, a pre-eminent osteopathic researcher and educator, wrote:

> *While the knowledge yielded by reductionist research is essential to osteopathic research, the latter requires, in effect, that the knowledge about the component structures and processes be reinserted into the total person whom it serves, where it is subject to the influence of all other parts through the communication systems of the body, and where it is affected by all the factors—physical, chemical, mental, emotional, social, and environmental—that render the human body distinct from all other species, and each human different from all other humans.* The reinsertion of the parts into the human context accomplishes the needed completion. *What is more, when the human is restored to its context, new light is cast on each part: Properties, functions, interaction emerge that are not evident in isolation and out of that context.* (Emphasis in original)[14]

"The art of clinical research is a fairly new endeavor; necessary new techniques and understandings must be developed."[15] Experiments designed for testing a drug or a technique's efficacy have, at times, been modified to test an osteopathic technique. Practicing osteopaths apply techniques with specific concepts in mind to restore normal anatomical, and therefore physiological, function to patients to allow their own inherent healing forces to correct the dysfunction. Every patient is different from the next, and every patient is different from one day to the next. Therefore, it would be an improper application of technique to use a specific maneuver for sinusitis, ear infections, headaches, back pain, or any other medical diagnosis. Such diagnoses describe the effect of a dysfunctional situation in the body rather than its cause. In Still's words, "Disease is the result of anatomical abnormalities followed by physiological discord."[16]

In the first half of the 20th century, Louisa Burns published a large volume of research and academic papers on osteopathic theory. Using the methods and instruments of her time, Burns performed experiments on animals by inducing strains (somatic dysfunction) and observing physiological as well as gross and microscopic anatomical changes in various organ systems, including the heart, gastrointestinal system, reproductive system, central nervous system, somatic structures, lungs, kidneys, and blood-forming structures.[17] She reported on the effect of bony lesions (somatic dysfunction) on behavior, on ways in which osteopathic lesions affect eye tissues, and on viscerosomatic and somatovisceral reflexes (organs affecting the body wall and vice versa, respectively).

John Stedman Denslow used electromyographic (EMG) studies, a new technology in the early 1940s, to study osteopathic lesions (somatic dysfunction) that he had diagnosed using his palpatory sense. He demonstrated areas in otherwise normal adults that had measurable overactive muscle activity. Further, he could show EMG changes in areas he had diagnosed as lesioned.[18]

Denslow's[19] first research paper, published in 1941 in the *Journal of Neurophysiology*, required the establishment of the Still Memorial Research Trust because refereed journals of that day would not consider publishing work from an osteopathic institution— osteopathy was too controversial. Through the Still Memorial Research Trust, Denslow could submit his paper from an institution that was not "tainted" by an association with osteopathy. Denslow continued to do research on the neuromuscular physiology involved in the osteopathic lesion and was joined in this research by Irvin M. Korr in 1947.

Korr's association with Denslow led to the development of a concept of segmental facilitation that is still being taught in osteopathic medical schools today. Korr has continued to conduct research that has supported osteopathic theory and practice from a neurophysiological perspective. He has also been instrumental in synthesizing basic science information to help explain osteopathic clinical observations.[20]

The concept of viscerosomatic reflexes has been attributed to Frank Chapman, who used reflex points in his practice in the 1920s.[21] Since that time, extensive work has been done on the relationship of the somatic and visceral systems. An extensive body of information now exists on a wide variety of organs and their associated somatic reflex regions. Myron Beal[22] performed a comprehensive review of the literature on viscerosomatic reflexes. In a long-term longitudinal study, William Johnston and Albert Kelso[23] have established that a pattern of somatic dysfunction, involving the 6th cervical, 2nd thoracic, and 6th thoracic vertebrae, is associated with hypertension.

Akio Sato and his associates have done extensive research in laboratory animals. This group has "employed various types of mechanical, thermal, and chemical stimulation of the skin, muscles, and joints at various spinal levels to produce reflex responses in . . . visceral organs."[24] This included stimulation to the skin in anesthetized animals, which caused increases in heart rate, increases and decreases in gastric motility, increased bladder tone, and inhibitory and excitatory input to sweat glands. They also demonstrated that such stimulation caused increases and decreases of adrenal medullary function, increases of adrenal cortical activity, and increases in cerebral blood flow. All these reflexes (including increases versus decreases) were site specific and demonstrated to be due to influence on the autonomic nervous system. Adrenal cortical activity was shown to be the result of increased amounts of corticotropin-releasing hormone from the hypothalamus, which causes release of adrenocorticotropic hormone from the anterior pituitary.

Research has also established the reliability of palpation of the thoracic vertebrae as being predictive of coronary atherosclerosis.[25] Patients in this study received a standardized musculoskeletal examination by qualified osteopathic physicians within a week of coronary angiography. Somatic dysfunction at the 4th thoracic vertebra had a 91 percent predictive value of at least 50 percent stenosis of one or more coronary arteries. Another study revealed that somatic dysfunction of the 1st through 4th thoracic vertebrae is highly correlated with patients diagnosed with acute myocardial infarction versus controls.[26] This was highly statistically significant ($p < .0001$).

The effect of osteopathic manipulation on respiration has been studied at length. Murphy[27,28] showed that mobilization of the thorax increased tidal volume and alveolar ventilation. She also showed an improvement of circulation to the lungs.[29] Murphy's research suggests that improved thoracic motion "[leads] to improved lung gas exchange."[30]

John W. Measel demonstrated that an osteopathic technique known as the "Miller lymphatic pump" produces a statistically significant increase in immune response to a specific antigen.[31] A more recent study by Kelly M. Jackson and colleagues[32] showed that use of the lymphatic and splenic pump produced an increase in antibody response to hepatitis B vaccine.

Viola Frymann[33] and colleagues have published research on the effect of osteopathic medical management on neurologic development in children. This study looked at children with and without neurologic problems, quantified by a standardized test, and measured development with and without osteopathic treatment. Children who had been diagnosed with neurologic problems significantly improved their performance in sensorimotor testing as well as on Houle's Profile of Development after osteopathic manipulative treatment. These positive changes were shown to last long after treatment had ended.

David Boesler and colleagues[34] showed that osteopathic manipulation performed on women with menstrual cramps and low back pain was successful in alleviating or reducing both symptoms. This study demonstrated a decrease in electromyographic activity in low back muscles after osteopathic manipulative treatment. Subjects also reported: "(1) more relaxed feeling; (2) ability to move with less resistance; (3) reduced or complete absence of low back pain; (4) alleviation or significant reduction of menstrual cramping."

Jane Carreiro[35] treated 18 children—ranging in age from 18 months to 5 years—suffering from chronic otitis media (middle ear infection) with effusion, using osteopathic manipulative treatment. Four children were on prophylactic antibiotics when they entered this study. These drugs were eventually discontinued by the referring physician. No antibiotics were added as an adjunct to osteopathic manipulative treatment. Sixteen of these children cleared these effusions with no recurrence of acute otitis media for an 18-month period.

Maxwell Fraval[36] evaluated a small number of infants with sucking dysfunction. Osteopathic treatment improved the efficiency of their suck. These otherwise normal infants had previously been seen by lactation consultants, who had exhausted their treatment options. Normal motion of the mouth, tongue, and pharynx requires clear communication via the glossopharyngeal and vagus nerves, which follow a course through the base of the skull and may be distorted through the strain of the birth process. Osteopathic physicians seek to reduce these strains in order to normalize function. Although this was only a pilot study, it validates clinical successes that have been achieved by osteopaths for more than 50 years.

Knowledge from Information

Still was a careful investigator of nature. He wrote: "Osteopathy walks hand in hand with nothing but nature's laws, and for this reason alone it marks the most significant progress in the history of scientific research."[37] Still's type of research, still practiced by some osteopaths today, relies on intense observation of anatomy and the natural world as well as an understanding of the laws of physics. Continuing research developments in physiology, pathology, and the various branches of medicine enhance our understanding of the human patient as a whole entity. Still was known for his continued study of human bones and once said, "To know all of a bone in its entirety would close both ends of an eternity."[38] It is in this tradition of study, with reverence for the elegance of God's creation, that many in this profession continue to dig for deeper understanding of the human condition and life in general.

Osteopath W. G. Sutherland performed tireless research in this spirit. While a student at the American School of Osteopathy between 1898 and 1900, he observed a skeleton mounted in a display case with a disarticulated skull. He later said:

> As I stood looking and thinking in the channel of Dr. Still's philosophy, my attention was called to the beveled articular surfaces of the sphenoid bone. Suddenly there came a thought—I call it a guiding thought—"beveled like the gills of a fish, indicating articular mobility for a respiratory mechanism."[39]

Sutherland initially rejected this notion of cranial bone mobility, citing the sound information of the textbooks he was studying. However, he was unable to get this thought out of his head and undertook the task of attempting to disprove this theory with arduous study over the next 30 years. The more he tried to disprove his idea, the more supportive information he gathered. Eventually this led to an understanding of *the primary respiratory mechanism*, a conceptual framework for a greater understanding of human health and physiology, applicable to osteopathic practice. Sutherland's cranial concept was tested clinically with remarkable results. In more recent years, the idea of cranial mobility has been substantiated by laboratory research using sophisticated instrumentation.[40,41,42] Sutherland's concept, a contribution to Still's philosophy, is seen as "one of the most innovative ideas to be advanced by a member of the osteopathic profession."[43]

There are many osteopathic physicians today who are in clinical practice and continue to gather information in an attempt to improve our understanding of the osteopathic concept. They are following in the footsteps of some great visionaries. Osteopaths gather knowledge by their senses and interpret with their intellect based on years of study in an attempt to understand the living human. In this way they are all researchers in the ever-expanding science of osteopathy.

Summary

Osteopathy is a science of infinite depth and boundless possibilities. It honors the life and health within each patient. It endeavors to facilitate the expression of health and eliminate the source of dysfunction. To the physician who practices osteopathy, it offers the rare privilege of being able, through the sense of touch, to feel and observe the process of the human body healing itself.

Still[44] wrote of the experience of the osteopath engaged in a clinical consultation: "Here you lay aside the long words, and use your mind in deep and silent earnestness; drink deep from the eternal fountain of reason, penetrate the forest of that law whose beauties are life and death." Those who practice osteopathy and those who are its patients inherit and benefit from this legacy of reverence and reason.

RESOURCES

American Academy of Osteopathy
3500 DePauw Blvd., Suite 1080
Indianapolis, IN 46268
Phone: (317) 879-1881

American Osteopathic Association
142 East Ontario St.
Chicago, IL 60611
Phone: (312) 202-8000

Still National Osteopathic Museum
800 W. Jefferson
Kirksville, MO 63501
Phone: (800) 626-5266, ext. 2359

REFERENCES

1. Still, AT: Autobiography of A.T. Still. Author, Kirksville, Mo., 1908.
2. 1998 American Osteopathic Association Yearbook and Directory, ed 89. American Osteopathic Association, Chicago, 1998, p 775.
3. Still, AT: Autobiography of A.T. Still. p 333.
4. Ibid, p 27.
5. Ibid, p 88.
6. Still, AT: Autobiography of A.T. Still. Author, Kirkesville, Mo., 1908, p 89.
7. Lay, E: In Ward, RC, et al (eds): Foundations for Osteopathic Medicine. Williams & Wilkins, Baltimore, 1997, pp 902-904.
8. Quoted in Webster, GV: Sage Sayings of Still. Wetzel Publishing, Los Angeles, 1935, p 26.
9. Still, AT: Autobiography of A.T. Still. Author, Kirkesville, Missouri, 1908, p 182.
10. Still, AT: Osteopathy Research and Practice, 1910. Reprinted: Eastland Press, Seattle, 1992, p 13.
11. Ibid at p 6.
12. Sutherland, WG, and Wales, AL (eds): Teachings in the Science of Osteopathy. Rudra Press, Portland, Ore., 1990, p 7.
13. Becker, RE, and Brooks, RE (eds): Life in Motion. Rudra Press, Portland, Ore., 1997, p 5.
14. Korr, IM: Osteopathic research: The needed paradigm shift. J Am Osteopath Assoc 91(2):156, 1991.
15. Patterson, MM: Osteopathic research—The future. In Ward, et al (eds): Foundations for Osteopathic Medicine. Williams & Wilkins, Baltimore, 1997, pp 1115–1124.
16. Still, AT: Osteopathy Research and Practice. Reprinted: Eastland Press, Seattle, 1992, p 9.
17. Cole, WV: Louisa Burns memorial lecture. In Louisa Burns, DO, Memorial, 1994 Yearbook. American Academy of Osteopathy, Indianapolis, 1994, p. 2.
18. Beal, MC (ed): In Selected papers of John Stedman Denslow, DO. 1993 Year Book, American Academy of Osteopathy, Indianapolis, 1993.
19. Denslow, JS, and Clough, GH: Reflex activity in the spinal extensors. J Neurophysiol 4:430-437,1941.
20. Peterson, B (ed): The Collected Papers of Irvin M. Korr. American Academy of Asteopathy, Colorado Springs, 1979.
21. Owens, C: An Endocrine Interpretation of Chapman's Reflexes, ed 2. Chattanooga Printing and Engraving, Chattanooga, Tenn., 1937.
22. Beal, MC: Viscerosomatic reflexes: A review. J Am Osteopath Assoc 85(12):786, 1985.
23. Johnston, WL, and Kelso, AF: Changes in presence of a segmental dysfunction pattern associated with hypertension: Part 2. A long-term longitudinal study. J Am Osteopath Assoc 95(5):315, 1995.
24. Sato, A: Reflex modulation of visceral functions by somatic afferent activity. In: Patterson, MM, and Howell, JN (eds.) The Central Connection: Somatovisceral/Viscerosomatic Interaction. College of Osteopathic Medicine, Ohio University, Columbus, 1989 p 53.

25. Cox, JM, et al: Palpable musculoskeletal findings in coronary artery disease. J Am Osteopath Assoc, 82(11):832, 1983.

26. Nicholas, AS, et al: A somatic component to myocardial infarction. BMJ. 29(16):13, 1985.

27. Murphy, AJ: Preliminary studies of the influence of pulmonary and thoracic mobilization procedures on pulmonary function. J Am Osteopath Assoc 64:951-952, 1995.

28. Murphy, AJ: Comparison of nitrogen washout curves from human experiments and from a mathematical model of the lung. J Am Osteopath Assoc 66:1023-1024, 1967.

29. Murphy, AJ: Continuation of the study of the effect of thoracic mobilation on the distribution of ^{131}I in the lungs. J Am Osteopath Assoc 70:1057-1058, 1971.

30. D'Alonzo, GE, and Krachman, SL: Respiratory Systems. In Ward, RC, et al (eds): Foundations for Osteopathic Medicine. Williams & Wilkins, Baltimore, 1997, p 453.

31. Measel, JW: The effect of the lymphatic pump on the immune response: Preliminary studies on the antibody response to pneumococcal polysaccharide assayed by bacterial agglutination and passive hemagglutination. J Am Osteopath Assoc 82(1):28, 1982.

32. Jackson, KM, et al: Effect of lymphatic and splenic pump techniques on the antibody response to hepatitis B vaccine: A pilot study. J Am Osteopath Assoc 98(3):155-160, 1998.

33. Frymann, VM, et al: Effect of osteopathic medical management on neurologic development in children. J Am Osteopath Assoc 92(6):729–744, 1992.

34. Boesler, D, et al: Efficacy of high-velocity low-amplitude manipulative technique I subjects with low back pain during menstrual cramping. J Am Osteopath Assoc 93(2):203, 1993.

35. Carriero, JE: Personal Communication, June 1998. Manuscript submitted for publication at the time of this writing.

36. Fraval, MM: A pilot study: Osteopathic treatment of infants with a sucking dysfunction. Am Acad Osteopath J, 8:2, 1998, p 25.

37. Still, AT: Autobiography of A.T. Still, 1908. Reprinted: American Academy of Osteopathy, Colorado Springs, 1981, p 298.

38. Ibid, p 152.

39. Sutherland, AS: With Thinking Fingers. The Cranial Academy, Kansas City, 1962, p 12.

40. Frymann, VM: A study of the rhythmic motions of the living cranium. J Am Osteopath Assoc 40: 928–945, 1971.

41. Zanakis, MF, et al: Cranial mobility in man: Objective measurements in normal subjects. J Am Osteopath Assoc 95(8):016, 1995.

42. Zanakis, MF, et al: Subjective and objective evaluations of the cranial rhythmic impulse in man. J Am Osteopath Assoc 95(8):017, 1995.

43. Northrup, GW (ed): Osteopathic Research: Growth and Development. American Osteopathic Association, Chicago, 1987, p 40.

44. Still, AT: Autobiography of A.T. Still. 1908, p152.

RECOMMENDED READING

Fulford, RC: Dr. Fulford's Touch of Life. Pocket Books, New York, 1996.

Still, AT: Autobiography of A.T. Still. Author, Kirksville, Mo., 1908. (Distributed by American Academy of Osteopathy)

Sutherland, AS: With Thinking Fingers: The Story of William Garner Sutherland, D.O., D.Sc. (Hon.). The Cranial Academy, Indianapolis, 1962.

Trowbridge, C: Andrew Taylor Still: 1828–1917. Thomas Jefferson University Press, Kirkland, Mo., 1991. (Distributed by Still National Osteopathic Museum)

Walter, G: The First School of Osteopathic Medicine. Thomas Jefferson University Press, Kirkland, Mo., 1992. (Distributed by Still National Osteopathic Museum)

Walter, G: Osteopathic Medicine: Past and Present. Kirksville College of Osteopathic Medicine, Kirksville, Mo., 1993. (Distributed by Still National Osteopathic Museum)

Walter, G: Women and Osteopathic Medicine. Kirksville College of Osteopathic Medicine, Kirksville, Mo., 1994. (Distributed by Still National Osteopathic Museum)

CHAPTER 17

Chiropractic

Vivian Roman and Andrea Callanan

Vivian Roman, DC, maintains a private practice in Massachusetts.
Andrea Callanan, DC, practices in Gainesville, Virginia.

The term *chiropractic* comes from the Greek word *chiropraktikos*, meaning "effective treatment by hand." *Dorland's Medical Dictionary*[1] defines chiropractic as "a system of therapeutics that attributes disease to irritation of the nervous system, and attempts to restore normal function by manipulation of the body structures, especially those of the vertebral column." According to Altman,[2] "Chiropractic deals with the vital relationship between the nervous system and the spinal column and the role of this relationship in the restoration and maintenance of health." Simply put, chiropractic is, in the words of Sportelli,[3] a health-care discipline based on the premise that "good health depends, in part, on a normally functioning nervous system. When body structures such as cells and organs are functioning normally, a state of heath or normal physiology exists. However, when the body's physiology is abnormal the potential for a disease state exists."

From the moment we are born, our bodies rely on the nervous system to function. This system is protected by the bones of the skull and 24 bones of the spine, called "vertebrae." In between the vertebrae are cartilaginous disks that together form the spinal column. Extending from the vertebrae are 31 pairs of spinal nerves branching off the spinal cord. These nerves go to the lungs, heart, ears, legs, and all the organs and muscles of the body. It is the nervous system that allows us to breathe, eat, move, see, think, and function, whether we are awake or asleep. So it is only natural that when there is any type of interference with the nervous system, our body fails, or parts of it fail, to function properly. This malfunction leads to pain, illness, disease, and possibly death.

There are many causes for nervous system dysfunction, such as trauma suffered from falls or auto accidents, or congenital defects such as scoliosis. Sometimes it can be due to a condition called "subluxation." This is the loss of proper position or motion of a joint in the body, most commonly the vertebral bones of the spinal column, which interferes with proper nervous system function.

Chiropractors work to remove the subluxation by realigning the bones, which allows the nerve impulses to flow without interruption, restoring proper function to the nervous system and improving health. The act of realigning the bones is called an "adjustment." This is performed without the use of drugs or surgery. The goal of chiropractic is to find and remove the cause of the symptom rather than cover up the symptom with drugs or alter the site of discomfort before treating the true cause. This allows the body to function optimally and to heal itself with its own abilities.

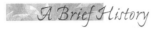 A Brief History

Chiropractic celebrated its 100th birthday in 1995. However, its roots can be traced back to the beginning of recorded history.[4] Tissue manipulation is described in an ancient Kong Fou document from China written in approximately 2700 BC. Descriptions of maneuvering the lower extremities to treat lower back conditions appear on a Greek papyrus dating to approximately 1500 BC.[5] But it was Hippocrates (c460–c375 BC), the father of medicine, who was the first physician to link spinal misalignments with ill health.[6] He advised his students to "get knowledge of the spine, for this is the requisite for many diseases."[7]

It was not until 1895 that a man named Daniel David Palmer employed the science of chiropractic. Palmer was the founder of chiropractic. He emigrated to the United states in 1865 from Port Perry, Ontario.[8] He was a self-educated man, as were most people in the 1800s, so he was always reading on his own to further his knowledge. He became interested in the new ideas of health and metaphysics.[9] In time he went on to study under a man named Paul Caster who taught magnetic healing, which was in vogue at the time.[10,11] In 1885 Palmer opened his own office in Davenport, Iowa, to practice magnetic healing and return to a lifelong interest in helping the sick.[12]

Throughout his years as a magnetic healer, Palmer helped many people. However, he knew there was much more involved in healing the human body and was constantly searching for a better way. Palmer was constantly reading books on anatomy and physiology. From studying the human spine extensively, he learned that the body receives nerve energy through the vertebral column, and he understood "that an impingement on the spinal nerves could inhibit the energy flowing from the brain through the nerves to various organs of the body."[13] It was this concept that led him to give the first chiropractic adjustment.

Palmer performed the first chiropractic adjustment on September 18, 1895.[14] The patient was Harvey Lillard, who told Palmer that for the past "seventeen years he had been so deaf that he could not hear the racket of a wagon on the street or the ticking of a watch."[15] He informed Palmer that once when he was exerting himself in a cramped, stooped position, he felt something give way in his back and immediately became deaf.[16] Palmer examined the man's back and noticed a vertebra out of its normal position. From his studies, he reasoned that if the vertebra were placed back in its normal position, Lillard's hearing would be restored. "[A] half-hour's talk persuaded Mr. Lillard to allow me to replace it. I racked it into position by using the spinous process as a lever and soon the man could hear as before."[17]

After this incident, Palmer claimed that he could cure deafness and other illnesses. It would have been nice if it were that simple. But he discovered that his "adjustment" did not work the same on everyone. His claims eventually created much controversy within the medical profession, but they also inspired the growth and development of chiropractic.

The philosophy of chiropractic teaches that "our ability to adapt to changes in our internal and external environment is essential to the maintenance of life and health. An unobstructed flow of nerve impulses from the brain through the spinal nerves and onward to every body cell will help achieve the balance, harmony and vitality we need to enjoy vibrant health and a long productive life."[18] The human body is designed to function on its own and heal itself, provided there is no interference with its physiological or physical mechanisms.

Applications

Chiropractic has brought relief to many people with back and neck pain. It has also helped relieve people of discomfort caused by neuralgia, sciatica, bursitis, tendonitis, disk problems, and muscle sprains.[19] And in many cases it has helped control such disorders as hypertension, arthritis, rheumatism, bronchial asthma, allergies, nervous tension, chronic fatigue, and heart trouble.[20] Many of these problems are related to subluxation, which is a clinical complex comprised of one or more of the following components: (1) kinesiopathology, which is an abnormal mobility or position; (2) neuropathology, which is abnormal function of the nervous system; (3) myopathology, which is abnormal muscle function; (4) histopathology, which is abnormal tissue function; and (5) pathophysiology, which is caused by biochemical abnormalities.[21]

Subluxations are brought on by everyday stresses such as poor posture, especially while working; fatigue or lack of proper rest; trauma or injury; sports; repetitive activities; sitting every day for long periods of time; and emotional stress, which keeps the body in a constant state of tension. These and other situations create an "unbalance" in the body and disrupt its homeostasis.[22] Homeostasis is the ability of a living system to control its internal environment.[23] When homeostasis is disrupted, the living system starts to break down, becoming vulnerable, and disease sets in because so much energy is being used to restore balance. The symptoms of this process include pain, decrease in motor and or organ function, lower immunity, illness, and eventual death of the system.

Clinical Practice

When a patient visits a chiropractor for treatment, the doctor first completes a chiropractic evaluation. This includes a complete health history, physical exam, and, in some cases, x-rays. X-rays are taken only if indicated by the health history or physical exam—to rule out fractures, tumors, and other pathologies. They also show any evidence of subluxations of the joints. After determining whether chiropractic treatment can help the patient, the doctor will begin an individualized treatment program to reduce any pain or discomfort and realign any subluxated joints.

A chiropractor removes or realigns a subluxation by performing an "adjustment," which usually involves placing his or her hands on the patient's spine and locating the area of subluxation. The area of subluxation is usually tender to the patient; the doctor can feel whether the muscles of the area are spasmed or hot from the irritation. A gentle force is then applied to the area in a specific direction, allowing the bone to return to its normal position. This is accompanied by decreasing spasm in the surrounding musculature and decreased irritation and symptomatology, allowing normal blood flow and nervous system function. (See Box 17–1.)

Common Chiropractic Techniques

There are a number of chiropractic techniques for performing an adjustment. These techniques involve manual manipulation of the skeletal structure to restore balance in the nervous system, joint mobility, and overall structure integrity. The patient is positioned by the chiropractor, who uses various methods of controlled pressure to realign the bones of the spine, the cranium, and the extremities.

Some practitioners also use other supportive therapies to help decrease patient discomfort, such as ice, heat, ultrasound, electrical muscle stimulation, traction, and massage. Nutritional advice is sometimes given to aid in the healing process. Relaxation techniques such as yoga and meditation may also be suggested to help alleviate stress.

BOX 17–1
The Growth of the Profession

In 1897, D. D. Palmer established the Palmer Infirmary and Chiropractic School in Davenport, Iowa.[1] This was the first chiropractic school. Students attending included men and women, medical doctors, osteopaths, and surgeons. In the first graduating class was Bartlett Joshua Palmer, son of D. D. Palmer. B. J. Palmer would go on to become the developer of chiropractic, helping to "elevate it to the second largest health care system in America by the time he died in 1961."[2]

More chiropractic schools opened, and chiropractic began to grow. By 1920 half the states had recognized chiropractic, and it became legalized in Kansas and North Dakota. To represent the profession, the American Chiropractic Association was established, as well as the International Chiropractors Association. The latter was founded by B. J. Palmer.

The medical profession was not comfortable with this new approach to primary health care, and the American Medical Association (AMA) tried to isolate it. Throughout the years many chiropractors were arrested and jailed for practicing medicine without a license. In 1933, in an attempt to discourage members from consulting with chiropractors or referring patients to them, the Judicial Council of the AMA stated that "the physician who maintains professional relations with cult practitioners would seem to exhibit a lack of faith in the correctness and efficacy of scientific medicine and to admit that there is merit to cult practitioners."[3]

The accusations and propaganda spread by the AMA were intended to discredit and condemn the chiropractic profession. In 1987, after an 11-year court battle, a federal court judge found the AMA guilty of having conspired to destroy the profession of chiropractic. This ruling was upheld by a three-judge federal appeals court and allowed to stand by the Supreme Court.[4] Many of these issues are beyond the scope of this text and further reading is recommended.

REFERENCES

1. Altman, N: The Chiropractic Alternative: A Spine Owner's Guide. JP Tarcher, Los Angeles, 1981.
2. Ibid, p 13.
3. Quoted in ibid.
4. Wilk v American Medical Association (1987) U.S. District Court (Northern District of Illinois), case 76C3777, August 27; affirmed by 7th Circuit Court of Appeals, February 7, 1990; ruling allowed to stand by the Supreme Court, November 28, 1990.

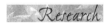

Research

Primary Benefits of Chiropractic

Research is continually being conducted to further enhance the benefits of chiropractic. In 1979 the government of New Zealand issued a report stating that "spinal manipulation in the hands of a doctor of chiropractic is both safe and effective."[24] An article in the *British Medical Journal*, reporting on a 10-year study comparing chiropractic care to traditional medical care for low back problems, found "chiropractic treatment to be significantly more effective than medical care and that the results were long term."[25]

Similarly, in 1993 the Ontario Ministry of Health reported that an independent study on low back pain treatment showed chiropractic care to be more effective, safer, and less costly than medical care. The ministry also reported that patients were more satisfied with chiropractic care and that injured workers returned to work much more quickly after chiropractic care.[26]

In 1994, after reviewing 10,000 medical abstracts and 4000 scientific articles, the U.S. Department of Health and Human Services issued guidelines that recommended spinal manipulation for low back pain rather then diathermy and ultrasound, prolonged bed rest and traction, acupuncture, biofeedback, transdermal electrical stimulation, oral steroids and muscle relaxants, epidural and trigger point injections, and spinal surgery—as long as no serious underlying conditions are present. Spinal manipulation was the only treatment recommended as being able to "relieve symptoms, increase function, and hasten recovery."[27]

Secondary Benefits of Chiropractic

Studies conducted by Browning and colleagues[28] show that many chiropractic patients experience health benefits in areas of the body not related to the musculoskeletal system. These benefits include improved breathing and digestion, and the resolution of pelvic, visual, and circulatory problems.[29] Other studies have shown the following results:

- R. F. Gorman,[30] an ophthalmologist working with chiropractors, reported 18 cases in which visual field loss was restored following spinal manipulation.
- K. Lewit,[31] a neurologist and manual medicine specialist, reported relief from chronic recurring tonsillitis in 37 children given manipulation for upper cervical spine dysfunction.
- D. Fitz-Ritson[32] and Bracher and colleagues[33] reported excellent results from chiropractic management of 112 and 16 patients, respectively, with vertigo secondary to cervical spine subluxation/dysfunction.

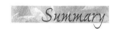 *Summary*

A growing number of people are turning to chiropractic because they are seeking less invasive, more natural, and holistic approaches to taking care of their health. (See Box 17–2.) Chiropractic benefits everyone, from infants to the elderly. Most individuals seek chiropractic initially to help relieve pain, but eventually they realize the benefits to their overall well-being.

Chiropractic has proven successful with a variety of ailments, such as headaches, backaches, sciatica, and jaw pain. Sports injuries are also benefited by chiropractic care. Proper joint alignment allows for maximum healing and lowers the risk for reinjury. Many professional sports teams maintain chiropractors on the sidelines.

Parents are beginning to realize that children can also benefit from chiropractic care to correct injuries from falls and mishaps when they are learning to walk. Children's constant activity and growth can sometimes create improper joint alignment and muscle imbalances. Chiropractic promotes correct posture and helps to decrease problems associated with scoliosis.

For the elderly, regular chiropractic care increases movement in the joints, which stimulates nerve function, blood flow, and transport of nutrients to the joints and muscles. This increases strength, function, and stability.

The scope of chiropractic may differ from state to state and from country to country, but the premise is the same: chiropractic is concerned with the relationship between structure (primarily that of the spine) and function (primarily that coordinated by the central nervous system) of the human body as that relationship may affect the restoration and preservation of health.[34]

No health-care approach can guarantee wellness, but chiropractic focuses on the body's ability to heal itself and "encourages us to take personal responsibility for our lives by teaching us to preserve our health rather than treating the symptoms of disease."[35]

BOX 17–2
Case Studies

Many individuals who seek less invasive, more natural, and holistic ways to take care of their health turn to chiropractic. Following are some examples.

Joe

Joe is a 52-year-old carpenter who has been "putting up sheet rock" for 20 years. He works with his hands overhead almost constantly and complains of pain in his lower neck, across his shoulders, and between his shoulder blades. An examination revealed multiple subluxations of the cervical and thoracic spine with associated hypertonic musculature. After being treated with chiropractic manipulations and ultrasound, he reported immediate relief.

Lisa

Lisa is a 6-year-old girl whose parents are concerned with her bed wetting, a persistent problem since infancy. Medical protocol has not helped. Lisa's right foot toes in, and she experiences tenderness over her right sacral iliac joint and lumbar spine. Her treatment consisted of spinal adjustments and nutritional advice to reduce soda intake. Lisa's mother noticed a decrease in bed wetting after the third treatment, with a significant decrease after the sixth treatment. Lisa remains under regular "maintenance" care and has not wet her bed in more than a year.

Carl

Carl is a 38-year-old store manager who complained of headaches, "clicking" in his left jaw joint, and pain in his right ear. Medical examination ruled out an ear infection, and Carl could not recall any accident or trauma. A dental evaluation led to a mouth appliance to help reduce his teeth grinding at night. Although this provided some relief, Carl still reported a high level of discomfort. A chiropractic evaluation revealed severely hypertonic cervical and thoracic musculature, minimal range of motion of the neck, and extreme tenderness upon palpation of musculature. X-rays revealed a decreased cervical curvature, with severe joint malposition (subluxation) of the 2nd and 3rd, as well as the 6th and 7th, cervical vertebral segments. No pathology or fracture was observed.

Treatment began with ultrasound of the trapezius musculature and chiropractic adjustments. In addition, the neck was taken through passive range of motion to help relax the muscles and gradually increase spinal motion. Carl did notice some relief after first treatment. By the third treatment, the pain had decreased and range of motion had increased. By the sixth treatment, Carl stated that the clicking in his jaw was minimal, as was the pain in his ear.

RESOURCES

Dynamic Chiropractic
P.O. Box 4109
Huntington Beach, CA 92605–4109
Phone: (714) 230-3150

Foundation for Chiropractic Education and Research
704 E. 4th St.
Des Moines, IA 50309
Phone: (800) 622-6809
Fax: (515) 282-3347
www.FCER.org

National Integrative Medicine Council (NIMC)
5151 E. Broadway, Suite 1095
Tucson, AZ 85711
Phone: (520) 571-1110
E-mail: *info@nimc.org*
www.Chiroweb.com

REFERENCES

1. Dorland's Pocket Medical Dictionary, ed 24. WB Saunders, Philadelphia, 1982.
2. Altman, N: The Chiropractic Alternative: A Spine Owner's Guide. JP Tarcher, Los Angeles, 1981.
3. Sportelli, L: A Natural Method of Health Care: Introduction to Chiropractic, Practice Makers Products, Palmerton, Philadelphia, 2000.
4. Altman, N: The Chiropractic Alternative: A Spine Owner's Guide. JP Tarcher, Los Angeles, 1981.
5. Ibid
6. Ibid
7. Ibid
8. Lawrence, DJ: Fundamentals of Chiropractic Diagnosis and Management. Williams & Wilkins, Baltimore, 1991.
9. Altman, N: The Chiropractic Alternative: A Spine Owner's Guide. JP Tarcher, Los Angeles, 1981.
10. Lawrence, DJ: Fundamentals of Chiropractic Diagnosis and Management. Williams & Wilkins, Baltimore, 1991.
11. Wilk, CA: Chiropractic Speaks Out: A Reply to Medical Propaganda, Bigotry and Ignorance. Wilk Publishing Company, Park Ridge, Ill 1976.
12. Lawrence, DJ: Fundamentals of Chiropractic Diagnosis and Management. Williams & Wilkins, Baltimore, 1991.
13. Altman, N: The Chiropractic Alternative: A Spine Owner's Guide. JP Tarcher, Los Angeles, 1981.
14. Ibid
15. Ibid
16. Palmer, DD: The Science, Art and Philosophy of Chiropractic. Portland Printing House Company; Portland, Ore., 1910.
17. Ibid
18. Altman, N: The Chiropractic Alternative: A Spine Owner's Guide. JP Tarcher, Los Angeles, 1981.
19. Ibid
20. Ibid
21. Schafer, RC, and Faye, LJ: Motion Palpation and Chiropractic Technique. Motion Palpation Institute, Huntington Beach, Calif., 1989.
22. Strang, VV: Essential Principles of Chiropractic. Palmer College of Chiropractic, Davenport, 1984.
23. Ibid
24. Commission of Inquiry, Chiropractic in New Zealand. PD Hasselberg, Government Printer, Wellington, New Zealand, 1979.
25. Meade, TW, Dyer, S, et al: Low Back Pain of Mechanical Origin and Hospital Outpatient Treatment. BMJ, 300(67137):1431-1437, 1990.
26. Manga, P; et al. Chiropractic Management of Low Back Pain. Pran Manga and Associates, Ontario, Canada, 1993.
27. Bigos, S, Bowyer, O, Braen, G, et al: Acute low back problems. In Adults: Clinical Practice Guideline No.14. AHCPR Publication No. 95-0642. Rockville, MD: Agency for Health Care Policy and Research, Public Health Service, U.S. Department of Health and Human Services. 1994.
28. The Chiropractic Report: Non-Musculoskeletal Benefits of Chiropractic Care, 14(2), March 2000.
29. Browning, JE: Chiropractic distractive decompression in the treatment of pelvic pain and organic dysfunction in patients with evidence of lower sacral nerve root compressioin. J Manip Physiol Ther 11: 436-32, 1988.
30. Gorman, RF: Monocular visual loss after closed head trauma: Immediate resolution associated with spinal manipulation. J Manip Physiol Ther 18: 308-14, 1995.
31. Lewit K. Manipulative Therapy and Rehabilitation of the Locomotor System, ed 2. Butterworth-Heineman, Oxford, England 1991.

32. Fitz-Ritson, D: Assessment of cervicogenic vertigo: J Manip Physiol Ther 14: 193–8, 1991.
33. Bracher, E, Bleggi, C, Almeida, C, et al: A Combined Approach for the Treatment of Cervical Vertigo. Proceedings of the 5th Biennial Congress of the World Federation of Chiropractic, 1999: 154–155. In print.
34. Palmer, DD: The Science, Art and Philosophy of Chiropractic. Portland Printing House Company, Portland Ore., 1910.
35. Altman, N: The Chiropractic Alternative: A Spine Owner's Guide. JP Tarcher, Los Angeles, 1981.
36. Ibid
37. Ibid
38. Ibid
39. Wilk v American Medical Association (1987) U.S. District Court (Northern District of Illinois), case 76C3777, August 27; affirmed by 7th Circuit Court of Appeals, February 7, 1990; ruling allowed to stand by U.S. Supreme Court, November, 1990.

Recommended Reading

American Chiropractic Association. Chiropractic: State of the Art. American Chiropractic Association, Arlington, Va., 1994.

Bigos, S, et al: Acute Low Back Problems in Adults. Clinical Practice Guideline No. 14 (AHCPR Publication No. 65-0642). U.S. Department of Health and Human Services, Public Health Service, Agency for Health Care Policy and Research, Rockville, Md., December 1994.

Langone, J; Chiropractors: A Consumer's Guide. Addison-Wesley, Reading, Mass., 1982.

Leach, RA: The Chiropractic Theories: A Synopsis of Scientific Research, ed. 2. Williams & Wilkins, Baltimore, 1986.

CHAPTER 18

Holistic Dentistry

Stephen M. Koral

Stephen M. Koral, DMD, maintains a private practice in Boulder, Colorado

Betty D. was convinced she knew exactly what her problem was. A 36-year-old homemaker with three small children, she had been experiencing tingling and numbness in her right foot and leg for about 4 years, in addition to night sweats and fatigue. Neurologists had formally ruled out multiple sclerosis and other known neuropathies, and oncologists had found no cancer. She believed her problem had something to do with the porcelain-fused-to-metal dental bridge that had been installed to replace two missing teeth the day the symptoms started. The dentistry was perfectly good—the bridge fit in every way, did not hurt or interfere with her bite—and no dentist could be convinced to remove it based on a layperson's suspicions. After all, these things just do not happen, and dentistry has been done exactly this way for generations. The onset of the patient's "medical" symptoms, which coincided so closely with her "dental" treatment, had to have been a coincidence.

Finally, Betty found a dentist adventurous enough to take seriously her request to remove the bridge. Sure enough, the numbness and tingling in her leg went away within 24 hours. The symptoms have not returned.

A case like this is very upsetting—it contradicts the wisdom of conventional dental practice. Could the materials in the bridge have caused an allergic reaction, which affected Betty's nervous system? Or could her nervous system have been affected by electrical currents generated by the metal substructure of the bridge; metals in the mouth often produce electricity at energies hundreds or thousands of times greater than that which occur naturally in the body? Or something else entirely? Does this sort of thing occur all the time, or is it a one-in-a-million fluke? Are those authorities right who say that dentistry as it is typically practiced is a triumph of art and science? Or is dentistry a minefield of unintended consequences, in which well-intentioned treatments frequently lead to health problems of an unpredictable nature in an unknown percentage of the population? Do we know enough about life and health to recognize when we are transgressing some physical, mental, or spiritual threshold in a given individual patient? This sort of moral crisis drives some dentists to question the ways of mainstream practice and look toward the holistic model.

Mainstream Dentistry

The universe of health care has been historically divided into separate professions, specialties, and subspecialties whose members too often know little, if anything, of what the others are doing. Dentistry reflects this condition. The profession is a micro-specialty of health care, a response to just two diseases—tooth decay and gum disease—that affect a large percentage of the population. (Management of a variety of growth anomalies complements the dental practice menu.) Dental methods, familiar to everyone, are among the most allopathic techniques imaginable. We treat tooth decay by grinding out diseased parts of teeth, and we reconstruct those teeth with synthetic materials. The use of fluoride dominates tooth decay prevention. We control gum disease by brushing and flossing away the irritating bacterial plaque that grows on our teeth daily, and every 6 months or so we scrape away tartar, the calcified fortifications those germs make. We strap teeth into wires, springs, and brackets to force them into more aesthetically pleasing positions, and we surgically remove wisdom teeth that may cause problems in the future.

Holistic Practice

The holistic ideal, in which the practitioner considers the totality of the patient—physical, emotional and spiritual—seems incongruous next to the mechanical technologies we are accustomed to in dentistry. But if we acknowledge that life and health cannot be adequately explained by any one school of thought or type of practice, we can only gain by striving toward the ideal of holism. At least we can employ a bigger tool box in our daily dealings with patients.

The Holistic Dental Association's book on standards of care includes chapters on myofascial release, classical homeopathy, dental kinesiology, dentocranial therapy, dental nutrition, oral myofunctional therapy, zone therapy, auricular therapy, interference fields and foci, classical acupuncture, biocompatibility testing, and neural therapy.[1] None of these topics is covered in dental schools, but all of them and others can add new dimensions to the way dentists see their patients and offer interesting techniques dentists can use to improve the quality of their work. Conversely, a person's dental condition affects each of the above areas of physiology. For example, irregularities in a person's bite will dramatically affect craniosacral mechanics, and infections of the teeth can be discerned in acupuncture meridians and may affect bodily structures on these meridians. How often are practitioners in these related fields aware of this?

The fundamentals of holistic practice can be said to derive from the proposition that "there are two causative factors of disease: one, the immediate, which may be bacterial, and two, the conditions that make it possible for the disease to flourish."[2] Allopathic medicine, of course, has made enormous progress in dealing with the first proposition, but it has paid little or no attention to the second. It has been left to the alternative/complementary community to deal with the factors involved in strengthening a person's defenses against disease.

The Role of Nutrition

Good nutrition is the primary factor in fortifying an individual's defenses against disease. Many of the great pioneers of clinical nutrition have, in fact, been dentists, although much of what was once considered very exciting has been forgotten and is no longer mentioned in dental schools.

Weston Price

In 1938, dentist Weston Price published his masterwork entitled *Nutrition and Physical Degeneration*.[3] Price reported on his years of travel around the globe during the 1920s and 1930s, searching for remnant groups of aboriginal people. He ultimately found 14 different ethnic groups, from isolated Swiss mountain families to Eskimos, Indians of northern Canada, Central Africans, and Pacific Islanders. He compared their health status to racially related groups that had been exposed to traders—and consequently the modern diet of white flour, sugar, and canned food. The uniform finding was that those people who were isolated enough to be eating only their traditional, aboriginal diet had full development of their jaws, with no crooked teeth and no tooth decay. They also had broad facial development. The men had wide shoulders and the women, wide hips. On the contrary, their ethnic relatives who lived near trading posts were plagued with tooth decay and malformed dental arches. They also had narrower skeletal development, which led to problems in childbirth for the women. A number of fascinating photographs, taken by Price, showed the development of these tendencies over generations in families. Grandparents with broad faces and perfect teeth sit next to their children and grandchildren, born after trade began, who have distinctly narrower faces and rotten teeth. Only one group, on an island in the South Pacific, had lost the market for their commodity a generation earlier and, consequently, their access to the trade diet. The young children, forced to eat only traditional foods, once again showed their ancestral pattern of broad skeletal development and lack of tooth decay.

Price's critics called his findings uncontrolled and unscientific, and more likely due to the transmission of bacterial species responsible for tooth decay, in a manner similar to the way tuberculosis and other European diseases had been transmitted. Price, though, ascribed these effects to the lack of nutritional value in the trade diet. He indicted the same dietary practices in industrial countries for contributing to the prevalence of tooth decay and other diseases. Many health commentators during his time and afterward have also expressed this belief.

Melvin Page

Melvin Page was a dentist, biochemist, and endocrinologist whose work was published predominantly in the 1950s. He expanded on a concept, originated by Price, that used the ratio of calcium and phosphorus in the blood as a measure of overall health in the regulation of body chemistry and correlated deviations in that ratio with the tendency toward illnesses of various types. This technique formed the basis for some current systems of examining body chemistry for imbalances at the level of functional regulation, before the condition progressed into frank disease. It led to a better understanding of how nutrition affects the regulation of body chemistry and increased understanding of how a person's underlying metabolism creates resistance or susceptibility to tooth decay and gum disease.

Page also pioneered the development of two other concepts important in functional medicine. "Microendocrinology" seeks to understand the impact on metabolism and overall health of deviations in hormone function that are too small to cause overt disease. The concept of "sympathetic versus parasympathetic dominance" is a paradigm for analyzing an individual patient's innate patterns of responding to stress.[4]

John Kelly

John Kelly, a dentist who developed a system of metabolic typing, branched out of dentistry with these ideas in the 1960s, when he began using nutritional methods of balancing body chemistry along with enzyme therapy to treat cancer. His methods underlie much of the nutritional cancer therapy in use today.

As with so many creative approaches to the "host susceptibility" side of the disease equation, these concepts were never applied on a grand scale. It is nearly impossible to encourage most people to change their diets, and we cannot send all the candy-eating children of the world to islands in the South Pacific and force them to eat aboriginal food to prevent tooth decay.

Fluoride

The work of Price, Page, and their allies coincided with the introduction of fluoride, a chemical that allegedly can make teeth more resistant to decay. Fluoride became the intervention of choice for the medical-dental-industrial establishment and has over-shadowed every other preventive technique since. Fluoride works as intended under some circumstances but has numerous disadvantages—it is quite toxic. Even in the small quantities used in community water supplies, fluoride has been shown to increase hip fractures in the elderly and has been implicated in an increase in bone cancer in young men as well as neurological damage and impaired brain function. Not only that, the efficacy of water fluoridation in preventing tooth decay has been strongly challenged. This large and acrimonious topic has been treated in many publications.[5–7]

Apart from the public health issues of fluoridation, its advent marked a philosophical crossroads for dentistry. Just as the profession was beginning to regard tooth decay as a systemic condition and to actively seek nutritional ways to prevent decay, fluoride drove thinking back into the reductionist, allopathic camp. Tooth decay was seen as a fluoride deficiency, and teeth, once again, would be treated in isolation from the rest of the body. Price, Page, and their generation of research disappeared from the journals and from the consciousness of dentists; they were forgotten by all but a fringe of "alternative" practitioners.

Mercury

Maintaining a vision of the health of the whole person in the face of a technological fix has always been hard. Nothing illustrates this problem for dentistry better than the long, difficult history of dental amalgam, the common "silver" filling material. The notion of scraping out the soft, decayed parts of teeth and restoring the shape of those teeth with some type of material goes back a long way. There is evidence that the ancient Egyptians and Romans poured molten gold or lead into dental cavities. The Chinese appear to have discovered the technique of mixing silver powder with liquid mercury to form a plastic mass that could be worked into a cavity, which would then set into a hardened state we call "amalgam." This silver-mercury amalgam process was introduced to the Western world in France at the beginning of the 19th century and spread to the United States by the early 1830s. Amalgam fillings quickly caught on because they were technically easy and relatively inexpensive.[8]

Medical science in the 19th century was fully aware of the toxic properties of mercury but found the economics of using amalgam fillings compelling; the only other viable material at the time was gold, which was then, as it is still, much more expensive to use. Tooth decay was rampant in the population, and amalgam fit the bill as a restorative material for the masses. It seemed that people tolerated amalgam well enough, and the fillings performed admirably.

Research: A History

Some dentists opposed the use of mercury in fillings from the beginning. In 1845 the National College of Dental Surgeons, citing the toxicity known at the time, demanded that its members sign an oath never to use mercury in people's mouths. There ensued a great schism among dentists over this issue, which led to the breakup of the National College. In 1872 the American Dental Association, the organization we know today, formed as the proamalgam faction of the time. By the turn of the 20th century, the manufacture and use of amalgam had been pretty well perfected under the leadership of Drs. G. V. Black, Elisha Townsend, and others, and the issue was considered settled. The materials and methods of that time, changed only in subtle ways over the century, are still in wide use today.[9] The dental establishment has continued to defend the safety record of amalgam. American Dental Association publications have averred that the mercury mixed in amalgam is stable and does not leach out—or if it does, it is in amounts too small to harm anyone—and that "mercury forms a biologically inactive substance when it combines with the other materials used to produce amalgam."[10] Amalgams have been referred to as "silver" fillings, and everyone else simply forgot that there was mercury in them.

In the 1930s, doubts about the safety of amalgam were raised again by Dr. Alfred Stock, a professor of chemistry in Berlin.[11] Himself a victim of mercury poisoning from his laboratory work, Stock claimed that many diseases of contemporary society were being caused by vapors of mercury released from the ubiquitous amalgam fillings. The interest raised by Stock ultimately died down for lack of corroboration, until the subject was revived in the late 1970s by Drs. Hal Huggins of Colorado Springs, and Olympio Pinto of Brazil.[12] By this time, instrumentation had been developed that could conveniently detect trace quantities of mercury vapor, and scientific corroboration of the suspicion that fillings were exposing people to real quantities of mercury began to accumulate rapidly. Amalgam fillings were found to emit mercury vapor continuously, and in even greater amounts after exposure to acids, hot foods, or friction from chewing. Radioactively labeled mercury included in fillings placed in the teeth of sheep and monkeys has been shown to spread rapidly to the brain, kidney, liver, intestines, jawbones, and endocrine glands, plus into fetal tissues and milk.[13] World Health Organization scientists have stated that amalgam fillings are the largest single source of mercury exposure in the general population.[14] Several countries have recommended restrictions or have partial bans of amalgam in place, and more such action is contemplated.[15]

Of course, people do not drop dead on the way out of their dentists' offices after being treated with amalgam fillings. Effective biochemical mechanisms protect most people from trace levels of toxins, including mercury. But it is increasingly clear that the universal use of amalgam fillings has resulted in widespread negative consequences for people's health. Table 18–1 summarizes the results of six different studies concerning the health effects of removing amalgam fillings. As can be seen, more than 1500 patients reported 54 to 97 percent relief from a wide range of symptoms after their fillings were removed. What this evidence implies for the overall population, though, still remains unclear. More recent research indicates that trace quantities of mercury in the brain may be one of the primary environmental factors leading to Alzheimer's disease.[16] Happily, newer filling materials of plastic and ceramic have been developed that are perhaps stronger and more reliable than amalgam. They also are more cosmetically pleasing. Toxicological risk assessment studies have demonstrated that these new "composite" materials are hundreds of times safer than amalgam.[17,18]

The tragedy, from a holistic perspective, is the fragmentation of health care that kept this problem from being clarified for more than 150 years. At least 80 percent of the

TABLE 18–1   Relief from Amalgam Filling Removal*

SYMPTOM	NUMBER REPORTING	PERCENTAGE REPORTING PARTIAL OR TOTAL IMPROVEMENT
Allergy	221	89
Anxiety	86	93
Bad temper	81	89
Bloating	88	88
Blood pressure problems	99	54
Chest pains	79	87
Depression	347	91
Dizziness	343	88
Fatigue	705	86
Gastrointestinal problems	231	83
Gum problems	129	94
Headaches	531	87
Migraine headaches	45	87
Insomnia	187	78
Irregular heartbeat	159	87
Irritability	132	90
Lack of concentration	270	80
Lack of energy	91	97
Memory loss	265	73
Metallic taste	260	95
Multiple sclerosis	113	76
Muscle tremor	126	83
Nervousness	158	83
Numbness (any location)	118	82
Skin problems	310	81
Sore throat	149	86
Tachycardia	97	70
Thyroid problems	56	79
Ulcers and sores in mouth	189	86
Urinary tract problems	115	76
Vision problems	462	63

*Summary analysis of health outcomes for 1569 symptomatic patients who underwent removal of amalgam fillings, as reported in six different studies from Europe, Canada, and the United States. Additional detoxification techniques varied among the studies cited.

Source: Bio-Probe Newsletter, Bio-Probe, Inc., Orlando, FL, March 1993, p 8, with permission.

population of the industrial world has amalgam fillings, so this condition forms the background—the population norm. A person who develops migraines, depression, or urinary tract problems as a result of mercury toxicity from fillings—and, of course, there are many other potential causes of all these symptoms—takes the complaint to a medical doctor, who has no idea of the source of the problem because the world outside of dentistry has forgotten that there is mercury in fillings. These complaints are not dental symptoms, so they do not come to the attention of the dentist, and the connection is never made. Dentists have been using amalgam all this time with the best of intentions for their patients, and, after all, most people seem to tolerate amalgam fillings.

But it is in the term *most people* that we find a significant breach of the tenets of holistic practice. Who fits into the category of "most people"? It is clear that people vary in their genetic capacity to perform all sorts of biological functions, from growing tall, to remembering facts in college, to utilizing antioxidant enzymes in their mitochondria. "Some people" are genetically susceptible to the effects of trace levels of toxins, whether it is mercury, pesticides, or air pollution. Every person is an individual, not a representative of a population statistic, and the holistic practitioner attempts to account for the unique susceptibilities of each one. Perhaps such practice is just good doctoring, but it is helped immensely by a broad knowledge of the different forms and traditions of health care. If we each knew more about what the other professions were doing, we would be less likely to forget such useful clues as the amalgam filling–mercury exposure connection.

The Holistic Approach

Holistic dentists strive to discover ways to relate their work to the health of the whole person and to assimilate that knowledge into practice. They are committed to the main agenda of dentistry, which is keeping the mouth healthy, and fixing and maintaining teeth whenever possible. The basic techniques, the nuts and bolts of working on teeth, are the same as in mainstream dentistry. The difference lies in a few specific disagreements with mainstream dentistry and in how much is brought in from other fields. Some clinical examples throughout the rest of the chapter will illustrate this.

John's Story

John J. was a 44-year-old physician who suffered from irritable bowel syndrome, an uncomfortable, annoying, and sometimes painful condition that falls into the awkward category of "functional disease," meaning that medicine does not really know what causes it. As a "functional" problem, it is not bad enough to be called colitis and require an operation, so there is no straightforward technological cure. John, a bit of a nonconformist, began searching the alternative/complementary side of the tracks for a solution to his problem. He tried careful manipulation of his diet but saw no real improvement. Various connections led him to a practitioner of electrodermal diagnosis, a branch of acupuncture, who just happened to be a dentist by training. He discovered that John had significant disturbances in the acupuncture meridians for the large intestine, disturbances coming from two molars associated with that meridian. He suggested that John have those teeth extracted. His former dentist had performed a root canal procedure on one and placed metallic crowns on both. There was no dental pain and the x-rays looked fine. Therefore the dentist would not extract them.

This is an example of a point at which mainstream and holistic dentistry part ways—the willingness to give at least some credit to information that comes from nontraditional sources. If acupuncture and electrodermal diagnosis are fraudulent, we are treading on dangerous territory by following the recommendation of the electrodermal practitioner. If, on the other hand, there is truth to these diagnoses, as a lot of experience would suggest,[19] we have powerful tools for exploring functional connections in the body.

In the electrodermal literature there is a chart of correspondence between individual teeth and particular acupuncture meridians that can be used to establish connections between problems in teeth and dysfunction in distant organs. (See Table 18–2.) This type of information might be very useful to dentists interested in the broader implications of their work. But we must be careful in our communication with patients at a point like this. It is crucial to be intellectually honest about the quality of the information we base our decisions on. Is it scientifically valid? Is it folklore, or supposition? Or is it somewhere in between, strongly suggested and supported by clinical experience but not yet fully supported by scientific research?

John's new dentist took the last approach, and although he was willing to give some credit to the electrodermal report, he shared his doubts with John. Sometimes these situations yield the hoped-for result, and sometimes they do not. For example, the patient may lose some teeth and still have an irritable bowel. There is mounting evidence that root canal treatments, even when they appear to have healed perfectly, can leave teeth inhabited

TABLE 18–2   Correspondence of Teeth to Acupuncture Meridians, According to the Voll System

KIDNEY/ BLADDER		LIVER/ GALLBLADDER	LUNG/LARGE INTESTINE		STOMACH/ SPLEEN		HEART/ SMALL INTESTINE
Upper central incisor	Upper lateral incisor	Upper canine	Upper first bicuspid	Upper second bicuspid	Upper first molar	Upper second molar	Upper third molar
Lower central incisor	Lower lateral incisor	Lower canine	Lower first bicuspid	Lower second bicuspid	Lower first molar	Lower second molar	Lower third molar
KIDNEY/ BLADDER		LIVER/ GALLBLADDER	STOMACH/ SPLEEN		LUNG/LARGE INTESTINE		HEART/ SMALL INTESTINE

Source: Adapted from Kramer, F: Electroacupuncture in Dental Practice in Germany. Karl F. Haug Verlag, Heidelberg, 1994.

by bacteria that excrete trace levels of powerful toxins and, therefore, may be hazardous to the overall health in unpredictable ways.[20–22] But no test yet devised can prove before extraction that a particular root-treated tooth is toxic. These are John's teeth and his bowels, and any decision would have to be his gamble.

John made his difficult choice to have the two teeth extracted. His bowels became distinctly more comfortable, but not completely. Other factors were at play, obviously, but John felt that the improvement in his abdomen adequately compensated for the dental loss.

Periodontal Disease

The Weston Price–Melvin Page philosophy of balancing body chemistry to improve a person's resistance to disease, mentioned earlier in this chapter, is utilized most often these days in the management of periodontal disease.[23] People who are susceptible to destructive gum disease have two problems: pathogenic bacteria live on the teeth under the gums, and their white blood cells function abnormally. This means that the germs are not killed effectively and that the chemicals liberated by both the germs and the defending white blood cells damage the surrounding tissue. Ultimately, this process destroys the bone and soft tissue structures that hold in the teeth.

Mainstream periodontal treatment aims exclusively at removing and killing the germs and surgically reconstructing damaged areas. This approach usually works well. But sometimes, by altering a patient's diet to reduce the load of metabolic acids, adding supplementary minerals and antioxidants such as vitamin C and coenzyme Q_{10}, using essential fatty acids to effect changes in prostaglandin metabolism, and using an individually customized nutritional program, the patient's underlying susceptibility to gum disease can be reduced. Could we be affecting that person's susceptibility to other diseases at the same time?

Data from several large-scale studies have shown that the presence of periodontal disease is a strong risk factor for heart attacks and strokes.[24,25] One theory to explain this phenomenon holds that the bacteria responsible for gum disease secrete toxins into a person's circulation that damage blood vessel walls and increase clotting, thus speeding up the pathological processes leading to cardiovascular disease. Another theory suggests that susceptibility to both gum disease and cardiovascular disease is a reflection of a common underlying metabolic defect.[26] It is tempting to speculate that the same nutritional manipulations we can use for periodontal conditions may have a preventive effect against cardiovascular diseases.

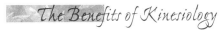

The Benefits of Kinesiology

Applied kinesiology—the study of mechanics and anatomy as they relate to the human body—can be useful in dentistry. Using tests of muscle strength, a practitioner can judge whether or not something is stressful to the patient at that moment. This technique is often used by holistic dentists to get a quick reading on which restorative material to use for an allergic patient or how to position the bite correctly for a patient with jaw muscle pain.

James's Story

James, 42, suffered from progressive, destructive periodontal disease. Despite treatment by a competent periodontist, he had had no significant reversal of this condition. Thinking there must be another way, he sought an opinion from a holistic dentist. The dentist ascertained that James had followed all the periodontist's advice diligently and, respecting the periodontist's abilities, concluded that there had to be systemic factors acting that could not be controlled with dental treatment alone. He immediately referred James to a doctor who specialized in applied kinesiology and clinical nutrition, with a good record of tracking down obscure influences on health. After several months of treatment with diet and specific supplements, James had less metabolic acid in his system and his antioxidant status had improved. As a result his gums were finally healthy enough to respond to hygienic treatment in the dental office. The condition of James's gums stabilized, a sign of success in a periodontal case treated hygienically. He still shows the scars of the old disease, but he is no longer losing attachment tissue around his teeth.

Elaine's Story

Elaine was a perfectly healthy woman of 34 until she was rear-ended at a stop sign and suffered a whiplash injury. Although neither her jaw nor her face was hit in the accident, within 2 weeks her jaw began to hurt. She would awaken every morning with her teeth tightly clenched and could neither chew without tiring nor open her mouth all the way. These symptoms are typical of whiplash, because pain in neck joints from the injury causes "recruitment" of muscle contraction in the whole region, including the jaw muscles. In essence, the brain says "immobilize that injured neck."

Elaine consulted her dentist, who constructed a splint, a plastic bite appliance designed to reposition the jaw when closing. The muscles and ligaments of the neck and jaw are so extensively interconnected that they may realistically be considered one structure (along with the rest of the body). Often, just changing the posture of the jaw under these circumstances will reduce the tendency of the jaw to clench and, therefore, reduce the constant painful contraction of the muscles. But this did not happen for Elaine. Her jaw clenched and hurt more than ever, and she developed headaches. Her primary physician, an osteopath, sent her to his own dentist, who had had some additional training in the mechanics of how the jaw, head, neck, and back work together.

The new dentist used a simple method of applied kinesiology, in which the strength of Elaine's shoulder muscle was employed as a stress gauge. He determined that although Elaine was biting evenly on her splint, the posture it imposed upon her jaw stressed her neck more than no splint at all. Checking her jaw posture with cervical and cranial criteria (which he had learned from the osteopath), he found a comfortable position for the bite that also relieved stresses in the head and neck. The solution was merely to grind down the splint and adjust it to this nonstressful position. The result was that Elaine's jaw muscles became much more relaxed within days and her headaches decreased.

It still took her 8 months to fully recover from the effects of the injury, but about that time she discovered that she no longer awoke with her teeth clenched in the morning when she forgot to sleep with the splint in her mouth. She put it in a drawer and forgot about it. Without a confluence of knowledge from dentistry, osteopathy, and chiropractic, the increase in symptoms Elaine experienced when she first received the splint would have remained a mystery. Her recovery would have been more uncomfortable and may have taken longer.

Some dentists use a more technological approach to the problem of balancing the jaw posture with the head and neck. They use a combination of transcutaneous electrical nerve stimulation (TENS) to relax the muscles of the head, face, and neck; electromyography (EMG) to measure and monitor the activity of those muscles; and computerized jaw movement tracking to help determine the ideal postural position of the jaw at closure. Both methods work, and, as in so many instances, they work even better when one technique can be used to verify the results of the other.

Chemical Sensitivity

Chemically sensitive patients present a challenge to dentists because of all the synthetic materials we install in people's mouths. No one knows exactly what percentage of the population is hyperreactive—made overtly sick by environmental chemicals—but their numbers seem to be increasing.[27] These people can be helped by detoxification treatments, improved nutrition, and antioxidants. They can reduce their reactivity to foods by rotation diets, in which a person consumes different foods each day on a rotating schedule. But how can they reduce their reactivity to chemically composed dental materials? You cannot rotate the materials in your fillings.

Mainstream dentistry has taken the position that "allergy" to dental materials, including silver-mercury amalgam, is exceedingly rare and that "most people" should have no difficulty with them. Therefore concern about individual testing for biocompatibility of dental materials in chemically sensitive patients has fallen to the holistic dentists.

Pamela's Story

No one would have any difficulty determining that Pamela was chemically sensitive. She lived in a chemical-free house in the mountains of Colorado. She could come into town only for brief periods of time, wearing a charcoal filter mask and breathing oxygen, because she could not tolerate auto exhaust. Any exposure to environmental chemicals would send her into deep fatigue that could take weeks to recover from. As with many other chemically sensitive people, her illness began with an acute exposure to pesticides, but she could look back to prior indications of reactions to chemicals. Luckily, she had a healthy and supportive husband, who saw her through several very difficult years. She was treated by a well-known environmental physician, who advised her that mercury exposure from her fillings was perpetuating the illness and recommended that they be removed.

Pamela's dentist was willing to remove the amalgam fillings, but what could they be replaced with? She might react to anything placed in her teeth; some chemically sensitive people never find dental materials that do not cause them to react. The dentist used several different techniques to find compatible filling materials—blood and skin allergy tests, applied kinesiology stress tests, electrodermal tests, homeopathic desensitization—and found a few likely candidates. Yet when she would hold a sample of a proposed filling material in her mouth, she would get sick. Finally, she and her dentist decided to forge ahead. The amalgams were removed all at once, with precautions to minimize her exposure to mercury vapor and particulates, and with intravenous vitamin C, provided by the environmental physician, to boost her antioxidant defenses during the procedure. Beeswax was used for just barely satisfactory temporary fillings. After a few weeks she reacted less and was able to tolerate one of the material samples the dentist provided for her. New fillings were made with that formula. Within a few months her health improved remarkably. Her recovery has lasted, although she continues to be careful about what she eats and gets herself exposed to. Biocompatible dentistry was certainly not the only avenue she took to recover her health, but she credits it with contributing a large piece of the puzzle for her. Unfortunately, not all cases of chemical sensitivity resolve this easily. Many such patients present a difficult tangle of biochemical, immunological, and psychological factors, and it is impossible for anyone to predict how much holistic dentistry might help.

It is important to note that removal of amalgam and other metal restorations from the teeth can expose the patient to increased amounts of toxic metals, if only transiently. The increased exposure can be very damaging to a person already suffering from a toxic burden, and the dentist must be trained in the various protocols and procedures for protecting the patient (and the dental staff) from toxic exposure. Physical barriers, such as a rubber dental dam, high-speed suction, and good ventilation, are a part of it. Physiological detoxification pathways in the body should be tested and supported with antioxidants and other nutrients prior to starting the dental procedures.

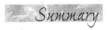

Summary

This chapter has briefly touched on some of the issues that face holistic dentists today. We have seen dentistry informed by acupuncture and electrodermal testing, dentistry using clinical nutrition and body chemistry balancing, dentistry combined with applied kinesiology, chiropractic, osteopathy, and environmental medicine. The range of subjects and possibilities for a holistic approach to dentistry is limited only by the imagination—and by the constraints of a dental license. The dental part—drilling and filling—is always going to be predominantly allopathic and must always be performed expertly and responsibly. But the context in which we perform that dentistry can be broadly informed, considerate of the whole, individual person, to the best of our abilities. That is the holistic way. It may not appeal to everyone, but for those with an expansive turn of mind, a holistic style of practice can keep the professional life ever interesting.

RESOURCES

American Academy of Biological Dentistry
P.O. Box 856
Carmel Valley, CA 93924

DAMS (dental amalgam mercury syndrome) patients' support network
P.O. Box 7249
Minneapolis, MN 55407
Phone: (800) 311-6265
www.amalgam.org

Holistic Dental Association
P.O. Box 5007
Durango, CO 81301
Fax: (970) 259-1091
www.holisticdental.org

International Academy of Oral Medicine and Toxicology
P.O. Box 608531
Orlando, FL 32860-8531
Phone: (407) 298-2450
www.iaomt.org

REFERENCES

1. Holistic Dental Association: Standards of Practice. Author, Durango, Colo., 1997.
2. Page, ME: Degeneration Regeneration. Price-Potter Nutrition Foundation, LaMesa, Calif., 1949, p 7.
3. Price, W: Nutrition and Physical Degeneration. Paul B. Hoeber, New York, 1938.
4. Page: Degeneration Regeneration.
5. Yamouyannis, J: Fluoride—The Aging Factor. Health Action Press, Delaware, Ohio, 1993.
6. Null, G: The fluoridation fiasco. Townsend Letter for Doctors and Patients, August/September 1996, p 56.
7. Banting, DE: The future of fluoride. J Am Dent Assoc 122;86, 1991.
8. Greener, EH: Amalgam—Yesterday, today and tomorrow. Oper Dent 4:24, 1979.
9. Mackert, JR: Dental amalgam and mercury. J Am Dent Assoc 122:54, 1991.
10. American Dental Association Divisions of Communication and Scientific Affairs: When your patients ask about mercury in amalgam. J Am Dent Assoc 120:395, 1990.
11. Mackert: Dental amalgam and mercury.
12. Ibid.
13. Lorscheider, FL, Vimy, MJ, and Summers, AO: Mercury exposure from "silver" tooth fillings: Emerging evidence questions a traditional dental paradigm. FASEB J 9:504, 1995.
14. World Health Organization: Environmental Health Criteria, vol 118. Inorganic Mercury. Author, Geneva, Switzerland, 1991, p 36.
15. The Safety of Dental Amalgam. Health Canada, Ottawa, 1996.
16. Pendergrass, JC, et al: Mercury vapor inhalation inhibits binding of GTP to tubulin in rat brain: Similarity to a molecular lesion in Alzheimer diseased brain. Neurotoxicology 18: 315, 1997.
17. Richardson, GM, and Allan, M: A Monte Carlo assessment of mercury exposure and risks from dental amalgam. Human and Ecological Risk Assessment 2:709, 1996.
18. Richardson, GM: An assessment of adult exposure and risks from components and degradation products of composite resin dental materials. Human and Ecological Risk Assessment 3:683, 1997.
19. Kramer, F: Electroacupuncture in Dental Practice [in German]. Karl F. Haug Verlag, Heidelberg, 1994.
20. Meinig, G: Canal Coverup. Bion Publishing Co., Ojai, Calif., 1996.
21. Debelian, GJ, Olsen, I, and Tronstad, L: Systemic diseases caused by oral microorganisms. Ended Dent Traumatol 10:57, 1994.
22. Pendergrass, JC: Personal communication.
23. Health Realities Newsletter 14:1, 1995.
24. De Stefano, F, et al: Dental disease and risk of coronary heart disease and mortality. BMJ 306:688, 1993.
25. Genco, R, et al: Periodontal disease is a predictor of cardiovascular disease in a Native American population. J Dent Res 76:408, 1997.
26. Beck, J, et al: Periodontal disease and cardiovascular disease. J Periodontol 67:1123, 1996.

Traditional Healing Systems

CHAPTER 19

Chinese Medicine

Joanne Ehret

Joanne Ehret, Dipl Ac, Dipl CH, FNAAOM, studied Chinese medicine at the Tri-State Institute of Traditional Chinese Acupuncture in New York City and at the Xi-Yuan Hospital of the China Academy of Traditional Chinese Medicine in Beijing, China. She is national-board certified in Chinese herbal medicine and acupuncture, and a fellow of the National Academy of Acupuncture and Oriental Medicine. She maintains a private practice, focusing on gynecology, internal medicine, and pediatrics, in Northampton, Massachusetts.

Used by one-quarter of the world's people, Chinese medicine is the oldest literate, professional, continuously practiced medicine in the world.[1] Traditional Chinese Medicine (TCM), a particular style of Chinese medicine, is based on writings originating between 200 BC and AD 200, with continuing commentaries, critiques, and many more original works since then. From the 1950s through to the 1970s, colloquia of TCM doctors in the People's Republic of China have codified and defined TCM into the style used today. TCM is based on a rational approach to medicine in the tradition of Confucian scholar-doctors, whose main modality of treatment was the administration of herbal medicinals to be taken internally. This systematic methodology is called *bian zheng lun zhi*, treatment based on a discrimination of patterns (literally, discrimination pattern determine treatment).[2] This means that any two patients with the same disease as defined in modern Western medical terminology are not likely to have the same *bian zheng*, or pattern discrimination in TCM. This is because the pattern is determined by gathering information about the signs and symptoms of all systems of the body, as well as constitution, physiognomy, and emotional state, even if the disease presenting itself seems to involve only one organ of the body.

In TCM, this means that two patients with the same disease will receive two different treatments if their patterns are different. It also means that two patients will receive the same treatment if their patterns are the same, even though their diseases may be different. The doctor of Chinese medicine thus follows this dictum: the same disease, different treatments; different diseases, the same treatment.[3] For example, one person who has been diagnosed with a common cold may be sneezing, have stiffness in the neck, and have copious, clear nasal mucus. Another person with the same diagnosis may have a sore throat, be very thirsty, and be perspiring lightly with a slight fever. These two patients' patterns are different and in Chinese medicine must receive different treatments despite the disease classification.

After recording the patient's particular pattern discrimination, the doctor chooses medicine according to certain treatment principles. Thus treatment is for the most part not empirical, but can be reasoned out precisely by following a series of steps. If signs or symptoms change even slightly over the course of treatment, the pattern, principles, and medicinals also change. Because each pattern can have several components, reflecting the complexity of the patient, and because there are so many ways of modifying Chinese medicinal formulas, this approach allows highly individualized treatment. The doctor can show the patient how his or her entire constellation of signs and symptoms creates the pattern being treated, and how any of them may change as the body rights itself.

The pattern reveals the etiology as well, describing disease causes and disease mechanisms. So the component parts of a pattern may add up to a discovery, such as this one, so commonly found in Chinese medicine: chronic sinus infections and bronchitis evolve from poor digestion that has been weakened by eating certain types of foods.

Knowing the cause and the mechanism by which one becomes ill, a practitioner can counsel the patient to change his or her diet in order to strengthen the digestion and therefore improve lung and sinus functions. In this way, the patient can be empowered to make the necessary changes to help prevent future diseases.[4]

Four Examinations

Practitioners of Chinese Medicine gather information by using the Four Examinations: Questioning, Looking, Palpation, and Listening/Smelling. Of these, Questioning involves the greatest amount of time. We ask the patient first to describe his or her experience of the chief complaint, such as details of the location of the problem, when discomfort occurs, duration of each incident, patterns of repetition, and history of the complaint. Then we cover each system: respiratory, cardiac, digestive, gynecological or urogenital; sleep, the extremities, sensations of heat or cold; history of past diseases, injuries, or surgery; life habits such as diet, exercise, work, and rest; and emotions. Objectively, the patient reports on what he or she sees, such as menstrual discharge or the nature of the stools.

The Looking examination involves noting physiognomy, facial color, eye color, and the tongue. We need to know, for instance, how height relates to body shape, whether the face is pale or reddish, and whether or not the eyes are red. The tongue's shape, size, color, and moisture, as well as the tongue's fur (also called "moss") location, color, thickness, and degree of dryness, add to an understanding of the duration, severity, location, and hot or cold nature of the disease.

Palpation is examination of the Chinese pulse. Feeling for any of the classic 28 pulse qualities on the six pulse positions, three on each wrist, as well as noting rate, gives the practitioner information on disease duration and depth in the system, strength or weakness of the body, relative heat or cold, and the state of fluids and blood.

Listening/Smelling includes listening to the sound of the voice and cough and noting any unusual smells coming from the mouth or body or smells that the patient reports, as of discharges or stools.

Treatment

Having determined the pattern discrimination and subsequent treatment principles, the practitioner chooses the treatment method. In TCM the primary modality is Chinese medicinals, consisting of plant, animal, and mineral substances used traditionally in their original, natural forms or prepared in specific ways, such as being stir-fried with honey, charred to an ash, or soaked in wine. After writing a prescription composed of anywhere from 4 to possibly 18 medicinals, the doctor gives the prescription to the pharmacist, who prepares packets, or *ji,* each one lasting from 1 to 4 days, which the patient decocts in water. The dosage the doctor will prescribe depends on the severity of the illness, the patient's constitution, and the body's sensitivity to the medicine. As time passes and the patient's condition changes or unwanted side effects occur, the doctor adjusts the formula to fit the patient's progress as closely as possible. For treatment of chronic or low-grade problems, tableted, granular, or tinctured formulas may be chosen.

Other modalities in TCM include acupuncture, the insertion of fine, sterile, stainless steel needles into specific points located along channels of energy in the body, and moxibustion, a form of heat treatment using the herb mugwort (*Artemisia vulgaris*). *Gua sya* is a technique of gentle scraping of the skin using the rounded edge of a ceramic or metal tool, and cupping uses glass cups with rounded edges to cause a gentle suction on the skin, once a vacuum has been created within the cup. These methods may be added to a medicinal treatment or used alone, particularly if blockages occur along these channels of energy, called "meridians." *Tui Na* is a type of massage, and *Qi Gong* and *Tai Ji* are exercises that build strength and calm the mind. Other self-help treatments include following dietary guidelines, getting adequate rest and proper exercise, and avoiding overworking. (See Box 19–1.)

Philosophy and History

The philosophical concepts most fundamental to Chinese medicine are those of yin and yang and the ways they interact with one another. The terms *yin* and *yang* express the idea of opposing, but complementary, phenomena that exist in a state of dynamic equilibrium. Yin and yang are always present simultaneously.[5] These concepts have been part of the Chinese worldview from ancient times to the present, and it is from this worldview that Chinese physicians organize their understanding of health, illness, and the individual's interrelationship with the environment.

The character for yin originally meant the shady side of a slope, and the character for yang, the sunny side. They are best described in relation to one another. Water is more yin, fire is more yang. Night is more yin, day is more yang. Winter is more yin, summer is more yang. The front, or softer, side of the body is more yin, and the back, because it is harder and stronger, is more yang. Sand inside a bucket is more yin because it is contained, soft, and held in place, while the bucket itself is more yang because it is hollow, harder, and facilitates movement of things in and out of it. A thing or state of being is never only yin or yang, because everything is in flux.[6] A person at the peak of strength is quite yang today, but tomorrow will be relatively more yin as he or she moves toward old age. Expanded into what we call the "Eight Principles," yin and yang, one continuously evolving into the other, explain virtually all the body's functions and how disease manifests itself. The Eight Principles are: Yin and Yang, Cold and Hot, Vacuity and Repletion (in some texts, Deficiency and Excess), and Interior and Exterior, each of the last three pairs expressing a yin/yang relationship. To understand their functions, we first need to know Chinese medical physiology and anatomy.

Chinese Physiology

The fundamental substances of the body are known as *qi, blood, jing, shen, and fluids.*

Qi

Qi is a concept so basic to Chinese medical thinking that it is only explained by what it does. Dr. Ted Kaptchuk says, "Chinese thought does not distinguish between matter and energy, but we can perhaps think of Qi as matter on the verge of becoming energy, or energy at the point of materializing."[7] Qi functions to direct all movement in the body, to protect the body, to govern transformation (e.g., to transform food into usable energy), to hold the organs and body fluids in their proper places, and to warm the body. All this activity makes qi relatively yang in nature.

BOX 19–1
Historical Context

As early as the Zhou Dynasty (1122–770 BC) the *Classic of Songs*[1] described specific medicinals used in the treatment of women's diseases and the *Mountain and Sea Classic*[2] discussed 120 types of Chinese medicinals. During the Warring States period (476–221 BC), the *Inner Classic of the Yellow Emperor*, the earliest known complete book on Chinese medical theory, was written.[3] Around the second century AD, the *Pharmacopoeia Classic of the Divine Husbandman*[4] described 365 medicines and divided them into upper, middle, and lower classes, the highest promoting longevity and the lowest treating disease. *The Discussion of Cold-Induced Disorders*,[5] written around AD 220, a foundation of clinical prescribing, described treatment of acute febrile diseases. Ted Kaptchuk, a scholar of Chinese medicine, describes scores of writings that, throughout Chinese history to the present, have critiqued and expanded on the literature.[6]

Since the founding of the People's Republic of China in 1949, TCM has been taught in medical schools, where, after learning individual medicinals and formulas, students go on to study the specialties of TCM, later concentrating on one: internal medicine, gynecology, pediatrics, traumatology, dermatology, tumerology (oncology), neurology and psychiatry, ophthalmology, otonasolaryngology, male urology, or geriatrics.[7] For each TCM disease, which is different from a Western disease, the student learns all representative patterns, treatment principles, formulas, and standard modifications of each formula. An example of a TCM disease in gynecology is early menstruation, which may have several causes, described as different patterns with names such as "replete heat," "qi vacuity," or "blood stasis." The TCM doctor will focus on treating the patterns. With each specialty, the holistic nature of the medicine requires the physician to know the state of the whole system and be able to tailor the formula to cover it: the gynecologist will add medicinals to help a respiratory or digestive issue that may exist coincidentally with a gynecological condition. In addition, Chinese doctors of TCM are fully trained in Western medicine, in which diseases, not patterns, are treated, and may practice both. Thus a gynecologist trained in surgery will know which Chinese medicinals to prescribe to speed postsurgical healing, combining the strength of both systems.

In the United States, training in TCM consists of a minimum of 3 years of study to qualify a practitioner for entry-level practice. Most schools focus on both Chinese medicinals and acupuncture, but practitioners who chooses to focus on medicinals must dedicate themselves to further study, particularly in order to specialize at the skill level of a doctor in a Chinese hospital, who has studied for 4 years before beginning several years of internship. Some practitioners in the United States practice acupuncture exclusively, some use medicinals alone, and some use both, depending on their training, specific interests, or the clinical situation.

REFERENCES

1. Flaws, B: TCM Gynecology Certification Program (vol 1). Blue Poppy Press, Boulder, Colo., 1995.
2. Ibid.
3. Ibid.
4. Kaptchuk, T: The Web That Has No Weaver. Congdon & Weed, New York, 1983.
5. Ibid.
6. Ibid.
7. Flaws, B: How to Write a TCM Herbal Formula. Blue Poppy Press, Boulder, Colo., 1993.

Blood

Blood in Chinese medicine is a concept that goes beyond the red fluid we know in the West, nourishing, maintaining, and moistening the entire body, and is yin in nature.

Jing

Jing, or essence, is a yin substance that governs the cycles of reproduction and sexual development, being responsible, for example, for the onset of puberty and menopause. Jing is said to be full or abundant at the height of a woman's most fertile years, and men are counseled against excessive sexual activity for fear of losing too much jing.

Shen

Shen is best understood as spirit, or the force of the human personality. A person who suffers from clinical depression in the West would be described as having a disorder of shen. "Shen is the awareness that shines out of our eyes when we are truly awake," medical philosophy states.[8]

Fluids

Fluids include bodily liquids other than blood: sweat, saliva, gastric juices, and urine; these substances moisten, nourish, lubricate, or cleanse the body.[9]

Chinese Anatomy

In Chinese medicine, anatomy is defined by functions rather than by physical organs, and physiology becomes the relationship of these functions to the fundamental substances outlined earlier. There are five yin organs, or *zang*, and six yang organs, or *fu*. These yin and yang "organs" are in reality functions, since the ancient Chinese did not see or manipulate the physical masses of tissue we know in the West as organs. The physical existence of organs, therefore, had no importance to the Chinese; only the activities that could be either felt by the patient or observed by the practitioner were taken into consideration. The yin organs include the heart, lungs, spleen, liver, and kidneys (some authors capitalize these and other terms to distinguish them as uniquely Chinese medical concepts). They function to produce, transform, regulate, and store the fundamental substances. They are yin in nature because they contain, secure, and protect qi, blood, jing, shen, and fluids. Under the yang organs we find the gallbladder, stomach, small intestine, large intestine, bladder, and triple burner. The triple burner describes the control of water metabolism throughout the upper, middle, and lower parts of the body. The yang organs are responsible for receiving, breaking down, and absorbing the part of food that will become the fundamental substances and then transporting and excreting the remaining part. They are yang in nature because, like a bucket, they allow substances to pass in and out without remaining very long. The activities of the yin organs are more complex than those of the yang organs, and so they receive more focus in theory and clinical practice.[10]

The Spleen

The Chinese spleen function illustrates perhaps one of the more striking differences between Chinese and Western medical thought. The spleen in Western medicine is a physical structure that stores red blood cells and acts as a blood filter. TCM uses the term *spleen* to mean the function that governs transformation and transportation, meaning it is the primary "organ" (meaning activity) of digestion, transforming the pure nutritive essences of food and drink into qi and blood. The spleen also produces and controls the blood (here it overlaps with the Western function), and diseases involving chronic or uncontrolled bleeding are treated by strengthening the spleen.[11]

Meridians and Acupuncture

Finally, the practitioner of TCM considers the meridians, channels of energy that traverse the body, carrying qi, blood, and, in some cases jing, throughout the body. There are 72 meridians in all, most of them not visible on the map found in acupuncture texts. Many have paths traveling deep into the body, and some connect meridians to one another. (See Fig. 19–1) Along each path are found several energetic "levels," accessed by choosing particular patterns of points that affect the level desired. For example, pain in the upper

FIGURE 19–1   Channel Distribution

According to practitioners of traditional Chinese medicine, the human body contains 72 meridians, or channels of energy, that traverses the body carrying qui, blood, and in some cases, jing.

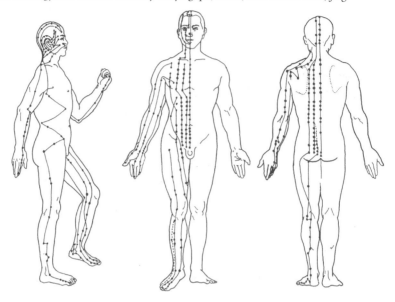

back may be treated with acupuncture needles inserted into points primarily in the area of pain or tightness. We may treat a digestive disorder, on the other hand, by stimulating points not only on the abdomen but also on the legs and arms. The former treatment, a tendino-muscular treatment, activates qi in the most superficial layers of the meridians, while the latter treats the spleen *zang* and the large intestine and stomach *fu*, deeper functions because they handle storage and transportation of qi, blood, jing, shen, and fluids. Acupuncture seems most effective in cases of qi stagnation. This includes cases in which there is discomfort such as pain or aching and in which bodily cycles are disrupted, as seen in irregular menstrual periods or bowel movements. Other examples of qi stagnation are nausea, abdominal bloating, and the wheezing of asthma. In 1997, the National Institutes of Health Consensus Development Statement on Acupuncture[12] presented the following conclusions from studies on the effectiveness of acupuncture:

> *[P]romising results have emerged, . . . [in the] efficacy of acupuncture in adult post-operative and chemotherapy nausea and vomiting and in post-operative dental pain. There are other situations such as addiction, stroke rehabilitation, headache, menstrual cramps, tennis elbow, fibromyalgia myofascial pain, osteoarthritis, low back pain, carpal tunnel syndrome, and asthma where acupuncture may be useful as an adjunct treatment or an acceptable alternative or be included in a comprehensive management program. Further research is likely to uncover additional areas where acupuncture interventions will be useful.*

The report goes on to say that the mechanisms of acupuncture seem to include the release of opioids and other peptides in the central nervous system and the periphery. In addition, the report says, acupuncture may activate the hypothalamus and the pituitary gland, leading to a broad range of systemic effects. It reports documentation of changes in the secretion of neurotransmitters and neurohormones and in blood flow, as well as evidence of alterations in immune functions. It concludes that there is "sufficient evidence of acupuncture's value to expand its use into conventional medicine and to encourage further studies of its physiology and clinical value."[13] This report confirms what practitioners and patients have experienced for two decades in the West and what Chinese practitioners have explained in Chinese medical terms for centuries. However, it is important to note that a limitation of this report is its emphasis on acupuncture and its omission of Chinese herbal medicine; as yet unstudied in the West is the broad effectiveness of Chinese herbal medicine, which, as emphasized earlier, is the primary modality of TCM in China. Its effectiveness has been clearly demonstrated in hundreds of medical journal articles reporting research in China.

Chinese Medicine's View of Six Excesses

The body becomes diseased if it is overexposed or vulnerable to the six external excesses: wind, cold, fire, summer heat, dampness, and dryness. Illness can arise from imbalance caused by an extreme of any of the seven affects or emotions: joy, anger, anxiety, thought (overthinking or worry), sorrow, fear, and fright (as with a sudden shock). Any of these influences can disrupt the balance between yin and yang, creating changes in the fundamental substances, the *zang* or *fu*, or the meridians. We then must apply the Eight Principles to determine if the pattern is Yin or Yang, Cold or Hot, Vacuous (Deficient) or Replete (Excess), Interior or Exterior, and which of the fundamental substances, *zang* or *fu*, or meridians are affected. Usually the pattern is a complex mix of one or more substances and one or more *zang* or *fu* described in a state of yin or yang, as guided by the Eight Principles.

To show how this works in practice, Ted Kaptchuk[14] clearly illustrates Chinese medicine's diagnostic method, pattern discrimination:

[The] difference between Western and Eastern perception can be illustrated by portions of recent clinical studies done in hospitals in China. In a typical study, a Western physician, using upper-gastrointestinal X-rays or endoscopy by means of a fiberscope, diagnoses six patients with stomach pain as having peptic ulcer disease. From the Western doctor's perspective, based on the analytic tendency to narrow diagnosis to an underlying entity, all these patients suffer from the same disorder. The physician then sends the patients to a Chinese doctor for examination. The following results are found.

Upon questioning and examining the first patient, the Chinese physician finds pain that increases at touch (by palpation) but diminishes with the application of cold compresses. The patient has a robust constitution, a reddish complexion, and a full, deep voice. He seems assertive and even aggressive. He is constipated and has dark yellow urine. His tongue has a greasy yellow coating; his pulse is "full" and "wiry." The Oriental physician characterizes this patient as having the pattern of disharmony called "Damp Heat Affecting the Spleen."

When the Chinese physician examines the second patient, he finds a different set of signs, which comprise another overall pattern. The patient is thin. Her complexion is ashen, though her cheeks are ruddy. She is constantly thirsty, her palms are sweaty, and she has a tendency toward constipation, insomnia, and night sweats. She seems nervous and fidgety. Her tongue is dry and slightly red, with no "moss"; her pulse is "thin" and also a bit "fast." This patient is said to have the pattern of "Deficient Yin Affecting the Stomach," a disharmony very different from that of the first patient. Accordingly, a different treatment would be prescribed.

The third patient reports that massage and heat somewhat alleviate his pain, which is experienced as a minor but persistent discomfort. He is temporarily relieved by eating. The patient fears cold [is easily chilled], has a pale face, sweats spontaneously in the daytime, and wants to sleep a lot. His urine is clear and his urination frequent; sometimes he has to get up in the middle of the night to empty his bladder. He appears timid, almost afraid. His tongue is moist and pale, his pulse "Empty." The patient's condition is diagnosed as the pattern of "Exhausted Fire of the Middle Burner," sometimes called "Deficient Cold Affecting the Spleen."

The fourth patient complains of very severe cramping pain; his movement and affect are ponderous and heavy. Hot-water bottles relieve the pain, but massaging the abdomen makes it worse. The patient has a bright white face and a tendency toward loose stools. His tongue has an especially thick, white, moist coating; his pulse is "tight" and "slippery." These signs lead to a diagnosis of the pattern of "Excess Cold Dampness Affecting the Spleen and Stomach."

The fifth patient experiences much sour belching and has headaches. Her pain is sharp, and although massaging the abdomen makes it diminish, heat and cold have no effect. She is very moody. Emotional distress, especially anger or melancholy, seems to precipitate attacks of pain; the pain is also worse during menses. Strangely enough, the patient's tongue is normal, but her pulse is particularly "wiry." The physician concludes that she is affected by the pattern of "disharmony of the Liver invading the Spleen."

The sixth patient has an extremely severe stabbing pain in the stomach that sometimes goes around to his back. The pain is much worse after eating and is aggravated by the slightest touch. He has had episodes of vomiting blood, and produces blackish stools. The patient is very thin and has a rather dark complexion. His tongue is a darkish purple and has markedly red eruptions on the sides. His pulse is "choppy." The Chinese physician describes the patient's problem as a "disharmony of Congealed Blood in the Stomach."

So the Chinese doctor, searching for and organizing signs and symptoms that a Western doctor might never heed, distinguishes six patterns of disharmony where Western medicine perceives only one disease. The patterns of disharmony are similar to what the West calls diseases in that their discovery tells the physician how to prescribe treatment. But they are different from diseases because they cannot be isolated from the patient in whom they occur. To Western medicine, understanding an illness means uncovering a distinct entity that is separate from the patient's being; to Chinese medicine, understanding means perceiving the relationships between all the patient's signs and symptoms. When confronted by a patient with stomach pain, the Western physician must look beyond the screen of symptoms for an underlying pathological mechanism—a peptic ulcer in this case, but it could have been an infection or a tumor or a nervous disorder. A Chinese physician examining the same patient must discern a pattern of disharmony made up of the entire accumulation of symptoms and signs.

The Chinese method is thus holistic, based on the idea that no single part can be understood except in its relation to the whole.

Research

Some 200 journals report research from medical schools and societies from many provinces in China. A sampling of this research follows.

Over a period of 1 year, the authors of one study treated 30 cases of gynecological cysts with a formula called *Xiao Nang Zhong Tang* with good results.[15] The women ranged in age from 19 to 47 years old. The longest duration of disease was more than 5 years and the shortest was 2 months. All these women had lower abdominal pain, low back soreness and pain, or irregular menstrual cycles. Ultrasonography revealed ovarian or pelvic cavity cysts in all cases, the largest being 7.5 by 3.3 cm and the smallest, 2.7 by 1.9 cm.

The medicinals prescribed were decocted in water and administered two times each day, 300 mL each time. One course of treatment lasted 15 days. If one course did not cure, then a second consecutive course was administered. Typically, cure did occur in two courses of treatment. All 30 women were cured. The number of medicinals ranged from 15 *ji* (a packet of medicinals lasting 1 day) to 50 *ji*.

In the case history example, the authors described a 47-year-old patient who for a year had been experiencing intermittent, left-sided, lower abdominal pain, low back soreness and pain, and irregular menstrual cycles. She had already been treated with Western medicine with no effect. Her tongue was moist with a white coating, and her pulse was deep and wiry. Ultrasound showed an abdominal cyst that was 5.4 by 3.6 cm. After 20 *ji* of *Xiao Nang Zhong Tang* were administered, ultrasound showed that the cyst had disappeared.

In the discussion section, the authors explained that gynecological cysts are categorized in Chinese medicine as concretions and conglomerations. The pattern discrimination here was phlegm congelation and blood stasis. The eight medicinals in the formula were chosen based on their abilities to work together to disperse swelling, scatter nodulation, eliminate dampness, transform phlegm, quicken the blood, and transform stasis. Ultrasound examination showed that in all 30 cases the cysts disappeared, demonstrating *Xiao Nang Zhong Tang's* effectiveness.

The researchers Li Xuejun and Liu Wenxi[16] gave one formula to 26 patients with ovarian cysts, adding two or three additional medicinals to fit each patient according to her symptoms of different patterns, such as qi stagnation–type pain, blood stasis–type pain, or cold-type pain. Of the total, 23 were cured within 5 to 36 days.

Fang Jian-ping[17] distinguished four patterns under a single diagnosis of (nonmalignant) breast lumps: liver depression, qi stagnation; liver depression, qi vacuity; liver depression, phlegm nodulation; and qi stagnation, blood stasis. (The "depression" here refers to a blockage of the free flow of liver qi.) Ages of the patients ranged from 15 to 50 years. Different medicinal formulas were given for each of the patterns, with some overlapping of certain medicinals experientially known to reduce breast lumps. Complete cure was defined as disappearance of the lumps, disappearance of the breast pain, and discontinuance of the medicinals after 3 months. Marked improvement was defined as diminishment of the size of the lumps by half and disappearance of the breast pain. Some improvement was defined as diminishment of the size of the lumps by less than half and reduction in the breast pain. No result was defined as no reduction in the size of the breast lumps. The number of cures was 72; marked improvement, 19; some improvement, 6; and no result, 3.

In another study reported, by Huang Suiping,[18] 30 patients diagnosed with irritable bowel syndrome, all having liver qi stagnation pattern, were given the same formula in pill form, in a blind cross-over method. Placebo pills were given to half the patients, whereas the remaining half took the Chinese medicinal formula for 3 weeks. After a 2-week break, the pills were then switched. With the medicinal formula, 28 patients showed improvements in bowel responses and fecal conditions, whereas during the placebo period only 9 patients improved. Other symptoms, such as abdominal pain, mucus in the feces, gurgling of the intestines, and insomnia, were similarly alleviated in about 92 percent of the patients while they were taking the active pills, whereas such improvements occurred in only about 30 percent of the patients while they were taking the placebo.

Fifty patients with cough caused by "accumulated fire," a pattern of chronic, severe heat in the body affecting the lungs, who had been suffering from 8 to 75 days, received the same formula of nine medicinals, consumed as a decoction taken in one dose per day, for up to 6 days.[19] All the patients had notable alleviation of coughing after one dose of the formula, with further improvement or complete cure with two more doses. Thirty-three of the cases were said to be cured in three doses, 21 of the cases in six doses, with 6 patients not cured by the treatment. (See Box 19–2).

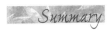

Summary

It is clear in the research literature, as well as in day-to-day practice, that Chinese medicine's strength lies in individualized diagnosis and treatment. If the *bian zheng*, the pattern discrimination,, is correct, and treatment follows faithfully from it, then treatment results are good. If results are poor, the physician must reexamine the patient's signs and symptoms to rediscover the correct pattern. In the clinical example in Box 19–2, this patient has more than one Western diagnosis. We can treat her quite well with one formula that is known to handle a clinical picture that *includes* dizziness, diarrhea, and cold extremities. Suddenly the different diseases dissolve into a single explainable clinical entity.

By following the theories of Chinese medicine on the fundamental influence of diet on asthma and allergies, patients have been given the power to radically change their health, leaving behind a lifetime of dependence on medications with unwanted side effects. A typical patient long plagued by allergies reported that she felt the best she has in a decade, after altering her diet and taking Chinese medicinals tailored to her pattern.

BOX 19–2
Case Study

In this clinical example from the author's practice, the patient, a woman, age 58, quite thin, was diagnosed with both Ménière's disease and Raynaud's disease. Ménière's disease is characterized[1] by attacks of vertigo that appear suddenly, lasting from a few to 24 hours, and associated with nausea and vomiting. There may be a sense of fullness or pressure, usually in one ear, with some progressive hearing loss and tinnitus (ringing). The cause is unknown. Raynaud's disease is characterized by impaired circulation to the extremities, leading to a sensation of severe cold in the hands and feet.

For several weeks before the first attack of dizziness and vertigo, the patient's ears felt blocked throughout the day. When the attack began (2 weeks before her initial appointment at the clinic), she lay down; the slightest movement, even of her eyes, led to a "falling" sensation. She felt nauseous and vomited. Her ears had a buzzing and feeling of water moving. This episode lasted 4 hours. One week later, she experienced another, milder attack. She had a long history of loose, watery stools, occurring within an hour after each meal.

Raynaud's disease manifested in her as extremely cold fingers that often turned white; this, too, was a long-standing condition. Her tongue was moist, tinged with purple, and showed slight teeth marks at the edges. Her pulse was slightly deep and slippery. These symptoms led to an identification of the patient's pattern: spleen and kidney yang vacuity and liver yin and blood vacuity. The spleen and kidney yang vacuities were revealed in the loose stools and cold fingers, as well as their chronic nature, the tongue, and pulse; the liver yin and blood vacuity accounted for the dizziness, the vertigo, and the lack of sufficient blood to the hands. Treatment principles focused on boosting and supplementing spleen and kidney yang, and nourishing and enriching liver yin and blood. The chosen medicinal formula addressed all aspects of this complex pattern.

In order to choose the correct combination of ingredients, the practitioner must draw on a knowledge of some 300 medicinals, which is the basic number that a TCM practitioner must learn. They are arranged by category, and in this case the most important ones were those that activate and warm the spleen and kidney yang and nourish and enrich the liver yin and blood. But the medicinals are not simply picked from these categories and combined into a formula. The practitioner determines which classic formula will best suit this patient, out of about 70 that he or she is required to know. The formula is then modified to fit the patient's pattern as closely as possible. The logic of TCM dictates choosing a formula that treats as much of the entire pattern as possible. Since these classic formulas have been modified and perfected over centuries, their combinations of ingredients have proven to be effective. The medicinals they contain work synergistically when decocted together. For a particular patient's pattern, medicinals that do not fit are deleted; for example, some may be too cold for the patient, so they would be removed, whereas the most fundamental ingredients in the formula are retained and other medicinals the patient needs are added. Chinese doctors call this keeping the "idea" of the formula, while tailoring it to the individual.

The dosage of each ingredient must be adjusted as well. For an acute problem, the doctor will see a patient once every 3 or 4 days in order to adjust the formula by as little as one or two ingredients, or to change the dosage of one or more medicinals, as the patient's system changes. For more chronic or milder problems, the doctor may only need to see the patient every week or two because the system, damaged over a longer period of time, recovers more slowly. Each time the patient is seen, the doctor recomposes the pattern discrimination to reflect the current condition and reconstitutes the formula. This is an art and science that the doctor perfects over the years. Thus the older that doctors are in China, the more they are respected for their years of experience.

In this case, the patient was given the medicinal formula in a granular form, in which the medicinals are decocted together and then dessicated, which is more convenient for some patients. She was instructed to eat a diet of mostly warm, cooked foods, adding a little meat to help build yang and blood (she had been a vegetarian). One week after beginning the medicine, the diarrhea was somewhat better, and she had experienced some pressure in one ear, but no dizziness. After making some dietary changes and taking the medicinals for 10 more days, she had no diarrhea and had had only one episode of relatively mild dizziness, with no ear pressure or nausea. As colder weather approached, I added ingredients that more strongly warmed yang and nourished blood, since she was so affected by the cold. As the winter continued, I added more warming ingredients and increased the dosage to help her

continued

BOX 19–2 continued
Case Study

hands stay as warm as possible. This aspect of the disorder was the most difficult to treat, as it often is in very lean people, whose constitutions are so yin. Her hands remained relatively cold. As long as she continued to take the medicine, she suffered no dizziness and only a rare bout of diarrhea related to eating unusual food. In this patient's case, the yang needed supplementing in an ongoing way because of the extremely yin constitution.

REFERENCE

1. The Merck Manual. Merck & Co., Whitehouse Station, N.J., 1996–1997.

She was finally without the constant facial pain and sinus blockage she had suffered for so long.

A patient in the author's practice has progressive kidney failure. For more than 2 years, only Chinese medicinals have kept him urinating regularly, avoiding the need for hemodialysis to clean his blood and preserve his life. One can only imagine how patients' quality of life would improve if each one with this diagnosis was given natural medicine free of side effects that could indefinitely delay the need for such extreme measures. With this medicine's ability to treat the entire person with his or her own unique needs, we might avoid the costs to both the patient and the medical system exacted by treating the disease alone.

In the West, the physician focuses on eliminating the disease in the same way in every body that enters the clinic, using medicines that work for some patients. The value of a medical system that treats the particular manifestation of a disease in an individual is that whatever weaknesses the body presents, we have the theoretical tools to support the needed changes so that healing can take place. In Chinese medicine, because we treat the way the disease lives in each individual, we must be prepared to craft a new formula for each patient and as each patient's clinical picture changes. By explaining to them how and why their illness has developed and how they can change their condition, we can help patients gain the understanding they need to preserve their health in the future.

RESOURCES

American Association of Oriental Medicine
433 Front St.
Catasauqua, PA 18032
Phone: (888) 500-7999 (toll-free); (610) 266-1433
Fax: (610) 264-2768
Website: *www.aaom.org*
E-mail: *aaom@aaom.org*
This is the main national organization of practitioners.

Blue Poppy Press
5441 Western Ave., #2
Boulder, CO 80301
Phone: (800) 487-9296 (toll-free); (303) 447-8372
Fax: (303) 245-8362
Website: *www.bluepoppy.com*
E-mail: *info@bluepoppy.com*
This press carries several books on various problems specifically for laypeople on such topics as menopause, breast disease, migraines, hay fever, and pediatrics.

REFERENCES

1. Flaws, B: What Is Chinese Medicine? Blue Poppy Press, Boulder, Colo., 1996.
2. Flaws, B: How to Write a TCM Herbal Formula. Blue Poppy Press, Boulder, Colo., 1993.
3. Ibid.
4. Ibid.
5. Micozzi, MS (ed): Fundamentals of Complementary and Alternative Medicine. Churchill Livingstone, New York, 1996.
6. Kaptchuk, T: The Web That Has No Weaver. Congdon & Weed, New York, 1983.
7. Ibid.
8. Ibid.
9. Ibid, p 46.
10. Ibid.
11. Ibid.
12. National Institutes of Health Consensus Development Statement on Acupuncture, Revised Draft, November 5, 1997, p 6.
13. Ibid.
14. Kaptchuk, The Web That Has No Weaver, pp 4–7.
15. Dong, B, and Zhang, X: A clinical survey of the treatment of 30 cases of gynecological cysts with *Xiao Nang Zhong Tang.* Shan Xi Zhong Yi [Shanxi Chinese Medicine] 5:23, 1995. In: TCM Gynecology Certification Program (B Flaws, trans; vol 3). Blue Poppy Press, Boulder, Colo., 1995.
16. Li, X, and Liu, W: Treatment of ovarian cyst with Chinese herb. In Kezhi, F, (trans-ed): Journal of Traditional Chinese Medicine. Reprinted in Dharmananda, S (ed), Straight from China newsletter, Institute for Traditional Medicine, Portland, Ore., 1993.
17. Fang, J: The pattern discrimination treatment of 100 cases of mammary hyperplasia. Jiang Su Zhong Yi [Jiang Su Chinese Medicine] 2:14, 1993. In: TCM Gynecology Certification Program (B Flaws, trans; vol 2). Blue Poppy Press, Boulder, Colo., 1995.
18. Huang, S: Treatment of irritable bowel syndrome with Chinese herbs. In Kezhi, F, (trans-ed): Journal of Traditional Chinese Medicine 31(3). Reprinted in Dharmananda, S (ed), Straight from China newsletter, Institute for Traditional Medicine, Portland, Ore., 1993.
19. Kezhi, F (trans-ed): Treatment of cough due to accumulated fire. Journal of Traditional Chinese Medicine 27(4):6, 1986. Reprinted in Dharmananda, S (ed), Straight from China newsletter, Institute for Traditional Medicine, Portland, Ore., 1993.

RECOMMENDED READING

Flaws, B: How to Write a TCM Herbal Formula. Blue Poppy Press, Boulder, Colo., 1993. A thorough explanation of b*ian zheng* diagnostic theory, written for students of TCM.

Flaws, B: The Tao of Healthy Eating. Blue Poppy Press, Boulder, Colo., 1989. A complete explanation of dietary theory according to the principles of TCM, written for patients.

Flaws, B: What Is Chinese Medicine? Blue Poppy Press, Boulder, Colo., 1996. A basic patient's pamphlet by one of the foremost teachers of TCM in the United States.

Kaptchuk, T: The Web That Has No Weaver. Congdon & Weed, New York, 1983. This is the best foundational book in the theories of TCM, for both laypeople and students of TCM.

CHAPTER 20

Ayurveda

Abbas Qutab

Abbas Qutab, MD, DC, PhD, DSc, is a practicing Ayurvedic physician and the director of the Twenty First Century Medical Center and Elan Vital Medical Centers and Spas. Qutab, who also founded the New England Institute of Ayurvedic Medicine (now called International Ayurvedic Institute), is the coauthor of Health and Disease in Ayurveda and Yoga *as well as* Pancha-Karma *and* Ayurvedic Massage.

Ayurveda, which originated in the Vedic civilization of ancient India, is one of the oldest scientific medical systems in the world. It is not only a system of medicine in the conventional sense of curing disease but also a way of life that teaches us how to maintain and protect health. Many throughout the world regard Ayurveda as one of the great gifts the ancient sages of India left to humankind.

The word *ayu* means "all aspects of life from birth to death." The word *veda* means "knowledge" or "learning." Thus *Ayurveda* denotes the science by which life in its totality is understood. It is a science of life that delineates the diet, medicines, and behaviors that are beneficial or harmful for life. Ayurveda considers that balance among people, the environment, and the larger cosmos is integral to human health.

Like other holistic modalities, Ayurveda shows us how to both cure disease and promote longevity. It treats each individual as a "whole," while at the same time viewing him or her as a combination of body, mind, and soul. Spiritual healing, or self-realization, is the ultimate goal of Ayurveda. A balance of physical, mental, and emotional health is the basis from which spiritual development evolves toward wholeness.

Ayurveda covers all aspects of health and wellness. Its inclusive healing methods encompass diet and healthy digestion, herbs, exercise, sleep, purification, the practices of yoga and meditation, and lifestyle recommendations. There is great emphasis on prevention of disease and the process of self-healing, which is fostered by sophisticated Ayurvedic therapeutics. An extensive materia medica of medicinal plants is the basis for prescribing therapeutic remedies. In addition, Ayurvedic physicians have a sophisticated understanding of biological rhythms, which form the basis for daily and seasonal behavioral routines to heal illness and to promote health. (See Box 20–1.)

Ayurveda's holistic and integral medical system is divided into eight branches. (See Table 20–1.) Ayurvedic medicine and health care can be translated into Western concepts, as seen in the clinical foci of Ayurvedic medical system branches and the corresponding "specialty" areas familiar to practitioners of Western health care. However, the principles on which Ayurveda is based go beyond Western concepts of health and illness in their connection to the Vedic understanding of the human life as being influenced by and being a part of the natural flow of the universe and the elements of which the universe is

BOX 20–1
Ayurveda and the Vedas

The Vedas are regarded as the oldest and most sacred written record of knowledge. The Vedas state that the Supreme Being, who created the universe out of love and concern for humanity, gave the divine Vedas to all humankind through the rishis, or seers of wisdom. The words of the Vedas were carefully memorized according to metrical chants and transmitted from generation to generation.

Thus the four Vedas—*Rig, Yajur, Sama,* and *Atharva*—have come down to us through several thousands of years of oral transmission before they were written down. The *Rig Veda* is the foundation of the other Vedas and contains, in 10 books called "mandalas," 1028 suktas, or hymns, with a total of 10,572 verses. The *Yajur Veda* has 1975 stanzas in 40 chapters of both verse and prose. The *Sama Veda* has 1800 verses repeated from the *Rig Veda* and 75 original verses. The *Atharva Veda* has 5977 verses, distributed among 731 suktas.

The *Rig Veda,* the oldest of the four, contains many concepts of Ayurveda. Its three great gods—Indra, Agni, and Soma—relate to the three biological humors of Ayurveda—vata, pitta, and kapha. References are found in it to organ transplants, in the case of an artificial limb that was made for Queen Vishpala, wife of King Khela. The *Rig Veda* also contains many hymns to Soma, a Vedic god as well as a great curative herbal preparation used to treat many diseases of the body and mind and to promote longevity.

Although all the Vedas contain references to Ayurvedic concepts, the *Atharva Veda* contains more of these, so much so that Ayurveda is considered to be an Upaveda, or a subsidiary teaching of the *Atharva Veda.* In the *Atharva* we find references to anatomical and physiological factors, the disease process, treatment of specific diseases, and other systematic knowledge about Ayurveda. In later ancient times, 1000–700 BC, Ayurveda developed into eight recognized branches or specialties and two prominent schools: Atreya, the school of physicians, and Dhanvantari, the school of surgeons.

The magico-religious aspect of medicine in the Vedas was gradually supplemented by observations based on scientific thinking. Ayurvedic scholars of subsequent generations gave a sound and logical philosophical foundation to Ayurveda. The material scattered in the Vedas was collected, subjected to rigid tests of efficacy, and systematically arranged. Such compilations were called "Samhitas." Many of these compilations no longer exist. Only three authentic works have stood the test of time and are available today—the *Charaka Samhita, Sushruta Samhita,* and *Ashtanga Hridaya Samhita.* This great trio—the *Brihatrayi,* as it is called—has enjoyed much popularity and respect for the last 2000 years. Although these texts have undergone some modification by various authors in subsequent periods, their present form is at least 1200 years old. They are all in the Sanskrit language.

comprised. A person is a small but whole representation of the universe and contains everything that makes up the surrounding world. Ayurveda recognizes the interconnectedness of individual, social, and environmental health.

This chapter presents an overview of the key Ayurvedic principles: tridosha theory (humors), constitution (parakti), and their relationship with aspects of the natural world.

TABLE 20–1   Ayurvedic Medical System

BRANCHES	CLINICAL FOCUS
1. Kaya chikitsa	Medicine
2. Shalya	Surgery
3. Agada tantra	Toxicology/treatment of poisoning
4. Budhtavidya	Psychology
5. Shalkya	Opthalmology and otorhinolaryngology
6. Kumar-Bhritya	Pediatrics
7. Rsayana	Rejuvenation geriatrics
8. Vajikaran	Aphrodisiacs/fertility/sterility

TABLE 20–2 Universal Correspondence with the Human Being

UNIVERSE		HUMAN BEING
Macrocosm		Microcosm
Three energy principles:	equivalent to	Three biological humors:
fire		pitta
air, space		vata
earth, water		kapha

Tridosha Theory: The Three Biological Humors

One of the key principles of Ayurvedic philosophy—and the aspect that most distinguishes it from other holistic modalities—is the perceived link between conditions in the body and phenomena in the physical universe. Ancient Indian scientists felt that changes in the sun, moon, and wind—the three main causative factors in the external universe—could have a profound effect on the workings of the human body.

These early scientists regarded the sun as the energy of conversion, represented as fire; the moon as the agency of cooling, represented by the combinations of earth and water; and wind as the principle of movement or propulsion, represented by the combination of air and ether. Table 20–2 depicts the body/universe equivalents.

These scientists also perceived all activities in the universe or in the human being as grouped into three basic functions: creation, preservation, and destruction. When these processes are balanced, health is the result. Imbalance results from excesses and deficiencies among these doshic qualities.

The tridosha theory, the foundation of Ayurvedic philosophy, relates these three functions of the physical universe to the three biological humors, or underlying metabolic principles, called "doshas." Through the doshas, the five basic elements—earth, air, fire, water, and space—interact to make up the human body. Kapha, the cohesive humor, is responsible for maintaining the creation. Pitta, the thermogenic humor, organizes body activities after transformation. Vata, the energetic humor, controls destruction. (See Table 20–3.)

Vata

Vata carries out many diverse functions in the human body and is responsible for all bodily movement and nervous functions. It is the principle of propulsion. It controls cell arrangement and division, the formation of different tissue layers, and the differentiation of organs and systems. It conducts impulses such as those from the sense organs to the brain and from the brain to the motor organs. Vata controls the expulsion of feces, urine, sweat, menstrual fluid, semen, and the fetus. It also controls respiratory, cardiac, and gastrointestinal movements, as well as all higher functions in the brain and spinal cord. Vata controls the mind and gives the energy to perform all bodily and mental activities. Disruption in vata is manifested in gas and pain.

TABLE 20–3 Universal Forces of the Tridoshas in the Human

UNIVERSE	HUMAN
Destruction	Vata
Preservation	Pitta
Creation	Kapha

Pitta

Pitta is responsible for the formation of tissues, waste products, and energy from the food, water, and air that we take in from the outside. It controls metabolic activities and is responsible for all the secretions in the gastrointestinal tract and for the secretion of enzymes and hormones from the ductless glands into the blood stream. It controls body temperature, hunger, thirst, fear, anxiety, anger, and sexual desire. Pitta is also responsible for courage and willpower, as well as assimilation of knowledge from the outside world. Disruption in pitta leads to inflammation.

Kapha

Kapha increases the deposits in the cell mass as well as being essential for the interlinking of cells, tissues, and organs. It is thus responsible for the growth of the body. It prevents destruction of tissues from wear and tear—resulting from friction and movement by vata—by maintaining the strength and immunity of the body. Capacities for reproductions, happiness, and retention of knowledge depend on the proper functioning of kapha. Disruption in kapha is seen in swelling, accumulation of fluid, and mucus formation.

Role of Equilibrium

Ayurveda attributes great importance to the equilibrium of the three humors, or tridosha. Although they are in a constant state of flux, because of the impact of internal and external factors, their equilibrium is usually maintained. When this equilibrium is disturbed, the disease process begins. According to the Indian system of medicine, all diseases are caused by aggravated humors, or vitiated doshas. Even traumatic diseases, which are not initially the result of an imbalance of these doshas, soon become accompanied by such an imbalance.

Constitution

The second key principle of Ayurvedic philosophy is the concept of a human's constitution, called "prakriti." The prakriti, or physical constitution of an individual, depends on the following:

The condition of the sperm and ovum at the time of conception
The nature of the season and the condition inside the uterus
Food and other regimens adopted by the mother during pregnancy
The nature of the doshic elements at the time of conception

The physical constitution of an individual is also influenced by social class, family traits, locality, time, age, and individuality. The predominance of elements determines the physical constitution. The predominance of gunas, which are the qualities of nature that bind the soul in the body, determines the psychological constitution. The predominance of humors (doshas) determines the prakriti energetic condition of the body. Of all the constitutions, the humoral dominance is most important in the examination of both health and disease.

Physical Constitution

The overall quality and functioning of the physical body are usually the result of a mix of the three doshic qualities. We now discuss the major characteristics of the three types of doshic, or humoral, constitutions.

Vata Constitution. Individuals of vata constitution usually have tall or thin body frames and less strength. Their body weight is low, and they have less resistance to disease. Their digestion and metabolism are changeable, and cannot form sturdy and stable tissues. Their life span is usually shorter than that of other individuals. Because of this variable nature in constitution, they cannot perform tasks steadily and continuously. Consequently, they may fail in achieving their goals. Such individuals should not have a job that demands strenuous physical activity, requires constant attention, or takes place in a cold or air-conditioned atmosphere. If they are forced to undertake such work, they are likely to develop diseases of the nerves and bones, suffer from constipation, and lose weight.

Pitta Constitution. Individuals of pitta constitution have rapid digestive and metabolic activity. Therefore they require constant food and drink that is cool and oily in nature. They are able to convert food quality to tissue, but because the total conversion rate in the body is very fast, they, too, usually have shorter life spans than others.

They have soft, smooth, and oily skin. Their hair becomes gray prematurely, and they tend to become bald at an early age. They have moderate strength and capacity to work, and they are often hot-tempered. They are very intelligent and possess an excellent capacity for conceptual comprehension. They usually possess good knowledge of any subject that interests them and are creative in nature. These persons require a job in a cool atmosphere, with some creative activity and intelligent work. They should not deal with chemicals, dyeing material, or petrochemical substances, nor work near heat.

Kapha Constitution. Individuals of kapha constitution have hefty, robust, and thick body frames with stout musculature. They naturally possess good strength, immunity, and vitality and have a longer life span with good health. They have smooth, deep voices and are often good-looking. The total digestive and metabolic rates are very slow; hence they require less food and drink. They are of a calm and quiet nature. Kapha types can carry out work that is heavy or strenuous. They are also good at maintaining public relations. However, they should not work in cold and damp atmospheres. They are likely to become obese and may fall victim to joint diseases and heart problems.

Humoral combinations result in seven constitution types:

1. Vata
2. Pitta
3. Kapha
4. Vata-pitta
5. Pitta-kapha
6. Kapha-vata
7. Vata-pitta-kapha

A single-dosha constitution is rare, and a balanced-dosha constitution (vata-pitta-kapha)—which is excellent—is also rare. A vata constitution is usually inferior in health and longevity, pitta is intermediate, and kapha is the most robust of doshic constitutions. The vata-pitta combination offers the most challenges to health. Vata-kapha-pitta in equal proportions is the ideal doshic state of health. (See Table 20–4.)

Psychological Constitution

A complete assessment of the person requires an understanding of the factors that make up psychological functioning as well as physical characteristics.

Mental states are based on qualities (gunas) of balance (sattva), energy (rajas), and inertia (tamas). The predominance of these three basic qualities at the time of birth

TABLE 20–4   Ayurvedic Constitutions

BODY CHARACTERISTIC	VATA (AIR)	PITTA (FIRE)	KAPHA (WATER)
Height	Tall or very short	Medium	Usually short but can be tall and large
Frame	Thin, bony, good muscles	Moderate, developed	Large, well-formed
Weight	Low, hard to maintain weight	Moderate	Heavy, hard to lose weight
Skin luster	Dull or dusky	Ruddy, lustrous	White or pale
Skin texture	Dry, rough, thin	Warm, oily	Cold, damp, thick
Eyes	Small, nervous	Piercing, easily inflamed	Large, white sclera
Hair	Dry, thin	Thin, oily	Thick, oily, wavy, lustrous
Teeth	Crooked, poorly formed	Moderate, bleeding gums	Large, well-formed
Nails	Tough, brittle	Soft, pink	Soft, white

Source: Frawley, D: Yoga and Ayurveda. Lotus Press, Twin Lakes, Wisc., 1999, with permission.

determines the psychological constitution of the person. Like doshic constitution, psychological constitution can be divided into seven types:

1. Sattva
2. Rajas
3. Tamas
4. Sattva-rajas
5. Sattva-tamas
6. Rajas-tamas
7. Sattva-rajas-tamas

Sattvic Constitution. Individuals of sattvic psychological constitution possess a good intellect and memory and have an inherent instinct for cleanliness. Although they usually have a good amount of knowledge, they always make efforts to improve their intellect. They possess goodwill and allow others to prosper well. They are polite and have faith in the divine and devotion to the good.

Rajasic Constitution. Individuals of rajasic psychological constitution have a nature that tries to overpower others. They have a propulsive and very dynamic energy. They are not satisfied with the positions and possessions they achieve and always strive for more. Hence they are ambitious and industrious in nature. Usually these people are hot-tempered and egoistic. They overexpress pain or pleasure. They have brave, but jealous and cruel, character.

Tamasic Constitution. Individuals of tamasic psychological constitution are lazy and ignorant—both physically and mentally. Consequently, they are not curious about anything. Usually they have lesser intelligence. They prefer not to work and are interested mainly, if not exclusively, in eating, drinking, and sleeping. They avoid cleanliness and are not health conscious. They are afraid of many things; hence they do not initiate any work on their own.

Importance of Constitution. If we observe different individuals as to their nutritional requirements, their tolerance to the atmosphere, or their particular behavior, we find that they have different needs for maintaining health. They prefer different types of drinks, foods, and activities.

Even though two persons are of identical weight and height, their nutritional requirements may be quite different. One may prefer large amounts of food or drink, whereas the other may prefer lesser quantities. If we analyze the serum, blood, and so forth in these individuals, we may not find any substantial differences. Yet differences clearly exist.

From this it becomes clear that the tolerance to food, drink, or environment cannot be discovered by the analytical study of body tissues alone. Instead, knowledge of comprehensive individual specificity or constitution is essential. By recognizing the constitution of any individual, we know which food and drink and which types of job and exercise are required for maintaining health.

Because there is a predominance of dosha in each type of constitution, all types require substances different from or opposite to their constitutional type to maintain health. For example, vata individuals possess the qualities of coldness, dryness, roughness, lightness, and so forth. Accordingly, a person of vata constitution requires food that is warm, hot, or oily. Otherwise there is always a tendency for vata to increase and give rise to vata diseases. To compensate for the vata in one's constitution, foods should be sweet, sour, and salty because these tastes possess such properties.

To maintain health, every person should know his or her constitution. If daily activities, diet, occupation, and behavior are not adjusted to balance the person, the constitutional humor will increase, giving rise to its characteristic disease. If the constitution is known, herbs, diet, and other regimens—including yogic postures—can be recommended to treat disease and to promote longevity.

Relationship to Natural World: Movement of Doshas through the Cycle of Time

The doshas reflect the rhythms of time. They show how the forces of nature discharge their effect according to the changes of time periods and developments of various processes of transformation. (See Table 20–5.)

In the cycle of the day, kapha is dominant in the morning and evening; pitta predominates at noon and midnight; and vata is highest at sunrise and sunset, the transitional points of the day. Seasonally, kapha is highest in late winter and early spring, the seasons of cold and dampness; pitta is highest in the late spring and summer, the seasons of heat; and vata is highest in the fall and early winter, the seasons of cold and dryness.

TABLE 20–5 Doshas and the Cycle of Time

TIME PERIOD	KAPHA	PITTA	VATA
Day	7 AM–11 AM	11 AM–3 PM	3 PM–7 PM
Night	7 PM–11 PM	11 PM–3 AM	3 AM–7 AM
Season	February 7–June 7	June 7–October 7	October 7–February 7
Digestion	First 1½ hour after eating	Second 1½ hour after eating	Third 1½ hour after eating

In the digestive process, kapha is highest immediately after eating. Hence nausea right after food intake indicates high kapha. Pitta is highest 2 or 3 hours after eating and manifested by symptoms such as gas or constipation. It is best to treat doshas at their respective times. Hence medicines to decrease kapha are given in the morning, for pitta in the afternoon, and for vata in the evening.

The drugs employed in medical sciences have been changing rapidly, whereas the nature of the human body has remained the same. When drugs used for a period of time become ineffective, it indicates that something is fundamentally wrong with our entire approach to healing.

Ayurvedic Consultation

An initial Ayurvedic consultation can last an hour or more. It includes a thorough history and physical examination. The history involves determining body constitution, pathological state, tissue vitality, physical build, and body measurement, as well as the patient's adaptability, psychological constitution, condition of digestion, capacity for exercise, and age.

The physical exam includes a general examination and systemic examination. The general exam is an eightfold examination that helps the Ayurvedic physician determine the imbalances in the body and mind. The eightfold exam is comprised of the following elements:

* Examination of the pulse.
* Examination of the tongue.
* Examination of the voice.
* Palpation, percussion, and auscultation.
* Examination of the general appearance.
* Urine analysis.
* Stool analysis.
* Systemic examination, which includes an examination and history of each system—digestive, respiratory, urinary, circulatory, and so forth. An Ayurvedic physician is interested in your lifestyle, eating habits, sleeping patterns, which season you prefer, which tastes you like or dislike, and even what kind of dreams you experience. Based on this comprehensive evaluation, treatment is devised for the patient.

Ayurvedic treatments consist of herbal medicine; dietary changes; specialized detoxification, purification, and rejuvenation therapies; meditation; yoga; sound and color therapy; and so forth. Ayurveda believes that, through proper metabolic cleansing and rejuvenation therapies, an individual can live a very long and healthy life, and avoid experiencing any age-related, chronic, and degenerative diseases.

Research: Clinical Effectiveness of Ayurvedic Herbs

Ashwaganda

Ashwaganda, also known as Indian ginseng, is an extract from the root of the plant *Withania somnifera* (family: Solanaceae) containing at least 1 percent alkaloids and 1.5 percent withanolides. Ashwaganda, described in the literature as an adaptogen or vitalizer, is used as a restorative and rejuvenative, particularly in the management of chronic disease. Experimental data show that ashwaganda increases physical and psychological endurance of stress. In technical terms, it increases the state of nonspecifically increased resistance (NSIR) of the human body by offering protection against the deleterious effect of stress.[1]

Ashwagandha has anti-inflammatory and analgesic properties; it lowers blood pressure, protects the liver from toxins, and protects the organism from the results of physical stress caused by chronic diseases such as diabetes. Ashwagandha decreases vata and kapha and increases pitta.

Boswellia with Curcumin

Boswellia is an extract from the *Boswellia serrata* gum (family: Burseraceae) containing at least 60 percent boswellic acids as the active ingredient. This ingredient is effective in treating various forms of arthritis. In a clinical trial performed on a mixed group of 175 rheumatoid arthritis patients, 97 percent reported considerable improvement. The treatment was effective in reducing pain and morning stiffness as well as improving grip strength and physical performance.[2]

In human studies, Boswellia has been found to improve blood supply to the joints and prevent the breakdown of tissues affected by arthritis. In general, it can be described as a nonsteroidal anti-inflammatory compound without the side effects caused by such nonsteroidal analgesics as aspirin. Boswellia balances kapha and vata and increases pitta.

Curcuminoids have been extracted from *Curcuma longa* (family: Zingiberaceae) and standardized to contain a minimum of 95 percent total curcuminoids. Curcumin, the most prevalent curcuminoid, has strong antioxidant properties, which helps prevent the formation of free radicals (highly toxic and destructive molecules) in food and body tissues. When curcumin was experimentally added to fats and oils, it prevented lipid peroxidation and resultant rancidity. Lipid peroxidation proceeds by the mechanism of free-radical formation and propagation. It is therefore believed that curcumin may prevent or slow down cardiovascular disease, neoplastic disease, chronic diseases such as arthritis, and viral infections by preventing free-radical formation.[3–5]

Deglycerrhizinated Licorice

Deglycerrhizinated licorice (DGL) is an extract from the root of *Glycyrrhiza glabra* (family: Leguminosae), with the glycyrrhizin component removed to avoid sodium and fluid retention. Clinical studies with DGL have proven its effectiveness in the treatment of gastrointestinal ulcers. One hundred patients with gastric ulcers were treated in a single-blind controlled trial to assess the efficacy of DGL in comparison to cimetidine. Both were equally effective, reducing pain and aiding in the healing. The healing process was confirmed by endoscopic evaluation. DGL seems to have a different mechanism of action from cimetidine. DGL increases blood flow to the stomach mucosa, whereas cimetidine decreases it. DGL is also known to increase the resistance of stomach and intestinal mucosa to drugs such as aspirin. DGL is clinically effective only in chewable form. DGL reduces vata and pitta and increases kapha.[6]

Gugul

Gugul, an extract from *Commiphora mukul* (wightii) (family: Burseraceae) standardized for 2.5 to 3.5 percent guggulsterones, has cholesterol-lowering properties combined with weight-loss properties. In a double-blind clinical study, gugul administered daily for 4 weeks to 60 overweight patients resulted in a significant decrease in total serum lipids, cholesterol, triglycerides, and beta lipoproteins. Gugul may also increase the metabolic process that generates energy, an effect called "thermogenesis," by stimulating thyroid functions and synthesis of neurohormones such as catecholamines, like norepinephrine, which decrease the amount of body fat without affecting food intake. Gugul balances kapha and vata and increases pitta.[7]

Summary

Ayurveda has been a sophisticated, effective natural health system for millions of people for more than two millennia. Its understanding of body-mind-spirit-environment unity predates the relatively recent trend in Western health care to treat the whole person. Ayurvedic physicians have known for centuries what we in the West consider new areas for investigative research—that is, that emotions, diet, and lifestyle behavior are insepara- ble from an understanding of health.

As the effectiveness of Ayurvedic treatments comes to the attention of the Western health-care system, people are demonstrating more interest in Ayervedic methods as complementary their Western medical care. Ayurvedic texts are slowly being translated from Sanskrit into other languages, making the gift of Ayurvedic knowledge and wisdom more generally available. Ayurvedic preparations are becoming more available in health food stores, although they should not be used as self-treatment remedies without the guidance of Ayurvedic consultation and education. Awareness of the benefits of this approach to individual and social health will continue to expand and contribute to human health.

RESOURCES

American Institute of Vedic Studies
P.O. Box 8357
Santa Fe, NM 87504-8357
Phone: (505) 982-3308
Training in Ayurveda, Ayurvedic lifestyle, or counseling.

Ayurvedic Institute
11311 Menaul NE
Albuquerque, NM 87112
Phone: 505-291-9698
Training in Ayurveda, Ayurvedic lifestyle, or counseling.

International Ayurvedic Institute
Administrative Offices
21 West Street
Worcester, MA 01609
Phone: (508) 753-0006
Fax: (508) 770-0618
ayurveda@hotmail.com
Training in Ayurveda, Ayurvedic lifestyle, and counseling.

LifeSpa
John Douillard
3065 Center Green Dr.
Boulder, CO 80301
Phone: (303) 442-1164
Fax: (303) 442-1240
Training in Ayurveda, Ayurvedic lifestyle, or counseling.

Maharishi Ayurveda
1068 Elkton Dr.
Colorado Springs, CO 80907-3538
Phone: (719) 260-5500
Ayurvedic herbs and information.

Sabinsa Corporation
121 Ethel Road West, Unit 6
Piscataway, NJ 08854
Phone: (732) 777-1111
Ayurvedic herbs and information.

Ultimate Health Center
21 West Street
Worcester, MA 01609
Phone: (508) 753-0006
Fax: (508) 770-0618
OR
Whittier Place, Suite 108
Charles River Park
Boston, MA 02114
Phone: (617) 227-6573
Training in Ayurveda, Ayurvedic lifestyle, or counseling.

REFERENCES

1. Sharma, K, and Dandiya, PC: *Withania somnifera* dunal: Present status. Indian Drugs 29(6):247–253, 1991.
2. Gupta, VN, et al: Chemistry and pharmacology of gum resin of *Boswellia serrara*. Indian Drugs 24(5):221–231, 1986.
3. Lin, JK, et al: Molecular mechanism of action of curcumin. In Food Phytochemicals II: Teas, spices, and herbs. Journal of American Chemical Society 20:196–203, 1994.
4. Schaich, KM, et al: Formation and reactivity of free radicals in curcuminoids. In Food Phytochemicals II: Tea, Spices, and Herbs. Journal of American Chemical Society 21:204, 1994.
5. Man-Ying, M., and Fong, D. In Anti-inflammatory and Cancer-Preventative Immunomodulations through Diet. American Chemical Society, 1994. Food Phytochemicals for Cancer Prevention II: Teas, Spices, and Herbs edited by C.-T. Ho, et al.
6. Morgan, AG, et al: Cimetidine and DGL in treatment of gastric ulceration. Gut. 23:545–551.
7. Satyavati, GV: Gugulipid: A promising hypolipidaemic agent from gum guggul (*Commiphora wightii*). In Economics and Medicinal Plant Research: vol 5. Plants and Traditional Medicine. Academic Press, New York, 1991.

RECOMMENDED READING

Charaka Samhita (Chowkhamba Sanskrit Series). Mysore Pub., Varanasi, India, 1976.

Dash, B, and Manfred, J: A Handbook of Ayurveda. Concept Publishing, New Delhi, India, 1983.

Frawley, D: Ayurvedic Healing—A Comprehensive Guide. Passage Press, Salt Lake City, Utah. 1989.

Lad,V, and Frawley, D: The Yoga of Herbs. Lotus Press, Santa Fe, N.M., 1986.

Lele, RD: Ayurveda and Modern Medicine. Bharatiya Vidya Bhavana, Bombay, India, 1986.

Qutab, A: Ayurvedic Notebook (vols II, IV). New England Institute of Ayurvedic Medicine, Worcester, Mass., 1996.

Qutab, A: Ayurvedic specific conditions review. The Protocol Journal of Botanical Medicine USA 1(3):187–193, 1996.

Qutab, A, and Ranade, S: Health and Disease in Ayurveda and Yoga. Anmol Prakasha, Pune, India, 1997.

Ranade, S: Natural Healing through Ayurveda. Passage Press, Salt Lake City, Utah, 1995.

Ranade, S, and Norbert, L: Ayurveda Science of Longevity [in German, English]. Anmol Prakashan, Pune, India, 1995.

Ranade, S, and Patkwardhan, BK: Handbook of Research Methods. Anmol Prakashana, Pune, India, 1989.

CHAPTER 21

Yoga

Lois Steinberg

Lois Steinberg, PhD, has more than 25 years of study, practice, and teaching experience in Iyengar Yoga. She is the director of the BKS Iyengar Yoga Institute of Champaign–Urbana, Illinois, and is a board member of the Iyengar Yoga National Association of the United States, where she chairs the Medical Research Committee. She studies annually at the Ramamani Iyengar Memorial Yoga Institute in Pune, India.

Yoga is a 5000-year-old traditional art, science, and philosophy that emphasizes a lifestyle of awareness, integrity, and compassion. When practiced regularly, it teaches one to explore and refine the subtle inner dimensions of existence—the mind, ego, intelligence, and consciousness. All aspects of one's life—work, play, relationships, decisions, and habits—can be enhanced by a dedicated practice of yoga.

While many people view yoga as merely another form of exercise, this is but one of its dimensions. "Yoga is based in moral observances; its trunk in ethical disciplines, the branches the various postures, the leaves the science of the breath, the sap the focusing of concentration, and the fruit the peace and freedom of the body, mind, and soul to unite in a state of absorption."[1]

History

Yoga has its roots in the Asian subcontinent of India. It first became known in the United States in the mid-19th century among literary circles when Henry David Thoreau and his colleagues read the *Bhagavad Gita*, the "Divine Song." This is an ancient sacred epic poem, whose author is reputed to be the sage Vyasa. The poem, which is about human moral dilemmas and the philosophy of yoga, affirms the inseparability of the spiritual and worldly life. The *Bhagavad Gita* accepts any path one takes to achieve awareness, integrity, and compassion.

In 1893 Swami Vivekananda (1863–1902) presented an aspect of yoga, known as meditation, at the World Parliament of Religions in Chicago. In the 1920s, Paramahansa Yogananda (1893–1952) founded the Self-Realization Fellowship in the United States, which still exists today. In the 1940s, the American Theos Bernard studied yoga in India and Tibet. His book *Hatha Yoga: The Report of a Personal Experience,* published in 1950 after his death, became the major reference about yoga in the 1950s.

Until the 1960s, however, the practice of yoga remained largely unknown to the general public until Richard Hittleman produced television programs on yoga that focused on flexibility and twisting positions. During this period, Swami Satchidananda opened the Woodstock Festival and the Beatles brought their meditation teacher, Maharishi Mahesh Yogi, to the West, which captured the public's attention.

The media embellished on images of candle gazing, incense burning, and immersing oneself into a cylinder filled with water while folded up into a pretzel-like position. Today, American culture continues to shift away from traditional yogic practices to use yoga as a "workout"—only a small piece of what yoga encompasses. However, yoga is not an exercise. It is an "innercise."

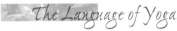 The Language of Yoga

Every science has its own language to facilitate communication within the field. Sanskrit, an ancient language that originated in India, is the language of yoga. The word *yoga* means to yoke, join, or integrate—body, mind, consciousness, emotions, and spirit.

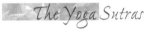 The Yoga Sutras

The Yoga Sutras are 196 aphorisms that guide the yoga practitioner to ultimate freedom from the shackles of the body, the tyranny of the mind, and the afflictions of life.[2,3] Patanjali, a learned scholar who lived approximately 2000 years ago, is credited with having written down the Yoga Sutras. The Yoga Sutras teach about the Ashtanga Yoga or the "eightfold path," the "limbs" of yoga. They are Yama, Niyama, Asana, Pranayama, Pratyahara, Dharana, Dhyana, and Samadhi. (See Table 21–1.) The eight limbs are not a linear path. In fact, all the limbs may be practiced and integrated into Asana, the third limb of Asthanga Yoga. For example, Dharana, concentration, requires complete attention, being in the present tense, thinking about neither the past nor the future, while focusing on the techniques of the pose to bring on the inner awareness. Yama, universal moral values, can also be understood within the practice of Asana. For example, when you ruthlessly "attack" your practice and go beyond your limit, you may end up creating an injury by acting in a violent manner toward yourself. The practice of Ahimsa, nonviolence, one of the Yamas, must be learned within your daily practice and transferred to your daily life, words, thoughts, and deeds.

The Practice of Yoga

A daily yoga practice enables one to experience the joy of self-discovery. According to the Yoga Sutras and the *Bhagavad Gita*, individuals—depending on their disposition—may practice yoga using one of three different approaches: Karma, Jnana, or Bhakti Yoga.

TABLE 21–1   Ashtanga Yoga—Eight Limbs of Yoga

Asana and Pranayama are the formal practices of Hatha Yoga.

1. *Yama*. The universal moral values: nonviolence, truth, nonstealing, continence, non-coveting
2. *Niyama*. Self-purification by discipline: cleanliness, contentment, burning desire, self-study, dedication of one's actions to the Divine
3. *Asana*. Postures, sequenced together to achieve a state of well-being of the body, mind, and soul
4. *Pranayama*. The regulation of the life force through channeling the breath
5. *Pratayahara*. Withdrawal of the mind from the domination of the senses
6. *Dharana*. Concentration, single-pointed attention
7. *Dhyana*. Meditation, attention focused internally and externally at the same time
8. *Samadhi*. The state of absorption in which the aspirant is one with the object of meditation

Karma Yoga is the yoga of action. It purifies the body, senses, and mind with self-discipline and the assumption of responsibility for one's actions, without any selfish motive. An inner sacrifice without attachment is part of every action. Selfless actions involve social duty and identity with society. *Karma* is a word that many are familiar with. One's actions should be without desire; the result of one's actions impacts one's destiny. Yama, Niyama, Asana, and Pranayama are the main practices of Karma Yoga.

Jnana Yoga is the yoga of knowledge and wisdom, encompassing intellectual, objective, intuitive, and personal experiences to discriminate between the real and nonreal. Study of the self and ancient texts is part of the practice involved in Jnana Yoga. Other practices include Asana, bringing the body and mind under control; Pratyahara, letting go of attachment to material objects by the senses (taste, sight, sound, touch, and smell); and Dharana, focusing concentration. Dhyana, meditation, is then possible when the practice is intense, freeing the body and mind from worldly preoccupation.

Bhakti Yoga is the yoga of selfless love and devotion to the Divine, which involves surrendering the pride of the ego and achieving humility through chanting, ritual, and Dhyana (meditation), opening the way to intense absorption with the Divine, Samadhi. These are the main practices of Bhakti Yoga. Karma, Jnana, and Bhakti come together and bring tranquillity.[4] The physical, mental, and spiritual are not divided in Eastern thought as they are in Western systems of philosophy.

Hatha Yoga

Hatha Yoga prepares the mind for intense meditation and self-surrender, with all the paths described earlier merged into one. Hatha Yoga is a rigorous discipline that involves daily practice of yoga postures, breathing exercises, meditation, and study. *Ha* means "sun" and *tha* means "moon." Thus Hatha Yoga involves the integration of opposites. The *Hatha Yoga Pradipika,* or *Light on Hatha Yoga,* by Swatmarama Yogendra, is one of the manuals on this type of yoga. Written in the 14th century, it deals with the physical and mental discipline needed to achieve liberation.

Iyengar Yoga

Iyengar Yoga, a type of Hatha Yoga and one of the popular systems of yoga currently practiced in the United States, is the method on which this chapter is based. This method is based on the teachings of the yoga master B. K. S. Iyengar, author of the classics *Light on Yoga* and *Light on Pranayama.* Iyengar's teachings are deeply grounded in the ancient yoga tradition. His intense practice and more than 60 years of teaching have produced significant innovations. Among the most noteworthy of these are (1) emphasis on standing poses to develop strength, stability, stamina, concentration, and body alignment, (2) the use of props to facilitate learning and to adjust poses for those who are inflexible, and (3) instruction on how to use yoga to ease various ailments and stress.

The Postures (Asanas) of Yoga

The word *Asana,* the term for a yoga position, means "posture" or "comfortable seat." However, yoga is an arduous discipline before the seat becomes comfortable. The Asana practice develops the necessary openness and internal awareness required for Pranayama, breathing exercises. Pratyahara, withdrawal of the senses, occurs through the inward consciousness developed while performing Asana. This leads to meditation, Dharana, in action while doing Asana.

Every name of a pose ends with *-asana.* For example, *tad* means mountain. *Tadasana,* which translates to "mountain pose," is the name for the basic standing pose. (See Figure

FIGURE 21–1   Tadasana

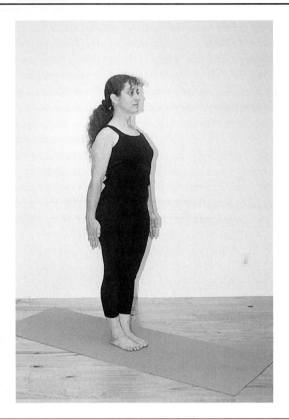

(Photo courtesy of Lois Steinberg)

21–1.) *Supta Padangusthasana* means "supine foot toe pose. (See Figure 21–2.) (Some Sanskrit words are similar to English ones, such as *supta* for "supine" and *pada* for "foot.")(See Table 21–2.)

Yoga Compared to Conventional Exercise

Yoga teaches one to observe and integrate the body, breath, mind, and spirit. Yoga does not require an individual to be flexible or in shape. In fact, those who are flexible are more difficult to teach because they tend to be unstable in their joints and muscles. Students such as these have to learn to "ground" or re-establish their bones, joints, and tissues in their natural place so that they do not injure themselves.

Individuals who tend to be stiff really feel what is going on inside their bodies and minds when they are learning and practicing; the understanding of the poses is within reach for them. However, whatever one's condition, he or she proceeds under the guidance of a qualified teacher. Iyengar Yoga has high standards of teacher certification, including intensive training in yoga philosophy, practice, and continuing education.

Yoga postures and breathing exercises are more directed in their approach than are conventional exercise, such as calisthenics or aerobics. Yoga is less goal oriented, not focused solely on achieving or completing a body position or set of exercises; rather, yoga develops the sensitivity needed to relax the brain cells while activating the cells of the bodily organs. This requires complete mental involvement and concentration. When yoga is performed correctly, attention is turned inward and engages the automatic feedback system of the mind and body. The mind and body become quiet and integrated, which leads to an awareness of postural alignment while strengthening and opening the body through the postures and breathing exercises.

Yoga encourages weak parts of the body to strengthen and stiff areas to lengthen, opening and aligning the body. Thus the body moves into better alignment, requiring less muscular work and increasing relaxation. A decrease in structural and organic difficulties may occur with improved alignment.

The body and mind nature of yoga involves moving parts to influence the whole, setting it further apart from conventional exercise that isolates body parts. In exercise, movement is repetitive, often jerky, and fast. In yoga it is nonrepetitive, smooth, and controlled. The effects of yoga are gentle, soothing, and rejuvenating. However, it is not necessarily slow. Depending on one's needs and capacities, the postures one can choose from range from either restorative/quiet poses to cardiovascular/jumping poses. Conventional exercise has its benefits, but it may overstimulate some of the body systems, ultimately resulting in fatigue. In exercise the intent is to develop muscles; in yoga it is to balance strength with flexibility as well as to increase coordination and endurance.

A regular yoga practice gives one the skills to cope with the stresses of life and ultimately permeates everything one does. Yoga influences practitioners in many ways—the way they walk, talk, and eat. For example, when learning the basic standing pose of Tadasana, students are taught to be aware of what parts of the body become unnecessarily tight. They learn to release the tongue to the lower palate, soften the mouth cavity, soften the eyes to the back of the head, and unclench the hands. Yoga practitioners learn to do the same during daily activities. They begin to recognize tendencies to create unnecessary tension in the body and, even at a cellular level, they can release the tensions, freeing themselves to deal with whatever comes their way.

FIGURE 21-2   Supta Padangusthasana

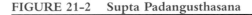

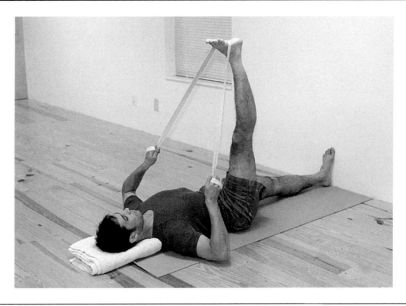

(Photo courtesy of Lois Steinberg)

TABLE 21–2   Primary Categories of Poses★

Standing poses. (See Figure 21–3.) Correct the method of standing, balance, and carriage. Tone, shape, and strengthen the leg and arm muscles. Decrease stiffness in the legs, hips, and shoulders. Relieve back and shoulder aches. The feet become supple, the ankles are strengthened, and the chest expands fully. Invigorate the abdominal organs, increase peristaltic activity, and aid elimination. Increase the blood supply to the spine. Create lightness of the body and agility of the mind. Mastery of the standing poses prepares the student for all the other categories of poses.

Forward bends. (See Figure 21–4.) Tone the liver, kidneys, intestines, and spleen. Aid digestion. Benefit the prostate gland. Blood is made to flow in the pelvis and benefits the reproductive organs. The abdominal organs are kept healthy. Tone the spine and abdominal organs. Relieve congestion in the pelvic organs, such as the prostate and gonads in men, the uterus and ovaries in women. Improve blood flow to the pituitary, pineal, thyroid, and parathyroid. Tone the adrenal glands and pancreas. Soothe the nerves and mind. Reduce stress and strain. Loosen joints of upper and lower extremities. Narrow the waist. Remove mental and physical fatigue.

Backward bends. (See Figure 21–5.) Tone the spine, keep the body alert and supple. The back feels strong and full of life. Strengthen the arms and wrists and have a soothing effect on the head. Create vitality, energy, and lightness. The pelvic region is opened and the reproductive organs are kept healthy. The diaphragm is opened and the heart is gently massaged to help to strengthen it. The abdominal muscles and chest lengthen and expand fully.

Inversions. (See Figure 21–6.) Facilitate healthy blood flow through the brain cells and the pituitary and pineal glands of the brain. Improve sleep, memory, and vitality when practiced regularly and correctly. Relieve constipation. Develop the body, give peace of mind, and lift the spirit. The endocrine and lymphatic systems are kept healthy. Healthy blood is allowed to circulate around the neck and chest. Bring back lost vitality.

Seated postures. (See Figure 21–7.) Benefit reproductive organs and urinary system. Relieve menstrual irregularities, pain in knee and hip joints, stiffness of ankles and feet. Quiet the mind and reduces anxiety, tension, and mental stress.

Twistings. (See Figure 21–8.) Increase lateral movement of the spine. Supply blood to the region of the disks. Relieve neck and shoulder tension and stiffness. Reduce fluid in the sinus passages and ear canal. Aches in the neck, shoulder, and back are relieved. Tone the liver, stomach, intestines, and kidneys.

★The benefits described are anecdotal, not yet thoroughly tested by conventional scientific research. They are also described in great detail in B. K. S. Iyengar's classic work, *Light on Yoga.*

The Role of Breathing in Yoga

Breathing exercises, Pranayama, a main component of a yoga practice, is merely a by-product of conventional exercise. *Pran* means "energy"; *ayama* means "movement, regulation, control." Pranayama is the movement of the energy through the body and mind. The Pranayama breathing exercises of yoga are practiced after some mastery of the Asana. In Asana, you first learn how to open and create space and at the same time release the force that you used to do that. The breath then, within Asana, starts to develop on its own as the chest is opened and the lungs become more elastic.

Pranayamic practice consists of first observing and equalizing the in-and-out breath in the nasal passages, throat, and lungs. With various breathing exercises, the practice develops to conscious lengthening of the exhalations, inhalations, as well as interruption and retention of the breath. Pranayama practice balances the nervous system, calms the brain, and helps the mind to concentrate, resulting in robust health.[5] It is best learned

Text continued on p. 294

FIGURE 21-3   **Standing Poses**

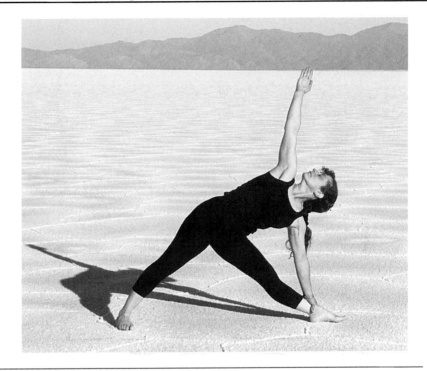

(Photo by Lucio Boschi)

FIGURE 21-4   **Forward Bends**

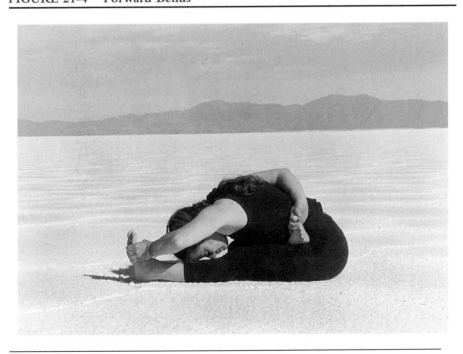

(Photo by Lucio Boschi)

FIGURE 21-5   Backward Bends

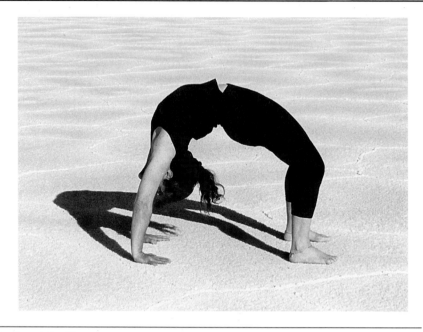

(Photo by Lucio Boschi)

FIGURE 21-6   Inversions

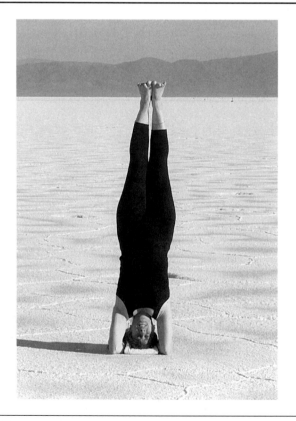

(Photo by Lucio Boschi)

FIGURE 21-7   Seated Postures

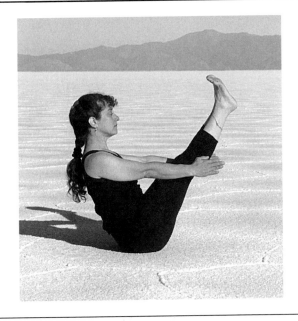

(Photo by Lucio Boschi)

FIGURE 21-8   Twistings

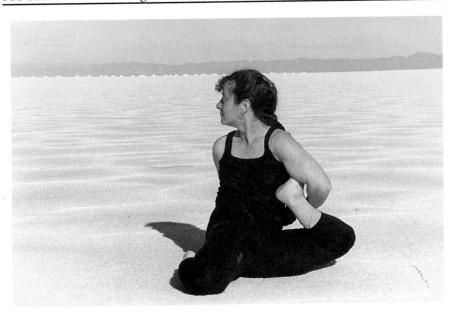

(Photo by Lucio Boschi)

under the guidance of an experienced teacher because improper practice may disturb the mind. For example, one may become light-headed. However, with correct practice, the benefits of Pranayma for bringing mental clarity and peace of mind cannot be overemphasized.

Meditation

Dhyana, meditation, is the discovery of the cosmic consciousness of which we are all one. Dhyana is not simply sitting, closing the eyes, and emptying the mind. Achieving harmony of the body and mind requires Asana and Pranayama, the basic foundation practices for the study of the self. Iyengar states that to start with only a meditation practice without Asana and Pranayama is like jumping into the ocean without a life preserver. One has to learn to be absolutely in the present tense, without being attracted to thoughts that tend to flood the mind. It is a demanding inward journey requiring years of uninterrupted practice of all the other limbs of Patanjali's yoga. Then the body and mind are calmed and balanced, and our realizations are applied to our daily lives.

Research

More than 5000 years of Eastern scientific traditions have shown that the practice of yoga can improve the muscular, skeletal, physiological, respiratory, cardiovascular, endocrine, and central nervous systems of the body and mind. Western scientific studies of yoga and yoga's healing techniques began in the 1920s. However, funding has been limited, resulting in a lack of available physiological and psychological research that passes rigorous scientific standards. Research has focused mostly on treatment of disease, yet yoga has a great deal to do with maintaining health and healthy lifestyle habits, and this aspect also needs to be examined.

Yoga provides the means to become physically fit in the context of a philosophy that encourages positive health practices and personality characteristics. Yoga practitioners cite changes in self-awareness and perspective as one of the benefits of yoga. Thomas, Tori, and Thomas[6] examined yoga practitioners with a sustained yoga practice of 10 or more years. The yoga practitioners achieved an optimal level of psychological adjustment and adaptation, functioning above normative levels as measured by five standardized tests. The practitioners were psychologically well adjusted, had developed the ability to concentrate, and had healthy lifestyle habits.

The practitioners were characterized as high functioning, confident, and independent, with a high level of vigor and physical energy combined with a keen interest in personal growth. They had positive and effective coping styles that emphasized the ability to control excessive emotion and adopt a more rational view of the world, seeking out the positive qualities of all situations. The authors concluded that yoga might be used as a method of psychological therapy to decrease stress and tension and reduce emotional liability.

Connor, Connor, and Lawrence[7] found yoga practitioners' eating habits and rates of illness over a 1-year time period to be compatible with better health. The researchers compared individuals who had practiced yoga for fewer than 6 months (beginning), 3 to 5 years (intermediate), and more than 10 years (advanced). The average number of sick days from work was significantly different. Beginners averaged 7.0 sick days, intermediates 1.2 days, and advanced practitioners 0.8 days. The advanced group reported low-fat, high-carbohydrate diets and ate less cholesterol and saturated fat, which was significantly different from the diet of the beginner and intermediate groups. The advanced group also rarely salted food at the table, drank less alcohol, ate out less often, made lower-fat choices in restaurants, and used low-fat recipes more often than the beginners and intermediates.

The beginners and intermediates had eating behaviors different from the typical American diet of 40 percent fat and 45 percent carbohydrates. They consumed a diet of 30 percent fat and 55 percent carbohydrates.

In another research project, Connor, Connor, and Lawrence[8] studied the psychosocial characteristics of people practicing yoga for the first time, for less than 2 years, and for more than 2 years. The authors did not give information on the latter group's average length of practice. It is interesting to note that 18 percent of the first-timers were vegetarians, whereas 43 percent of those who had practiced yoga for fewer than 2 years and 47 percent of those who had practiced yoga for more than 2 years were vegetarians. The authors concluded that the benefits of yoga are greater for those who have practiced it longer.

DiCarlo and colleagues[9] compared the responses of beginning students when doing Iyengar Yoga standing poses, the base of the Asana practice, to their responses when walking on a treadmill. Heart rate, blood pressure, and perceived level of exertion were higher during yoga than during walking, while oxygen consumption was higher during walking than during yoga. The study set a good standard for future studies comparing physical and physiological effects as well as perceived level of difficulty between the two regimens in a normal, healthy population. However, the sample size of 10 was small, and the methods did not give an accurate picture of how the effects of yoga would evolve over time.

The other problem with this study is that Virabhadrasana II, the pose targeted for measurements of heart rate, blood pressure, and oxygen consumption, automatically raises blood pressure when the arms are taken out to the sides, especially in beginners holding the pose for 40 seconds. (See Figure 21–9.) Generally, the pose is held for 1 minute by an advanced practitioner but for only 20 to 30 seconds by beginners and intermediates. This pose is one of the more challenging of standing poses. It is not dangerous to do, but to

FIGURE 21-9   Virabhadrasana II

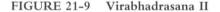

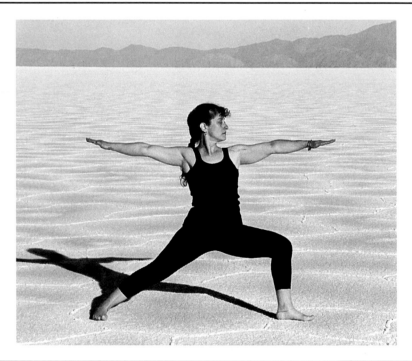

(Photo by Lucio Boschi)

FIGURE 21-10   Ardha Uttanasana (carpal tunnel syndrome)

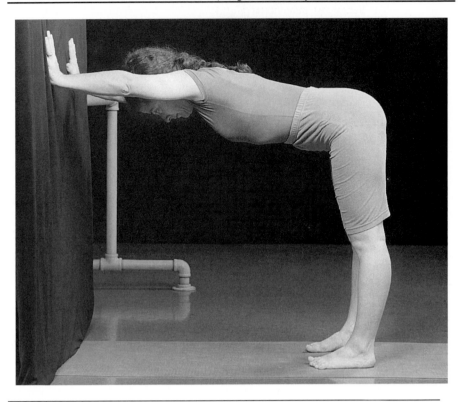

(Photo by Lucio Boschi)

hold it for 40 seconds on each side, repeating it four times in a sequence of standing poses, while having measurements taken by the examiners, would be very demanding even for a seasoned practitioner.

Trained teachers ask their students who have high blood pressure not controlled by medication to keep their hands on their hips when doing Virabhadrasana II, which makes it safer for them to perform. It would have been interesting if the researchers had recorded the measurements using a less demanding standing pose and also had assessed intermediate and advanced practitioners. At that level of practice, one has learned how to lower one's blood pressure and heart rate even when challenged. The authors did have a good basic design and the sequencing of Asanas was appropriate, but the length of time of the measurements would need to be field tested and re-evaluated for future studies to determine the effects of these poses.

Garfinkel and colleagues[10] conducted an excellent randomized, single-blind, controlled clinical study of the effects of yoga on carpal tunnel syndrome. They used an Iyengar sequence, including *Ardha Uttanasana*, that provided pain relief and improved grip strength in individuals with the syndrome when compared to those who used a wrist splint or underwent no treatment at all. (See Figure 21–10.)

Garfinkel and a different set of colleagues[11] used the same research design for evaluating treatment of osteoarthritis of the hands with an Iyengar Yoga–based regimen. The study demonstrated a significant reduction in pain and tenderness in the hands and increase in finger range of motion during activity in the yoga-treated subjects compared to controls who received no yoga treatment. The authors also noted the importance of the psychosocial benefit and supportive group format of yoga therapy. However, as the authors reported, the study group was small, the length of treatment was short, and comparison to other treatments was lacking. Future studies addressing these shortcomings will help to evaluate which aspects of the yoga therapy were most significant. Also, the subjects of these studies were receiving drug-based treatment. It would be interesting to evaluate yoga therapy before commencement of such drug treatment.

Many different methods of yoga exist, and each has its own technique with respect to preventing and treating disease. The efficacy of yoga as a way to optimal health or as a healing treatment has to be evaluated by scientists using consistent methods so that replication of the studies is possible to validate its long-claimed therapeutic benefit. The studies cited earlier were all conducted within the framework of Iyengar Yoga. More research is needed. Using one standard in research studying the effects of yoga would be the ideal method. At best, the yogic training given to subjects in research projects should be described in more detail than has been done in past publications.

Other studies on the effects of yoga cited in the literature do not include an accurate description of the yoga postures and/or breathing exercises. However, some of the studies are provocative. They are briefly summarized here to inspire similar undertakings in future research.

Raju and colleagues[12] found that athletes who practiced Pranayama breathing exercises achieved higher aerobic efficiency, with reduced oxygen consumption without an increase in blood lactic acid concentrations, compared to athletes who did not practice the breathing exercises. Lactic acid is produced by skeletal muscle during intense activity and may cause the shakiness one feels after strenuous exercise. An improvement in aerobic capacity was observed in 16- to 18-year-old students after 6 weeks of yoga when compared to controls who did not practice yoga.[13] Another study showed that 1 year of yogic training improved aerobic capacity, body weight, body density, and endurance in high school students compared to those who did not train.[14]

Bowman and colleagues[15] studied elderly people during bicycling, an aerobic training, to those doing yoga postures that were of a nonaerobic nature. The findings showed that aerobic training did not decrease heart rate but that yoga did. The authors suggested a future study to determine whether this effect is directly related to yoga itself by comparing it to a nonaerobic control intervention.

Many well-intentioned people think yoga is about relaxation, and they may embark on a program of yoga to manage stress. However, focusing strictly on relaxation made subjects in one study significantly more sleepy and sluggish than after a yoga session of Asanas.[16] Visualization also made subjects more sluggish as well as more upset and less content. Yoga made the subjects feel invigorated and resulted in a greater increase in perceptions of mental and physical energy and feelings of alertness and enthusiasm than did the other two procedures. The authors suggested that yoga may be useful for decreasing fatigue.

In a comparison of yoga and swimming,[17] both activities were correlated to decreased scores on anger, confusion, tension, and depression in college students when compared to control subjects. The authors concluded that aerobic conditioning such as swimming may not be necessary to enhance mood states. The authors did not exactly define the yoga training, although it must have been of a nonaerobic nature. As described earlier, yoga can be aerobic when practiced in a kinetic way.

Jain and colleagues[18] found that yoga training improved blood glucose control, with a resulting decrease in oral therapy, for patients with non-insulin-dependent diabetes. Schmidt and colleagues[19]evaluated a 3-month residential yogic training program, including low-fat vegetarian meals, for healthy, young male and female adults. The program resulted in a reduction of cardiovascular risk factors: smoking cessation, decreased body-mass index, decreased low-density lipoproteins concentrations, and lowered blood pressure. Also of note is that most women ceased menstruation during the course of the study. The methods do not reveal which yoga practices the women performed during

FIGURE 21-11   Supta Baddha Konasana (menstruation)

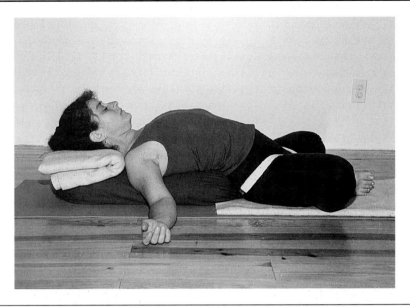

(Photo courtesy of Lois Steinberg)

menstruation. Inversions should not to be done during menstruation, partly because they may stop the normal flow and they stress uterine ligaments during this time.[20] Women should do a menstrual sequence during their monthly cycle. (See Figure 21–11.)[21]

The use of yoga in the treatment of asthma, resulting in decreased use of drug treatments when compared to control subjects,[22–24] has generated an interest in further studies to understand in more detail the physiological and psychological basis for this phenomenon.

Iyengar Yoga as Therapy

As stated earlier in the chapter, Asanas are designed to regulate the life force in the body in order to balance and strengthen it. The by-product of the practice of yoga is health and well-being. This leads to its therapeutic dimension. Yoga can serve as a therapeutic treatment in many situations. It preserves and enhances the sensitivity of the body and may increase its response to conventional medical treatment.

A student with a physical, physiological, or psychological problem may not be able to perform certain classical Asanas and Pranayamas. Yoga therapy is based on using the classical yoga poses in a modified fashion—sometimes with props—to achieve the appropriate benefit. As the practice progresses, the student reduces the level of modification and may advance from a remedial/recovering practice to a strengthening practice.

Yoga therapeutics includes a range of practices from active-dynamic to recuperative-passive yoga postures. It also includes breathing exercises. The purpose of yoga treatment is to bring individuals into balance to correct inner malfunction. For example, when an individual suffers from knock-knee, not only is the leg crooked but also the inner organic body does not receive full support from the structure of the legs. Figures 21–12A and 21–12B show a person with knock-knee performing a yoga pose therapeutically to help straighten the knees, thereby providing more balanced support to the pelvic organs.

General principles of a yoga practice assist the yoga teacher in designing a program for a student with a presenting condition or concern involving structural, organic-hormonal, or emotional needs. Most introductory-level yoga instructors understand how to work with basic conditions such as knee problems, high blood pressure, and normal pregnancy. The instructor will consider aspects of a student's history, current circumstances, concerns, and physical, psychological, and emotional levels of tolerance in determining a sequence of Asanas and Pranayamas. It is critical for all yoga instructors to understand the classic Asanas and Pranayamas in order to understand alternatives for use in remedial work. It is also essential for instructors to recognize their limitations and to refer students with specific problems to a specialist who has been trained in yoga therapy.

Unlike conventional medicine, a "prescription" for an individual's treatment is very specific. General guidelines exist, but, as can be seen in the case studies that follow, a student's practice has to be guided by the teacher in such a way that all the nuances of the student are taken into account. Often a person has multiple areas of concern. The treatment sequence for women has to be adjusted for the cycle of life she is in, from menarche to postmenopause.

A therapeutic sequence of yoga postures is often modified as the student improves or goes through bouts of difficult periods. Teachers ask their students to report any undesirable effects within the first 48 hours after a practice. Sometimes students may feel great immediately after a session, but worse the following day. Students are responsible for reporting these events to their teacher in order for the teacher to assess what modifications can be made to their sequence. Just as in medicine, yoga can be a trial-and-error process. Not all people react the same way to a yoga program, and it often needs to be changed to suit their individual needs and capacities.

FIGURE 21-12(A,B)   Tadasana (leg deformities)

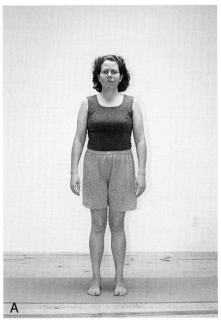
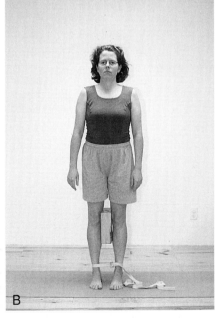

(Photos courtesy of Lois Steinberg)

The initial period of a yoga treatment program includes a sequence of yoga postures and breathing exercises that are fully supported with the use of yoga props, such as bolsters and wooden furniture. The supported postures are recuperative, conducive to learning, and easy for people to do. Over time, the sequence is augmented or changed from the original program. According to their capacity, students may be able to add poses that develop their strength and build their endurance.

When students' health concerns are resolved consistently, a maintenance period is initiated. They may be able to do the classic unsupported Asanas but continue to practice their recuperative sequence for 1 to 3 days of their weekly practice to maintain their newfound health. Students are responsible for learning to develop sensitivity to what their body and mind need in choosing their daily practice.

Novice practitioners and nonpractitioners may sometimes regard yoga healing as a miraculous event without reason behind it. For example, when a person has suffered from severe headaches for years and has been through medical treatment without relief, then becomes free of headaches after a few yoga sessions, it seems to be a miracle. It is not. Yoga is a sophisticated system grounded in solid science through which the body and mind are directed to "cure that which you cannot endure, and endure that which you cannot cure."[25] Three case studies illustrate how yoga can be used to help people with organic-hormonal, structural, or emotional needs.

Case Study 1

Maria

Maria, 18 years old, suffers from irritable bowel syndrome and frequent mild headaches. Her menstrual cycle is regular, but she tends to get heavy cramping. She had a regular regimen of jogging, but she changed to walking with the encouragement of her yoga instructor. She is a serious student in school and works part-time. She often does not get enough sleep in order to keep up with her schedule. Maria is of normal body weight, is somewhat flexible in her joints, but is very stiff in her legs. She tried drug treatment for her irritable bowel syndrome, but it was not effective and made her feel worse. She discontinued the drug treatment with the knowledge of her physician.

Maria decided to try yoga and liked the initial results. Although she often came to class with a mild headache, it would usually disappear after the first pose. She reported that the day after her first session, her abdominal tenderness and bloating were greatly reduced and she had had a normal stool, the first that she could remember. On her own initiative, Maria also started modifying her diet by eating out less frequently and cooking fresh foods more often.

Maria continued to come to class regularly. She learned the yoga postures for relieving menstrual cramps, and it helped. Forward bends, part of the basic menstrual sequence, are contraindicated for irritable bowel syndrome. However, Maria modified this pose by doing the forward bends as a forward extension. This allowed her to keep her back in a concave position so as not to irritate the bowel and, at the same time, experience relief from menstrual discomfort.

After the fourth session, Maria came in quite distraught. She reported that the day after the previous yoga session, she had become quite ill. While she was in class at school, she started to get a headache that made her feel nauseous and shaky. She went home and continued to feel worse. The next day she vomited from the intensity of the pain in her head. She had never had a migraine headache. She didn't consult a doctor. She "braved it out" and slowly started to return to a normal state after 2 days. The yoga instructor advised her to consult a physician, but she did not.

Maria continued with her regular sequence and did not experience migraines again. Her stools are normal, but sometimes she tends to get bloated and uses the yoga to reduce the swelling. The headaches have disappeared. If Maria's progress continues and she is not in an acute phase of gastrointestinal flare-up, she will be able to do forward bending poses. Although these poses may irritate a person with gastrointestinal problems, these same poses will strengthen and tone the intestines. She will still be advised to practice her specific sequence two to three times a week to maintain her health, or more frequently if her gastrointestinal system "tells" her she needs it.

Discussion. Maria may have experienced what many traditional therapies call a "healing crisis." After an initial improvement, she regressed and went through a period of extreme discomfort during which the symptoms worsened before they improved consistently. She had made many changes at once—walking instead of running, eating home-cooked meals instead of restaurant food, and practicing a yoga sequence designed specifically for her areas of concern. It would have been better if Maria had gone to a physician for a diagnosis to determine if conventional medical treatment was necessary for her. Fortunately, she improved and has not had an episode of this nature again. Maria's case is typical of how yoga therapy cannot include a simple prescription for the main presenting problem. Her headaches, menstrual cycle, and fatigue from overwork have to be evaluated each session to determine how her sequence of Asanas needs to be modified for that session.

Case Study 2

Mohammed

Mohammed is so athletic, he would play soccer every day if he could. The sport requires bursts of intense physical activity, with frequent starts and stops. This is hard on the feet, ankles, knees, and legs. The activity also shortens the calf and hamstring muscles, and after a game Mohammed's legs often feel excessively shaky. Sometimes his foot hits a rough patch of dirt and he sprains his ankle. At other times he pulls groin or leg muscles.

He loved the sport and did not want to give it up, but his injuries were getting the better of him. He found a yoga teacher who devised a sequence of poses to prevent and/or heal injuries for him that took 15 minutes. Some of the poses he did before he played, some after. He learned therapeutic use of the poses for times when he was injured. Mohammed attributed some of his great soccer games to his yoga practice. He also learned that he would have a longer soccer career if he practiced yoga consistently. During periods when he did not practice yoga, he would get injured more frequently.

Discussion. Like Mohammed, those who enjoy athletic endeavors will benefit from a regular yoga practice, which will help prevent injuries and allow them to continue playing their sport for a longer period of time. Mohammed loved soccer and became committed more fully to practicing yoga so he could continue in his sport.

Case Study 3

Conrad

Conrad was unable to maintain good grades in school because of his depressive mood, which was often exacerbated by anxiety attacks. He did not want to go the conven-

FIGURE 21-13   Prasarita Padottanasana (fatigue)

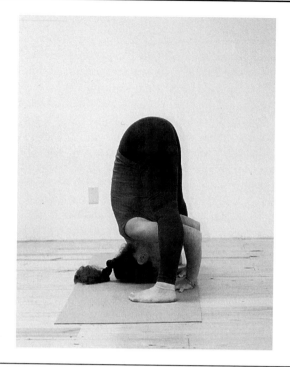

(Photo courtesy of Lois Steinberg)

tional medical route and decided to give yoga a try. His sequence started with a series of standing poses—getting into them quickly, holding them for short timings, and coming out of them quickly. The standing poses, as stated earlier, help one to get grounded. Done rapidly, they also help one to get "out of one's head" and into the moment.

Conrad was initially fearful about some of the "topsy-turvy" poses that would help to uplift his spirits and bring about a balance to his endocrine system. His teacher would stand him on his hands quickly before he knew what was happening, and he was made to repeat the handstand three times in rapid succession. He became exhilarated and overcame his fear. During the next class, he asked to do the handstands again because they made him feel so good. Occasionally when Conrad came to class, he reported he was in the midst of a panic attack.

He was instructed to perform Tratakam, a technique that aids concentration. To help him calm his nerves, he kept his eyes open and gazed upward. This was done while in Tadasana, mountain pose, with his back body supported by a countertop. His hands were placed on the counter in such a way as to support his back, raise his chest up, and "unfreeze" his diaphragm. At the same time, his feet were rooted downward. He reported that both these techniques relieved his panic state and he was ready to proceed with his regular sequence.

Prasarita Padottanasana is another good pose to perform prior to study or exams. (See Figure 21–13.) This semi-inverted posture increases oxygen supply to the brain.

Discussion. As we see from Conrad's experience, yoga can also improve one's mood. After practicing yoga, Conrad found that his depression was relieved and that he functioned better at school. In his case, the yoga worked quickly. For others, it might not be as effective. If depression is life-threatening, treatment from a medical doctor is required.

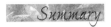 Summary

Yoga, specifically Iyengar Yoga, encompasses a broad spectrum of Asana and Pranayama techniques, including recuperative-therapeutic poses, holding of static positions, and a kinetic component linking the poses in a fast pace. Yoga study also involves understanding the philosophy of yoga in order to deepen one's understanding of how the practice of yoga leads to the path of freedom.

In the video entitled *The Ultimate Freedom*,[26] after demonstrating all the categories of poses from basic standing positions to advanced backbends, Iyengar states, "Some people may think after observing me that my body is in pieces, but my mind is in one piece. Others, their bodies are in one piece, but their minds are in pieces!" Yoga brings not only peace of mind but also joy, beauty, and personal fulfillment. It also brings determination and skill to one's daily activities.

Although there is a lack of research about the effects of yoga, several studies have been reported in the literature with respect to treating carpal tunnel syndrome and osteoarthritis as well as evaluating the differences between yoga practitioners and nonpractitioners. Future studies need to include larger sample sizes and focus on one system of yoga so that their results can be compared and replicated. Using yoga as a preventive tool in at-risk populations with work-related syndromes or injuries is an important area for researchers to explore.

Currently, this author is compiling a registry of yoga therapeutics to be evaluated epidemiologically. Participating Iyengar Yoga instructors in North America are gathering information from students, including their conditions, background, characteristics, the sequences given by the instructor, their use of other traditional and conventional treatments, the amount of time they practice yoga, and evaluation of their physical and mental states before and after each session. The large sample size will provide a global picture of how students use yoga therapy, how they comply with the prescribed sequences, and how yoga has helped or not helped them to resolve their condition.

REFERENCES

1. Iyengar, BKS: The Tree of Yoga. Shambala, Boston, 1989, p 41.
2. Iyengar, BKS: Light on the Yoga Sutras of Patanjali. Thorsons, San Francisco, 1996.
3. Taimni, IK: The Science of Yoga. Vasanta Press, Madras, India, 1986.
4. Iyengar, BKS: Light on Yoga. Schocken, New York, 1980.
5. Iyengar, BKS: Light on Pranayama. Crossroad Publishing, New York, 1981.
6. Thomas, T, Tori, CD, and Thomas, BA: Assessing the benefits of practicing Iyengar Yoga. Yoga Rahasya 5(2):30, 1998.
7. Connor, WE, Connor, SL, and Lawrence, J: Rates of illness and eating habits of yoga practitioners. Unpublished abstract.
8. Connor, WE, Connor, SL, and Lawrence, J: Psychosocial characteristics of yoga practitioners. Unpublished abstract.
9. DiCarlo, LJ, et al: Cardiovascular, metabolic, and perceptual responses to Hatha Yoga standing poses. Med Exerc Nutr Health 5(4):107, 1995.
10. Garfinkel, MS, et al: Yoga-based intervention for carpal tunnel syndrome: A randomized trial. JAMA 280:1601, 1998.
11. Garfinkel, MS, et al: Evaluation of a yoga based regimen for treatment of osteoarthritis of the hands. J Rheumatol 21:2341, 1994.
12. Raju, PS, et al: Comparison of effects of yoga and physical exercise in athletes. Indian J Med Res 100:81, 1994.

13. Balasubramanian, B, and Pansare, MS: Effect of yoga on aerobic and anaerobic power of muscle. Indian J Physiol Pharmacol 35(4):281–282, 1991.
14. Bera, TK, and Rajapurkar, MV: Body composition, cardiovascular endurance and anaerobic power of yogic practitioner. Indian J Physiol Pharmacol 37(3):225, 1993.
15. Bowman, AJ, et al: Effects of aerobic exercise training and yoga on the baro reflex in healthy elderly persons. Eur J Clin Invest 27:443, 1997.
16. Wood, C: Mood change and perceptions of vitality: A comparison of the effects of relaxation, visualization and yoga. J R Soc Med 86:254, 1993.
17. Berger, BG, and Owen, DR: Mood alteration with yoga and swimming: Aerobic exercise may not necessary. Percept Mot Skills 75:1331,1992.
18. Jain, SC, et al: A study of response pattern of non–insulin dependent diabetics to yoga therapy. Diabetes Res Clin Pract 19:69, 1993.
19. Schmidt, T, et al: Changes in cardiovascular risk factors and hormones during a comprehensive residential three month kriya yoga training and vegetarian nutrition. Acta Physiol Scand 640(suppl 161):158, 1997.
20. Schultz, MP: A woman's balance: Inversions and menstruation. Yoga Journal November/December, 1983, p 30.
21. Iyengar, GS: Yoga: A Gem for Women. Timeless Books, Spokane, Wash., 1990.
22. Nagarathna, R, and Nagendra, HR: Yoga for bronchial asthma: A controlled study. BMJ 291:1077, 1985.
23. Khanam, AA, et al: Study of pulmonary and autonomic functions of asthma patients after yoga training. Indian J Physiol Pharmacol 40(4):318, 1996.
24. Fluge, T, et al: Long-term effects of breathing exercises and yoga in patients suffering from bronchial asthma. Pneumologie 48:484, 1994.
25. Iyengar, BKS: Yoga Rahasya. Light on Yoga Research Trust, Bombay, 1999.
26. Ann Arbor "Y" (producer): The Ultimate Freedom [video]. Ann Arbor, Mich., 1976.

RECOMMENDED READING

Feuerstein, G: The Yoga Tradition: Its History, Literature, Philosophy and Practice. Hohm Press, Prescott, Ariz., 1998.

Iyengar, BKS: Light on Pranayama. Crossroad Publishing, New York, 1981.

Iyengar, BKS: Light on Yoga. Unwin Hyman, London, 1988.

Iyengar, BKS: Light on the Yoga Sutras of Patanjali. Aquarian Press, London, 1993.

Iyengar, BKS: The Tree of Yoga. Shambhala, Boston, 1989.

Iyengar, GS: Yoga: A Gem for Women. Allied Publishers, New Delhi, India, 1983.

Mehta, M: How to Use Yoga. Smithmark, New York, 1994.

Mehta, S, Mehta, M, and Mehta, S: Yoga the Iyengar Way. Knopf, New York, 1990.

Miller, BS (trans): The Bhagavad Gita: Krishna's Counsel in Time of War. Bantam Books, New York, 1986.

Radhakrishnan, S (trans): The Bhagavadgita. Indus, New Delhi, India, 1993.

Raman, K: A Matter of Health: Integration of Yoga and Western Medicine for Prevention and Cure. Eastwest Books, Madras, India, 1998.

Rieker, H (trans): Hatha Yoga Pradipika: Yoga Swami Svatmarama. Thorsons, London, 1992.

Taimni, IK: The Science of Yoga. Theosophical Publishing House, Wheaton, Ill., 1986.

CHAPTER 22

T'ai Chi

Dan Ogrydziak and Robert Levine

Dan Ogrydziak is a certified T'ai Chi instructor who has taught T'ai Chi for the past 15 years at the University of Massachusetts–Amherst.

Robert Levine is the director of The Balance Institute in Baltimore, Maryland, and an instructor at Villa Julie College School of Nursing, also in Baltimore.

At sunrise in every park, garden, or parking lot in China, hundreds of people, mostly elderly, meet to practice the graceful movements of T'ai Chi Ch'uan. They begin as one large group, breathing, shifting weight, and gently doing self-massage in unison. After about 15 or 20 minutes of this warm-up, the group disperses and gathers with friends and teachers in reserved areas. There, they practice a wide variety of T'ai Chi forms, push-hands routines (practitioners work to sense the imbalances of partners while maintaining their own balance), and sword forms. Other people are holding postures until their legs tremble, attempting to maintain their equilibrium by breathing in a deep and relaxed manner. After focusing and breathing to center scattered thoughts, and exercising the body by relaxing all muscles except those needed for each movement of T'ai Chi, the practitioners leave to begin their workday.

What Is T'ai Chi?

T'ai Chi Ch'uan is a nonaggressive Chinese martial art based on the principles of relaxation and yielding rather than force, bravery, and technique. Classic Chinese literature shows that from early times, martial arts were linked to external strength and physical courage.[1] To understand the role of martial arts, or T'ai Chi, in promoting health, one must first understand that the Chinese view of health is holistic, unifying body, mind, and spirit. T'ai Chi can be a way to find health and balance in the physical, emotional, mental, and spiritual realms. This integral approach to health makes T'ai Chi an important option for Western medical practitioners willing to explore the mind-body connection. (See Box 22–1.)

The Healing Process—A Holistic Perspective

In China, T'ai Chi Chuan is considered more than a physical exercise and relaxation routine. The balance, muscular relaxation, movements that lubricate joints (hips, knees, ankles, etc.), and physical alignments provide the conditions for the concentration, flow,

BOX 22-1
What Is Chi?

Oscar Ichazo,[1] founder of the Arica Institute and friend of Cheng Man-Ching, expressed the concept of chi and its relationship to health and exercise as follows:

[Chi is] the healthy result of all three parameters (diet, exercise, and vital energy) in balance. In accordance with traditional Chinese medicine, vital energy is stored from food and from the air. . . . But it is also equally important to promote vital energy by activating our organism in a determined way that includes physical exercises and mental exercises. . . . The first two parameters (food and air) are provided by nature, but the third parameter has to be awakened by our intentional activities. In a way, it is more like having a secret treasure of which we are not aware. In the moment we discover our fortune, our life is transformed and enriched by the constant motion of the most precious element of life: vital energy.

The cultivation of chi forms the basis of the possibility of rejuvenation, the strengthening of the bones, the development of softness, and the interruption of the degenerative process associated with aging. According to Ichazo,[2] When this element (vital energy) is not considered, the other two parameters alone, diet and exercise, are a great help, but they will not produce the regeneration that is the exclusive quality of vital energy when circulating unobtrusively between organs, glands, and tissues.

REFERENCES

1. Ichazo, O: Master Level Psychocalisthenics. Sequoia Press, New Rochelle, N.Y., 1993, p 18.
2. Ibid, p 19.

and projection of vital energy (chi), allowing for health and the raising of spirits. Chi flows through and across the body via subtle pathways (commonly referred to as acupuncture meridians) that connect all of the organs of the body. When there is a block in one of the pathways, less energy is delivered to a given organ and consequently more is delivered to the others, creating an imbalance that can manifest as either physical or psychological symptoms. Left uncorrected, this condition may become a progressively serious disease and possibly threaten life.

Traditional Chinese Medicine (TCM) combines a variety of health practices to affect the healing process. The first stage of health maintenance involves a balanced diet and T'ai Chi exercises. If the first stage fails and a person becomes ill or continues to be ill, herbs are used. Acupuncture would then be used if the first and second stages fail to bring the person back to a balanced state (health). In China, allopathic medicine is also utilized, although it is quite separate from TCM. Allopathic practitioners do, however, use T'ai Chi and dietary instructions in combination with Western-style treatments.

For example, Lei Bingjun[2] of the West China University of Medical Sciences used the scenario of a patient with a liver inflammation to describe how allopathic doctors use T'ai Chi. After prescribing appropriate medication and suggesting foods that should be avoided, Dr. Lei referred the patient to a T'ai Chi practitioner at the hospital. The T'ai Chi practitioner prescribed specific movements and standing positions with focused breathing patterns in order to "reduce the energy to the liver," thus optimizing the effect of the medication.

Although a Western doctor would prescribe medication, dietary advice, rest, and exercise, the Chinese approach is different in that it is based on an understanding of the dynamic interaction of subtle energies that affect health and vitality. The TCM practitioner, on the other hand, is more interested in the underlying imbalance of energy that causes illness.

A Brief History

In China, T'ai Chi developed in several family lineages. The most influential lineage in America is the Yang-style short form developed by the late Cheng Man-Ching, and this chapter is primarily based on the Yang family of T'ai Chi tradition.

T'ai Chi Ch'uan is rooted in the development of martial arts in China. In the 6th century AD, Bhodi Dharma brought Zen Buddhism to China. The monks needed self-defense as well as exercise to offset the long periods of seated meditation. Monks, dedicated to spiritual practice, were naturally drawn to the study of movements commensurate with a spiritual goal. The result was the Shao-Lin martial arts, based on two fundamental pillars: strength and courage.

The best estimated date of T'ai Chi Ch'uan's origin is the latter half of the 14th century. The most widely accepted version of T'ai Chi Ch'uan's beginnings is a legend: A Taoist hermit named Chang San-Feng of Wu Tang Mountain witnessed a battle for survival between a bird and a snake. The bird was the aggressor, whereas the snake defended itself using suppleness and yielding to overcome the bird's hard force.

The insight of this legendary conflict, coupled with the wisdom of Lao Tzu (author of the *Tao Teh Ching*), Huang Ti (the Yellow Emperor, mythical author of *Yellow Emperor's Classic of Internal Medicine*), and the *I Ching* (Book of Changes), inspired Chang San-Feng to develop T'ai Chi Ch'uan, based not on strength and ferocity but on pliability, relaxation, and yielding.

The next important link in T'ai Chi history is Cheng Man-Ching, who became serious about the study of T'ai Chi Ch'uan because of his deteriorating health. Professor Cheng was the last disciple of the Yang family's teachings of Tai Chi, and after 6 years of intensive study, he emerged with the tremendous health, vitality, and martial skill that he would retain for the rest of his life.

Cheng's teaching of T'ai Chi was deeply influenced by his compassion toward the illness and suffering he encountered as a physician. Cheng told his students: "For the sake of the nation or social order, or even for one's kith and kin, or neighbors, often one is prepared to dedicate one's whole life. How thoughtless it would be, therefore, to grudge oneself the ten-minutes-a-day-for-the-sake-of-physical-well-being! Without sound health, as without education, what good can one do for one's nation or social order, kith and kin, or neighbors?"[3] (One practice round of the T'ai Chi form in the morning and evening takes about 10 minutes, the minimum time investment recommended for accruing the health benefits of T'ai Chi). Cheng said that T'ai Chi was useful for "health, relaxation, and self-defense in that order of importance."[4]

East Meets West

In 1992, Bill Moyers produced a PBS series entitled *Healing and the Mind*,[5] which introduced T'ai Chi Chuan and other Eastern healing methods as possible complements to established Western medical treatments. Since that time, several institutions have focused on T'ai Chi to see whether it could effect changes in the condition of people with psychiatric problems, neurotrauma, blindness, and essentially untreatable conditions such as multiple sclerosis and Parkinson's disease. These institutions include the Multiple Sclerosis Association, the Brain Injury Association, the Blind Industries of America, the National Center for Institutions and Alternatives, and the University of Maryland's Montebello Rehabilitation Hospital.[6]

The results of these early studies inspired serious scientific research to measure the effectiveness of T'ai Chi. Beginning in 1996, results of these studies reached the health community as articles and editorials appeared in established journals such as the *Journal of qualities .*

the American Medical Association and the *Journal of the American Geriatric Society*. The positive results of these quantitative studies were consistent with the findings of anecdotal research done by the Institutes of Traditional Chinese Medicine and the Chinese Medical Association. As a result, the National Institutes of Health created a division to specifically study alternative medicine. Major medical institutions have begun to offer courses and continuing education seminars in complementary medicine to educate doctors on these various approaches.

There is currently little structure, however, for using Chinese healing therapies in the Western health-care system. For example, there are not enough qualified T'ai Chi practitioners in enough locations to provide services through health-care establishments.[7] There is also the question of whether individuals trained in T'ai Chi have any place in a hospital environment, because they are not trained in hospital protocols. In addition, if an institution employs a T'ai Chi practitioner only once or twice a week, there is frequently no compliance between visits, reducing the benefits to the patient.

A form of T'ai Chi therapy called Psycho-Physical Balance Therapy™, approved by the T'ai Chi Foundation, a nonprofit organization devoted to research, was developed by Robert Levine, a T'ai Chi practitioner for 25 years. Psycho-Physical Balance Therapy™ has a curriculum intended to be taught to health-care professionals. Using a nursing education format (nurses were the original practitioners of complementary medicine) as its model, the curriculum provides a balance between classroom learning and clinical evaluation. This intervention does not rely on a nonmedical staff of T'ai Chi professionals; instead, it trains hospital staff to deliver the program and achieve the results.

Psycho-Physical Balance Therapy™ is currently part of the nursing curriculum at Villa Julie College in Baltimore, Maryland, and has been approved as a continuing education program for physical therapists, occupational therapists, and recreational therapists throughout the United States. It has been promoted by the Federation Suisse des Physiotherapeutes as a postgraduate course.

Research

A number of research projects have compared the benefits of T'ai Chi with those of normal exercise as possible preventive interventions for populations with limited capacities: the elderly, people with compromised immune systems, people at risk for cardiac problems, people in rehabilitation, and so forth. The most sophisticated research done was in relation to injury prevention and maintenance of viability in the elderly. According to Province and colleagues,[8] "Each year, approximately 30% of persons over 65 years of age sustain a fall. . . . Over 6% of all medical care dollars for persons aged 65 and older were spent on unintentional injury, with the majority spent for fall injuries. This was estimated to have reached $3.7 billion by 1984." More recently, it has been estimated that there will be 350,000 fractures by the year 2000. The annual cost will have risen by $20.2 billion, with hip fractures (averaging $35,000 per patient) accounting for the bulk of the cost. While 25 percent of hip fracture patients fully recover, 40 percent require nursing home admission, 50 percent will need to rely on a cane or a walker for ambulation, and 20 percent will die each year.[9] The increase in the number of falls is occurring at a rate that cannot be explained solely by the increase in population.[10]

Fitness programs normally recommended for the elderly have been shown to exacerbate the incidence of fall injuries. In a 1998 news conference, Dr. Nicholas DiNubile, spokesman for the American Academy of Orthopedic Surgeons, warned that improperly done exercise had resulted in a 54 percent increase in sports-related injuries to older Americans. "Paradoxically, the riskiest categories seemed to include . . . aerobic activity and weight training," he stated.[11]

This situation prompted the initiation of the Frailty and Injuries: Cooperative Studies of Intervention Techniques (FICSIT), the most extensive study to date involving T'ai Chi and other movement methods.[12] Conducted by the National Institute on Aging and the National Center for Nursing Research, the FICSIT trials ran from 1990 to 1994 at seven university sites. The trials aimed to reduce frailty and maintain postural integrity in persons aged 70 and older who were still living in the community (people with serious illness or dementia were excluded). Steve Wolf[13] of Emory University, the director of the T'ai Chi study, believes T'ai Chi to be a valuable intervention:

> [P]rogressively greater movement is seen, the knees are flexed, and body weight shifts . . . head and trunk are aligned in a straight and extended position. All the movement patterns usually associated with older individuals (a rounded posture, slightly flexed trunk, and limited base of support) appear to be counteracted within the components of T'ai Chi Quan.

Researchers examined frequency of falls, fear of falling, maintenance of upper-body strength, and blood pressure. A comparison was done of three groups—one practicing a distilled form of T'ai Chi, one using computerized balance equipment, and one receiving an education program. The T'ai Chi practitioners had 47.5 percent fewer falls. After the T'ai Chi intervention, only 8 percent of the participants still reported a fear of falling, as opposed to 23 percent prior to the intervention.

There was less loss of upper-body strength in the T'ai Chi group during the course of the study, as measured by left hand grip strength. The T'ai Chi group had lowered systolic blood pressure after a 12-minute walk.

At another FICSIT site, balance training and weight training were used. This was followed by 6 months of T'ai Chi instruction. The strength and balance gained during the training were maintained successfully using only one session per week of T'ai Chi.[14]

The T'ai Chi groups did so well in all these clinical trials that an article in the *Journal of the American Geriatric Society* recommended T'ai Chi as a low-technology approach to conditioning that can be implemented at relatively low cost in widely distributed facilities throughout the community.[15]

Other research studies have indicated that T'ai Chi can significantly enhance the immune system,[16] suggesting that future research could benefit populations with lupus, AIDS, and other immunodeficiency ailments. A positive reduction of systolic blood pressure was reported by Johns Hopkins University researcher Deborah Young in a 1998 speech to an American Heart Association conference.[17] Another cardiovascular study comparing elderly T'ai Chi practitioners with a sedentary group found that "the T'ai Chi group showed 19% higher peak oxygen uptake in comparison with their sedentary counterparts."[18]

Summary

The uniqueness of T'ai Chi emerges from its conscious focus on the fundamental principles of movement, while minimizing the energy needed to accomplish any task. This approach defines T'ai Chi as a martial art based on relaxation and yielding and easily adapted as a health exercise that both rehabilitates and conditions.

Modern research has shown that when T'ai Chi is practiced on a regular basis, the immune, cardiovascular, and musculoskeletal systems receive significant benefit. Because of its gentle nature, T'ai Chi is an excellent choice as a lifelong health activity and an appropriate choice for people whose health is challenged. (See Box 22–2.)

BOX 22–2

Case Study

Michael was a 53-year-old Caucasian male with neurologic injuries resulting from an automobile accident. He had been a pediatrician prior to the accident, but he had since been unable to practice his profession because of the extent of the resulting disabilities. His neurologist had referred him for T'ai Chi therapies because his lack of balance had resulted in frequent falls with serious injuries (16 broken bones).

For Michael's T'ai Chi therapy evaluation, a history was taken, documenting the events leading up to and following the accident, including medical and rehabilitation interventions. Michael was also asked to perform certain kinesthetic tasks to determine the extent to which the brain injury had affected his gait, posture, and reactions and also to determine his compensatory mechanisms. In addition, Michael was asked a series of questions to determine how he was coping emotionally with his condition. This evaluation was followed by seven 1-hour treatment sessions scheduled about 1 week apart. His medical diagnoses included cortical blindness (he could see but he did not know what he was seeing), cerebellar contusion, spastic right hemiplegia of the lower extremities, spastic left hemiplegia of the upper extremities, and hyperclonus in the right leg and occasionally in the left.

Physically, he reported limited use of his left and right hands; his left leg felt normal, but his right leg was spastic. Emotionally, he said he was depressed and considering suicide. He tended to get upset and emotional without provocation. Intellectually, he described himself as sharp, with a thirst for information. He had figured out how to sign his name and was trying to solve the problem of his vision loss. He had had extensive physical rehabilitation, and his neurologist had prescribed lorazepam q4h prn and amitriptyline bid 75 mg for anxiety and depression, respectively.

Michael sat in a wheelchair, his spine curved, his neck craned, and his head hanging down. His chest and abdomen showed little movement as he breathed. The muscles in his thighs and calves were weak and undeveloped, but he could correctly identify where he was touched, tapped, and squeezed.

When walking behind his wheelchair, Michael leaned forward, moving his legs without bending his knees. He moved his legs in rapid, small, spastic steps. There was a great deal of back-and-forth movement in both the torso and the arms. His upper-body tension, lack of strength in the legs, and leaning posture accentuated the lack of balance and contributed to his tendency to fall.

A treatment plan was designed and implemented over the course of several years. Michael was taught to use methods of T'ai Chi practice and related tools of self-recognition to address all his physical, emotional, and intellectual disabilities. Because of his inability to control his spasticity or prevent falls by stepping back in time to catch himself, the first step was to teach him to fall in such a way that he could protect himself from injury. Michael reported falling every day for the duration of the treatment, but he suffered no serious injury. This apparently gave him the confidence to try other methods aimed at increasing his walking capabilities.

T'ai Chi breathing techniques were taught to help him get more oxygen to his brain and to relax his chest and abdomen. He learned how to change his posture for optimal breathing. His mood improved when he breathed deeply, and his intellectual focus also improved. Michael was taught the T'ai Chi method of pouring weight from one leg to the other slowly, focusing on emptying the weight from one leg as it is shifted to the other. The therapist molded Michael's body to straighten his posture and head when he shifted his weight and when he sat in his wheelchair. Michael was also taught T'ai Chi exercises that helped coordinate the upper and lower body, strengthen his legs, and allow him to move with his knees bent and his upper body relaxed. They also served to focus his thoughts on his points of balance, giving him some power over his tendency to fall.

He practiced diligently, and his legs strengthened to the point where he could walk slowly but confidently when an assistant held both his hands. He was able to get out of his wheelchair and come gracefully to a standing position (previously he had had to go down to the ground on his knees and pull himself up, using the side of his wheelchair).

Michael was taught a method of emotional self-recognition to help him deal with his emotions. This was a gradual process. At first he was asked to keep a diary of every time he had an emotional outburst and to identify it (e.g., anger, joy, etc.). Then he was asked to notice the muscular tension accompanying the outburst (e.g., tightness in a particular location or facial tension). Finally, he was taught to use the breathing and other T'ai Chi techniques he had learned to relax any tension and observe how it affected the outburst. Eventually the outbursts stopped.

References

1. Cheng, M-C: T'ai Chi Chuan. North Atlantic Books, Berkeley, Calif., 1981, p 4.
2. Dr. Bingjun is director of infectious medicine. His comments were made in an informal discussion with delegates to the First Symposium on Sexology: East and West, held in Beijing, October 12–26, 1993.
3. Cheng: T'ai Chi Chuan.
4. Lowenthal, W: Gateway to the Miraculous. Frog Ltd, Berkeley, Calif., 1994.
5. Moyers, B: Healing and the Mind. Doubleday, New York, 1993. (Also published as an audiocassette by Doubleday)
6. All these projects were conducted by the T'ai Chi Foundation between 1993 and 1997, using an adapted and simplified form of T'ai Chi that maintains all of the T'ai Chi principles.
7. Most T'ai Chi teachers work with able-bodied people and exclude participants who have medical problems (for liability reasons). With few exceptions, they have not gone through any training to enable them to work with frail or ill populations.
8. Province, A, et al: The effects of exercise on falls in elderly patients: A preplanned meta-analysis of the FICSIT trials. JAMA 273:1341–1347, 1995.
9. American Academy of Orthopaedic Surgeons. Don't let a fall be your last trip. Rosemont, Ill., 1998.
10. Pekka, K, et al: Fall induced injuries and deaths among older adults. JAMA 28(20), 1998.
11. Associated Press report, May 3, 1998.
12. Province et al: The effects of exercise on falls in elderly patients.
13. Wolf, S: Exploring novel interventions to reduce falls in older individuals. In Apple, DF, and Hayes, WC: Prevention of Falls and Hip Fractures in the Elderly. American Academy of Orthopaedics, Rosemont, Ill., 1994.
14. Wolfson, L: et al: Balance and strength training in older adults: Intervention gains and T'ai Chi maintenance. J Am Geriatr Soc 44:498–506, 1996.
15. Blair, SN, and Garcia, ME: Get up and move: A call to action for older men and women. J Am Geriatr Soc 44:599–600, 1996.
16. Xushing, S, Yugi, X, and Yunjian, X: Determination of e-rosette-forming lymphocytes in aged subjects with T'ai Chi exercise. Int J Sports Med 10:217–219, 1989.
17. Reported in Krucoff, C: T'ai Chi as effective as aerobics in study on hypertension. Los Angeles Times, May 11, 1998.
18. Lan, C, et al: Cardiovascular function, flexibility, and body composition among geriatric T'ai Chi Chuan practitioners. Arch Phys Med Rehabil 77:612–616, 1996.

Index

Page numbers followed by f indicate figures; page numbers followed by t indicate tables; page numbers followed by b indicate boxes.

Active imagery, defined, 114
Acupuncture, in Chinese medicine, 265–267, 266f
  holistic dentistry and, 254t
Acute illness, biomedicine and, 3
Ader, as mind-body connection pioneer, 57t, 67b
Adjustments, in chiropractic, 239–241
Agriculture, nutrition and, 123–124
Alcohol consumption, culture and, 74–75
Allergy, food, 128, 128t
  immune system and, 59
Alternative medicine *See* Complementary and alternative medicine
Alternative systems of medical practice, as NCCAM category, 9
Alternative therapy *See also* Complementary and alternative medicine
  defined, 7
Amalgam fillings, holistic dentistry and, 250–253, 252t, 256–257
American Holistic Nurses Association, founding of, 41
American Medical Association, chiropractic and, 13, 242b
  homeopathy and, 200b
  naturopathy and, 190b
American Naturopathic Association, 190b
Amhara, cultural considerations in, 73
Amino acids, in nutrition, 122
Anesthetics, herbal interactions with, 142t
Animal magnetism, Mesmer's theory of, 39
Anthroposophic medicine, 213–223
  clinical example of, 223b
  defined, 213
  imbalance as cause of illness in, 217
  origin of, 214b–215b
  other therapies and, 218f–220f, 218–219, 221
  physiology in, 215–217, 216f
  research into, 221–222
  spiritual anatomy in, 217–218
  training for, 215b
Anticholinergics, herbal interactions with, 142t

Anticoagulants, herbal interactions with, 142t
Anticonvulsants, herbal interactions with, 142t
Antidiabetes drugs, herbal interactions with, 146t
Antigen presentation, in immune system, 58, 58f
Antihistamines, herbal interactions with, 142t
Antihypertensives, herbal interactions with, 143t
Antioxidants, in nutrition, 130–131, 131t
Anxiety, Therapeutic Touch in, 175
  yoga in, 301–303
Appropriation, complementary and alternative medicine and, 12–13
Armoring, bioenergetics and, 48–49, 50b
Art therapies, in anthroposophism, 221
Asanas, in yoga, 287–288, 288f–289f, 290t
Asclepius, herbs and, 135
Ashen, ISM system of, 116
Ashtanga yoga, 286, 286t
Ashwaganda, in Ayurveda, 280–281
Aspirin, history of, 137–138
Assessment, in Therapeutic Touch, 176
Asthma, imagery in, 118–119
Astragalus, in nutrition, 132
Astral body, in anthroposophism, 218
Atomic bomb, ecological movement and, 81–82
Attitude, cancer survival and, 65
Aurobindo, life cycle model of, 35, 35t
Ayurveda, 273–282
  biological humors in, 275t, 275–276
  constitution in, 276–279, 278t
  consultation in, 280
  doshas and, 279t, 279–280
  herbs in, 137, 280–281
  origin of, 273, 274b
  principles of, 273–274, 274t–275t

B cells, in immune system, 56, 57f
Balance with nature, global health issues and, 85
Becker and Selden, energy research of, 172
Belladonna, in homeopathy, 199, 201
Bendit, dis-ease defined by, 35

Benson, Mind-Body Medical Institute founded by, 107
Benveniste, research of, 202
Berry, on death, 36
Bhakti yoga, 287
Bhavagad Gita, 285–286
Bible, herbs mentioned in, 137
Biocentrism, in deep ecology, 93–94
Bioelectromagnetic therapy, as NCCAM category, 9
Bioenergetic analysis, armor and, 48–49, 50b
  character and, 51, 52b
  exercises and, 53b
  grounding and, 52–53, 53b
  rhythm of life and, 51
  sexuality and, 49–51, 50t
Bioenergetic basis of health, 47–54
  bioenergetic analysis and, 47–48, 48t
  criteria for, 54t
  energetic functioning and, 48–53, 50b, 50t, 52b–53b
Biological humors, in Ayurveda, 275t, 275–276
Biomedicine *See also* Conventional medicine
  Chinese medicine *versus,* 83, 84f
  global health issues and, 83–85
  principles of, 3–4
Blair, views of, 82
Blanket roll, bioenergetics and, 53b
Blood, in Chinese medicine, 264
Blood group diet, 127
Blood pressure, yoga and, 295–296
Blood pressure, herbal interactions with, 143t
Boesler, osteopathic research of, 234
Bohm, holographic theory of, 33–34
Boswellia, in Ayurveda, 281
Brain injury, homeopathic treatment of, 203–207, 205f
Brain theories, of imagery, 115b
Breast cancer, imagery and, 117–118
Breast lesions, Chinese medical treatment of, 269
Breast-feeding, imagery in, 119
Breathing, in anthroposophism, 216f, 216–217
  in yoga, 290, 294
Buddhism, meditation in, 107
Burkhardt, on spirituality, 40
Burns, osteopathic research of, 233
Burr, energy field described by, 172

Calcium, herbal interactions with, 143t
  in nutrition, 122
Calories, defined, 122
  formula for calculating required, 124

Cancer, antioxidants and, 131
  imagery and, 117–118
  immune system and, 64–65
  mistletoe in, 221–222
Cannon, as mind-body connection pioneer, 57t, 67b
Capitalism, global health issues and, 89–90
  radical ecology and, 100
Carbohydrate-protein balance, in nutrition, 126–127
Cardiac drugs, herbal interactions with, 143t–145t
Carman, views of, 86
Carreiro, osteopathic research of, 234
Carson, views of, 82
Centering, in Therapeutic Touch, 175–176, 177b
Central nervous system drugs, herbal interactions with, 145t
Change, models of, 15–24
  at organizational level, 22–24
  resistance to, 21–22
Character, bioenergetics and, 51, 52b
Chemical sensitivity, holistic dentistry and, 256–257
Chemotherapy, herbal interactions with, 145t
Cheng, in T'ai chi, 307
Chinese medicine, 261–271
  anatomy in, 265
  case study of, 270b–271b
  early herbal, 137
  examinations in, 262
  meridians and acupuncture in, 265–267, 266f
  philosophy and history of, 263, 264b
  physiology in, 263–265
  principles of, 261–262
  research into, 268–269
  six excesses in, 267–268
  treatments used in, 262–263
  Western medicine *versus,* 83, 84f
Chiropractic medicine, 239–244
  AMA *versus,* 13, 242b
  applications of, 241
  benefits of, 242–243
  case studies of, 244b
  changing attitudes on, 7–8
  defined, 239
  effectiveness of, 13
  growth of, 242b
  history of, 240
  principles of, 239–240
  research into, 242–243
  techniques of, 241
Cholesterol-lowering drugs, herbal interactions with, 145t

Chronic fatigue syndrome, Therapeutic Touch in, 178
Chronic illness, biomedicine and, 3
  imagery and, 117–119, 118b
  massage and, 166–167
  naturopathy in, 188b, 189, 193b–195b
  Therapeutic Touch in, 178
Chronic pain, imagery and, 118b
Circular causality and circular logic models, in Worldview Hypotheses, 25t, 27
Circulation, massage and, 162
Civil rights movement, holistic perspective and, 10b
Client, patient versus, 10b
Clients, holistic, 14
Clonal expansion, in immune system, 59f
Colby, views of, 82
Commission E, herbs and, 150, 151t–155t
Complementary and alternative medicine, environmental issues and, 91
  history of, 8–9
  paradigm shifts in, 7–14, 10b–11b See also Paradigm shifts in medicine
  politics of, 12–14
    evolution of, 10b–11b
    regulation and appropriation and, 12–13
  rise of, 5
  sources of information on, 6, 8
  statistics on use of, 5
  terminology of, 7–8
Complementary therapy See also Complementary and alternative medicine; specific techniques
  anthroposophic, 213–223
  chiropractic, 239–244
  defined, 7
  holistic dental, 247–257
  homeopathic, 197–209
  naturopathic, 183–195
  osteopathic, 227–235
Complexity, culture and, 72
Concentration meditation, defined, 106
Connectedness, global health issues and, 87–88
  holism and, 32, 34
  indigenous perspectives on, 86–87
Consciousness, in holistic health model, 38b
  in radical ecology, 97, 98f
Constitution, in Ayurveda, 276–279, 278t
Consumer capitalism, global health issues and, 89–90
Consumer rights movement, holistic perspective and, 10b
Consumers, defined, 10b
  FDA regulation of herbs and, 150, 155–156
Contextual models, in Worldview Hypotheses, 25t, 26

Contraction, bioenergetics and, 51
Conventional medicine See also Biomedicine
  homeopathy versus, 197
  paradigm shifts in, 3–28 See also Paradigm shifts in medicine
  principles of, 3–4
Conventionals, in Personal Theories of Health Model, 17
Corticosteroids, herbal interactions with, 146t
Cosmology, global health issues and, 87–88
Cost-containment strategies, holistic medicine and, 12–13
Creative unfolding and intentional models, in Worldview Hypotheses, 25t, 27
Cultural competence, defined, 75
  ethnocentrism and, 76b
  steps toward, 75–79
Cultural diversity, in holistic health model, 38b
Cultural movements, holistic perspective and, 10b–11b
Culture, competence and, 75–79, 76b
  defined, 72
  environmental interaction and, 74–75, 75b
  holistic nursing and, 71–79
    case study of, 71, 75–79
  incompatible meaning and, 75b
  intracultural variation and, 73–74
  point of view and, 73
Curcumin, in Ayurveda, 281
Cytokines, in immune system, 57, 60t

D'Adamo blood group diet, 127
Death, holistic view of, 36
  spirituality and, 40
Deep ecology, global health issues and, 93–94, 94t
Deglycerrhizinated licorice, in Ayurveda, 281
Denslow, osteopathic research of, 233
Dentistry, holistic, 247–257 See also Holistic dentistry
Depression, yoga in, 301–303
Dhyana, in yoga, 294
Diet See also Nutrition
  ideal, 125–126, 126t
  Mediterranean, 125–126
  nutrition and, as NCCAM category, 9
  paleolithic, 123, 123t
  Pritiken, 126–127
  traditional versus modern, 122–123, 123t
  For Your Type, 127
Dilution, in homeopathy, 198–199
Dioscorides, on herbs, 137
Disease, in Chinese medicine, 267–268
  as focus of conventional medicine, 4–5
  in naturopathy, 186f, 186–188

Dis-ease, defined, 35–36
Diuretics, herbal interactions with, 146t
Doshas, in Ayurveda, 279t, 279–280
Dossey, Barbara, 36, 44t
    Larry, 40
Drug interactions, with herbs, 141,
        142t–149t, 150
Drugs, plant-based, 137–139, 138t
        See also Herbal medicine

Eastern medicine, Western *versus,* 83, 84f
Echinacea, in nutrition, 132
Ecofeminism, global issues and, 94–95
Ecology *See also* Global health issues
        deep, 93–94, 94t
        feminism and, 94–95
        radical, 97–100, 98f
Ecology movement, atomic bomb and,
        81–82
        holistic perspective and, 10b
Economic debt, global health issues and, 89
Ego, in anthroposophism, 218
Egyptian medicine, ancient herbal, 137
Einstein, on connectedness, 32
        relativity theory of, 33
Elderly patients, chiropractic in, 243
        massage in, 166
        T'ai chi in, 308–309
Emergent paradigm of health, 6t
Emotional health, Vithoulkas on, 35
Emotions, bioenergetics and, 51
        immune system and, 61–63
        mind-body healing and, 55
Energy, bioenergetics and, 51
        Einstein's view of, 33
        holism and, 38
        Therapeutic Touch and, 171–172, 172b
Environment, global health issues and,
        81–82 *See also* Global health issues
        interaction of culture with, 74–75, 75b
        recent changes in, 88–90, 89t
Essential fatty acids, in nutrition, 122
Essential amino acids, in nutrition, 122
Etheric body, in anthroposophism, 217–218
Ethics, Therapeutic Touch and, 176b
Ethnocentrism, cultural competence and, 76b
Eurythmy, in anthroposophism, 221
Exercise, bioenergetic, 53b
        massage and, 164–165
        yoga and, 288–289
Expansion, bioenergetics and, 51
Expenditures, for alternative medicine, 5
Experiential imagery, defined, 114

Faraday, field theory of, 32
Fatty acids, in nutrition, 122
Feminism, global issues and, 94–95

Fertility and culture, case study of, 71,
        75–79
Fertilizers, nutrition and, 123–124
Fiber, in nutrition, 130
Field theory, holism and, 32
First- and second-order models of change,
        in paradigm shifts in medicine,
        18f–19f, 18–24, 21t
Fitzgerald, reflexology and, 166
Fluids, in Chinese medicine, 265
Fluoride, holistic dentistry and, 250
Food allergy, 128, 128t
Food and Drug Administration, herbs and,
        150, 155–156
Food pyramid, 125
For Your Type Diet, 127
Formistic models, in Worldview Hypotheses,
        25, 25t
Fraval, osteopathic research of, 234
Frejka aprons, Navajo rejection of, 72
Freud, bioenergetic analysis and, 48
        sexuality and, 49
Frymann, osteopathic research of, 234
Functional theories of imagery, 115b–116b

Gamma linolenic acid, in nutrition, 122
Gandhi, naturopathy of, 184b
Gerber, observations of, 36, 41
German Commission E, herbs and, 150,
        151t–155t
Ginseng, in Ayurveda, 280–281
Global health issues, 81–100
        balance with nature and, 85
        biomedicine and, 83–85, 84f
        complementary medicine and, 90–91
        deep ecology as, 93–94, 94t
        ecofeminism as, 94–95
        effective response to, 92–93
        environmental changes and, 88–90, 89t
        impediments to change in, 91–92
        indigenous perspectives and, 86–87
        mechanistic worldview in, 95–97
        new consciousness in, 95
        outlandish premises in, 87–88
        practitioners and, 82–83
        radical ecology as, 97–100, 98f
Glucocorticoids, herbal interactions with,
        147t
Gore, environmental strategy of, 93
Grace, bioenergetics and, 52
Graham, homeopathy of, 200b
Granulocytes, in immune system, 56f
Grief, imagery in, 114
Grounding, bioenergetics and, 52–53, 53b
Growth, massage and, 166
Gugul, in Ayurveda, 281
Guha, on environmental consciousness, 95

Guided imagery, defined, 114
Gynecological cysts, Chinese medical
　　treatment of, 268–269

Hahnemann, as homeopathy founder,
　　8, 197, 200b
Hand-warming visualization, 118
Hatha yoga, 287
Headache, foods triggering, 128, 128t
Healing, evolving understanding of, 36
　　in naturopathy, 188b, 188–189
　　in osteopathy, 228
　　psychophysiology of, 55–68
　　in T'ai chi, 305–306
Healing crisis, in naturopathy, 188, 188b
　　in yoga, 301
Health, in anthroposophism, 215
　　bioenergetic basis of, 47–54
　　defined, 32
　　　bioenergetic analysis and, 48t
　　emergent paradigm of, 6t
　　emotions and, 61–66
　　global issues in, 81–100 See also Global
　　　health issues
　　in holistic health model, 37b
　　spirituality and, 40–41
　　Steiner on, 34–35
　　Vithoulkas on, 35
Health Belief Model, components of,
　　15t, 15–16
　　environmental issues and, 90–91
Health-care professionals See also
　　Practitioners
　　herbs and, 157, 158t
Health models, Health Belief Model as,
　　15t, 15–16
　　Personal Theories of Health Model as,
　　16–17
Heart drugs, herbal interactions with,
　　143t–145t
Helplessness, immune system and, 63–64
Hepatotoxic drugs, herbal interactions with,
　　147t
Heraclitus, observations of, 3, 28
Herbal medicine, 135–159
　　in Ayurveda, 280–281
　　as basis for modern pharmacology,
　　137–139, 138t
　　future of, 157, 159
　　history of, 135–137
　　as NCCAM category, 9
　　popularity of, 156–157
　　practitioners and, 157, 158t
　　problems with, 141
　　　drug interactions as, 141, 142t–149t, 150
　　　nomenclature as, 141
　　pros and cons of, 140t, 141

rationale for, 139
　　regulation of, 150, 151t–155t, 155–156
　　sources of, 157, 158t
Hippocrates, on chiropractic, 240
　　massage and, 161
　　overview of, 135–136
Hmong, cultural considerations in, 73
Holism, death and, 36
　　defined, 32
　　in holistic health model, 37b
　　love and, 34
　　philosophical and theoretical basis of,
　　32–34
　　placebo response and, 39
　　spirituality and, 40–41
　　in T'ai chi, 305–306
Holistic dentistry, 247–257
　　acupuncture and, 254t
　　case studies of, 247, 253–257
　　chemical sensitivity and, 256
　　fluoride and, 250
　　kinesiology and, 255–256
　　mainstream dentistry versus, 248
　　mercury and, 250
　　nutrition in, 248–249
　　periodontal disease and, 254–255
　　pioneers in, 249–250
　　principles of, 248
　　research into, 251–253, 252t
Holistic medicine See also Complementary
　　and alternative medicine; specific
　　modalities
　　clients of, 14
　　constraints against, 12–13
　　defined, 7, 14
　　dental, 247–257
　　herbal, 135–159
　　imagery in, 113–119
　　meditation in, 105–111
　　nutrition in, 121–132
　　practitioners of, 14
　　sociopolitical evolution of, 10b–11b
　　therapeutic massage in, 161–167
　　therapeutic touch in, 171–179
Holistic movement, sociopolitical evolution
　　of, 11b
Holistic nursing, case study of, 43b
　　common interventions in, 44t
　　culture and, 71–79
　　principles of, 41, 41b, 42
　　theories of, 42–43
Holistic theories, of imagery, 115b–116b
Holographic theories, 33–34
　　of imagery, 115b
Homeopathy, 197–209
　　anthroposophism versus, 218
　　clinical example of, 203–207, 205f

defined, 197
effectiveness of, 208
history of, 8, 200b–201b
law of similars in, 197
provings in, 199, 201
research into, 202–203
single remedy in, 201–202
treatment principles of, 198–199
Vithoulkas in, 35
Homeostasis, chiropractic in, 241
in naturopathy, 186
Hora, metapsychiatry of, 41
Hormones, herbal interactions with, 147t
Horowitz, on imagery, 116
Hufeland, in vitalist lineage, 192b
Human immunodeficiency virus, herbal
interactions with therapy for, 147t
Humors, in Ayurveda, 275t, 275–276
Hygeia, 135
Hypothalamic-pituitary-adrenal axis,
immune system and, 63f

Ichazo, T'ai chi defined by, 306b
Illness *See also* Disease
as focus of conventional medicine, 4–5
Imagery, 113–120
classification of systems of, 116
defined, 113
research into, 116–120
case study of, 118b
theories of, 115b–116b
therapeutic uses of, 114, 119b
types of, 114
Imbalance, as cause of illness in
anthroposophism, 217
Immune system, 55–68
acquired, 56–57, 57f, 57t
components of, 56f–59f, 56–59
defined, 55–56
functioning of, 59–60
imagery and, 117–118, 118b
innate, 56, 56f
nervous system and, 60–61, 61f,
62b, 63f
research into, 61–66
on feeling helpless, 63–64
on social support, 65–66
on stress, infections, and cancer,
64–65
on thoughts and emotions, 61–63
suppression of, 60–61, 61f
Immunomodifiers, herbal interactions
with, 148t
Implicit process and information energy
models, in Worldview Hypotheses,
25t, 26
Impotence, orgastic, 49–51

Indigenous perspectives, on global issues,
86–87
on imagery, 113
Individual responsibility, in holistic health
model, 37b
Infections, anthroposophic treatment of,
223b
immune system and, 64–65
Inflammatory illness, in anthroposophism, 217
Ingram, reflexology and, 166
Insurance companies, holistic medicine
constrained by, 12–13
Integration, culture and, 72
Integrative care, defined, 9, 11
holistic and, 11–12
Integrative diversity and interconnected
models, in Worldview Hypotheses,
25t, 27–28
Intention, in Therapeutic Touch, 176
International Institute for Bioenergetic
Analysis, 50b
Intracultural variation, in culture definitions,
73–74
Iron supplements, in nutrition, 132
Irritable bowel syndrome, Chinese medical
treatment of, 269
yoga in, 300–301
ISM system of imagery, 116
Iyengar yoga, principles of, 287
therapy with, 298–303, 299f, 302f

Jing, in Chinese medicine, 264
Jnana yoga, 287

Kabat-Zinn, work and views on meditation of,
105–109
Kapha, in Ayurveda, 275t, 276–277, 278t
Kaptchuk, on Chinese medicine, 267–268
Karma yoga, 287
Keegan, philosophy of nursing of, 42
Kelly, holistic dentistry of, 249–250
Kent, homeopathy of, 200b
Kicking, bioenergetics and, 53b
Kinesiology, holistic dentistry and, 255–256
King, views of, 94
Kleinman, explpanatory models of,
77–78
Kniepp, naturopathy of, 183, 184b, 190b
Korr, osteopathic research of, 232–233
Krieger/Kunz, Method of Therapeutic
Touch, 173

Lactobacillus, in nutrition, 130
Lao Tzu, on centering, 175
Law of similars, in homeopathy, 197
Laxatives, herbal interactions with, 148t
Lei, T'ai chi practiced by, 306

Levine, on illness, 40
  T'ai chi method of, 308
Licorice, in Ayurveda, 281
Life cycle stages, Aurobindo model of, 35, 35t
Life force, Therapeutic Touch and, 173
Lifestyles, naturopathy and, 193b–194b
  radical ecology and, 99–100
Ling, massage practiced by, 161
Lo, research of, 202
Love, holism and, 34
Lowen, bioenergetics and, 50b
Lust, naturopathy founded by, 183, 190b–191b
Lymphatic system, massage and, 161–162
Lymphedema, massage for, 164
Lymphocytes, in immune system, 56–59,
  57f–59f

Macrophages, in immune system, 56f
Magnetic therapy, 172
Maimonides, in vitalist lineage, 192b
Mal de ojo, as cultural consideration, 74
Managed care, holistic medicine constrained
  by, 12–13
Manipulation, chiropractic, 239–244
  in osteopathy, 231–232
Manual healing, as NCCAM category, 9
Marglin, views of, 95–96
Massage, therapeutic, 161–167 See also
  Therapeutic massage
Materialism, radical ecology and, 99
Matter, Einstein's view of, 33
Mead, views of, 72
Measel, osteopathic research of, 234
Mechanism, global issues and, 95–97
  vitalism versus, 187
  in Worldview Hypotheses, 25, 25t
Medical anthropology, emergence of, 8
Medications, plant-based, 137–139, 138t
  See also Herbal medicine
Meditation, 105–111
  awakening to reality with, 106, 107b–108b
  case study of, 110b–111b
  categories of, 106
  defined, 105
  medical effects of, 108–109, 110b–111b
  research into, 106–109, 110b–111b
  in yoga, 294
Mediterranean diet, 125–126
Memory of water theory, in homeopathy, 199
Meniere's disease, Chinese medical treatment
  of, 270b–271b
Merchant, radical ecology of, 97–99, 98f
Mercury fillings, holistic dentistry and,
  250–253, 252t
Meridians, in Chinese medicine, 265–267,
  266f
Mesmer, magnetic healing theory of, 8, 39

Metabolic-limb system, in anthroposophism,
  215–216, 216f, 219, 220f
Metapsychiatry, Hora and, 41
Mexican-Americans, cultural considerations
  in, 74
Migraine, foods triggering, 128, 128t
  herbal interactions with therapy for, 148t
Migration, global health issues and, 89
Mind-body healing, meditation in, 105–111
  pioneers in, 57t, 67b
  psychophysiology of, 55–68
Mind-body interventions, as NCCAM
  category, 9
Mind-Body Medical Institute, founding
  of, 107
Mindfulness meditation, defined, 106
Mindfulness-Based Stress Reduction, 107, 109
Mineral supplements, in nutrition,
  128–129, 129t
Mineralocorticoids, herbal interactions
  with, 149t
Mistletoe, in anthroposophism, 221–222
Models of change, in paradigm shifts
  in medicine, 15–24
  first- and second-order models as,
  18f–19f, 18–24
  Health Belief Model as, 15t, 15–17
Monoamine oxidase inhibitors, herbal inter-
  actions with, 148t
Monte, on health-care crisis, 4
Moyers, T'ai chi and, 307
Multiple sclerosis, imagery in, 119
Murphy, osteopathic research of, 234
Muscles, massage and, 162–163
Myofascial release, 165

Naess, deep ecology of, 93
National Center for Complementary and
  Alternative Medicine, categories
  recognized by, 9
  establishment of, 9, 85
National Institutes of Health, National Center
  for Complementary and Alternative
  Medicine of, 9
Native Americans, herbs used by, 136
Natural killer cells, in immune system, 56, 56f
  research into, 62b, 64–65
Natural versus synthetic drugs, 138–139
Nature, global health issues and, 85
  healing power of, 184–185 See also
  Naturopathy
Naturopathy, 183–195
  case study of, 193b–195b
  defined, 183
  disease continuum in, 186, 186f
  healing responses in, 188b, 188–189
  history of, 8, 190b–191b

lineage of, 184b, 192b
mail-order degrees in, 191b
meaning of disease in, 187–188
mechanism *versus* vitalism and, 187
philosophy and theory of, 186
principles of, 183–185
professional organizations of, 191b,
    191–192
research into, 189, 191–192
Navajos, cultural considerations in, 72
Nerve-sense system, in anthroposophism,
    215–216, 216f, 219, 220f
Nervous system, chiropractic and, 239
    immune system and, 60–61, 61f, 62b, 63f
Neurochemicals, in immune system, 60t,
    60–61, 61f
Neuroendocrine factors *See also* Immune
    system
    in immune system, 68t
Neurologic injury, T'ai chi in, 310b
New conventionals, in Personal Theories
    of Health Model, 17
Newman, theories of, 36, 42
Nightingale, as holistic nurse, 42
Nine-dot problem, in change model, 18f–19f,
    18–19
Nonsteroidal anti-inflammatory drugs,
    herbal interactions with, 148t–149t
Nursing, cultural biases in, 75–76
    holistic *See* Holistic nursing
Nutrient density, defined, 124
    examples of, 124–125, 125t
Nutrients, calories of, 122
    composition of, 121–122
Nutrition, 121–132
    carbohydrate-protein balance and,
        126–127
    ideal diet and, 125–126, 126t
    nutrient density in, 124–125, 125t
    nutrients in, 121–122
    soil degeneration and, 123–124
    supplementation in, 128–132, 129t, 131t
    traditional *versus* modern, 122–123, 123t
    trigger foods and allergies and, 128, 128t
Nutrition Labeling and Education Act of
    1990, herbs and, 156
Nux vomica, in homeopathy, 205–207

Office of Alternative Medicine, establishment
    of, 8–9, 203
Office of Minority Health, culture defined
    by, 72
Oldways nutritional guidelines, 125
Omega-3 fatty acids, in nutrition, 123,
    127–129
Organ transplant rejection therapy, herbal
    interactions with, 149t

Organismic and relationship models, in
    Worldview Hypotheses, 25t, 26
Organizational change, models of, 22–24
Orgastic impotence, bioenergetics and,
    49–51
Ornish, naturopathy and, 189
Osteopathy, 227–235
    case study of, 230–231
    changing attitudes about, 7–8
    dynamic unit of function in, 227–228
    history of, 229b
    information gathering in, 235
    manipulation in, 231–232
    rational treatment in, 230–231
    research into, 232–234
    self-regulation in, 228
    structure-function interrelation in, 228, 230
Over-the-counter medications, FDA
    regulation of, 156
    use of, 139
Oyster shell, in anthroposophism, 221

Page, holistic dentistry of, 249
Pain, imagery and, 118b
    meditation and, 108–109
Paleolithic diet, 123, 123t
Palmer, chiropractic founded by, 240, 242b
Paracelsus, aura described by, 38, 173
    in vitalist lineage, 192b
Paradigm shifts in medicine, 3–28
    biomedicine's promise and, 4–5, 7
    complementary health care in, approach
        integration and, 9, 11–12
        political implications of, 12–14
        rise of, 7–9, 10b–11b
        types of, 9
    models of change and, 15t, 15–24,
        18f–19f, 21t
        old *versus* new assumptions in, 6t
        world hypotheses in, 24–28, 25t
Patient, client *versus,* 10b
Pepper, Worldview Hypotheses of, 24–28, 25t
Perceptions, in Health Belief Model,
    15t, 15–16
Periodontal disease, holistic dentistry and,
    254–255
Perlman, views and writings of, 81–82, 100
Personal Theories of Health Model, 16–17
Pharmacodynamics, defined, 141
Pharmacokinetics, defined, 141
Pharmacologic and biological treatments,
    as NCCAM category, 9
Pharmacology, plant-based medicine in,
    138–139 *See also* Herbal medicine
Philosophical basis of holism, 32–34
Photosensitizers, herbal interactions with,
    149t

Pitta, in Ayurveda, 275t, 276–277, 278t
Placebo, defined, 39
Placebo response, holism and, 39
Plants, medicinal, 135–159 *See also* Herbal
    medicine
    in anthroposophism, 218–219,
        219f–220f
Politics of complementary and alternative
    medicine, 12–14
    evolution of, 10b–11b
Pollution, global health issues and, 90
Pop holism, true holism *versus,* 40–41
Population explosion, global health issues
    and, 89
Post-traumatic stress disorder, immune system
    and, 60
Postures, in yoga, 287–288, 288f–289f, 290t,
    291f–293f
Potency, in homeopathy, 198–199
Practitioners, cultural biases of, 75–76
    global health issues and, 82–83
    herbs and, 157, 158t
    holistic, 14
    in holistic health model, 37b–38b
    of naturopathy, 185
    osteopathic, 227
Prakriti, in Ayurveda, 276–279, 278t
Pranayama, in yoga, 290, 294
Pregnancy, herbal interactions with, 149t
    massage during, 164
Preissnitz, naturopathy of, 184b
Prevention, in naturopathy, 185
Pribam, holographic theory of, 33
Price, holistic dentistry of, 249
Primary respiratory mechanism, in osteopathy,
    228, 235
Pritiken diet, 126–127
Process imagery, defined, 114
Production, in radical ecology, 97, 98f
Protein, in Mediterranean diet, 126
Protein-carbohydrate balance, in nutrition,
    126–127
Provings, in homeopathy, 199, 201
Psychiatric conditions, massage and, 166
Psychoanalytic theory, of imagery, 115b
Psychological stress, in immune system,
    64–65
Psychoneuroimmunology, mind-body healing
    and, 55–68, 67b
Psycho-Physical Balance Therapy,
    in T'ai chi, 308
Psychophysiology of mind-body healing,
    55–68
    emotions and, 55
    immune system and, 55–66
Puerto Ricans, cultural considerations in,
    74–75, 77–78

Pulsation, bioenergetics and, 51
Pythagoras, on energy, 38, 173

Qi, in Chinese medicine, 263

Radical ecology, global health issues and,
    97–100, 98f
Radioisotopes, herbal interactions with,
    149t
Rational treatment, in osteopathy, 230–231
Raynaud's disease, Chinese medical treatment
    of, 270b–271b
Receptive imagery, defined, 114
Recovery, immune system and, 65–66
Reflexology, 165–166
Regulation, of complementary and alternative
    medicine, 12–13
Reich, theory of, 49–50, 50b
Relativity theory, of Einstein, 33
Relaxation Response, defined, 107
Religion, holism and, 40–41
Reproduction, in radical ecology, 97, 98f
Rhythmical massage, in anthroposophism, 221
Robbins, on problems of Western medicine, 4
Rogers, theory of, 42
Rogers' Science of Unitary Human
    Beings, 174
Rubik, energy theory of, 39
    observations of, 174

Salicylic acid, history of, 137–138
Saluretics, herbal interactions with, 149t
Sampson, observations of, 85
Sato, osteopathic research of, 233–234
Schroth, naturopathy of, 184b
Sclerotic illness, in anthroposophism, 217
Seager, views of, 94–95
Self-medication, drugs in, 139
    herbs in, 139, 141
        pros and cons of, 140t
Self-regulation, in osteopathy, 228
Selye, as mind-body connection pioneer,
    57t, 67b
Setir, culture and, 73
Shamanism, imagery in, 113
Shen, in Chinese medicine, 265
Shiatsu massage, 165
Silver-mercury tooth fillings, holistic dentistry
    and, 250–253, 252t, 256–257
Sinusitis, osteopathic treatment of, 231
Smoking cessation, in change model, 19–21
Smuts, holistic movement and, 11b
Social acquisition, culture and, 72
Social support, immune system and, 65–66
Sociopolitical evolution of holistic perspective,
    10b–11b
Soil quality, nutrition and, 123–124

Solomon, as mind-body connection pioneer, 57t, 67b

Spiegel, imagery research of, 117

Spinal manipulation, in chiropractic, 239–244

Spiritual anatomy, in anthroposophism, 217–218

Spirituality, holism and, 40–41

Spirituals, in Personal Theories of Health Model, 17

Spleen, in Chinese medicine, 265

Sports massage, 164–165

State medical boards, holistic care regulated by, 12–13

Steiner, anthroposophism founded by, 214b
  views of, 34–35

Stereotyping, culture and, 74

Still, osteopathy founded by, 227, 229b, 232, 235

Stimulants, herbal interactions with, 149t

Stock, holistic dentistry of, 251

Stress, imagery in reduction of, 119
  immune system and, 64–65

Stress Reduction Program, meditation in, 107, 109, 110b–111b

Subluxation, chiropractic in, 239, 241

Supplements, dietary, 128–132, 129t, 131t

Susceptibility, in naturopathy, 186

Sutherland, osteopathic work of, 228, 235

Sutras, in yoga, 286, 286t

Swedish massage, 161, 164

Sympathomimetics, herbal interactions with, 149t

Synthetic *versus* natural drugs, 138–139

T cells, in immune system, 56–57, 57f, 64

T'ai chi, 305–310
  case study of, 310b
  defined, 305, 306b
  healing in, 305–306
  history of, 307
  research into, 308–309
  Western interest in, 307–308

Tallbull, views of, 86–87

Tavis, wellness movement and, 11b

Teilhard de Chardin, views of, 34

Theoretical basis of holism, 32–34

Therapeutic imagery, defined, 114

Therapeutic massage, 161–167
  applications of, 163–164
  methods of, 164–166
  research into, 166–167
  techniques of, 162f–163f, 162–163

Therapeutic Touch, 171–179
  case studies of, 177–178
  effects of, 174
  energy field and, 171–172, 172b
  ethics and, 176b

method of, 175–177, 177b
  practice of, 173
  research into, 174–175
  vitalism and, 173

Thich Nhat Hanh, interbeing concept of, 10b

Thompsonism, history of, 8, 136

Thoughts, immune system and, 61–63

Time cycle, in Ayurveda, 279t, 279–280

Tooth fillings, holistic dentistry and, 250–253, 252t, 256–257

Touch, Therapeutic, 171–179 *See also* Therapeutic Touch

Toxic shock syndrome, immune system and, 59

Traditional Chinese medicine *See* Chinese medicine

Traditional cultures, cultural competence and, 77
  global health issues and, 86–87

Traditional healing systems *See also* specific entities
  ayurveda as, 273–282
  Chinese, 261–271
  t'ai chi as, 305–310
  yoga as, 285–303

Transcendental Meditation Society, research sponsored by, 108

Trauma, chiropractic in, 239

Traumatic brain injury, homeopathic treatment of, 203–207, 205f

Trestman, imagery research of, 117

Tridosha theory, in Ayurveda, 275t, 275–276

Trigger foods, in food allergy, 128, 128t

Tylor, definition of culture of, 72

Unconventionals, in Personal Theories of Health Model, 17

United Nations Environmental Program, recommendation of, 90

Urban density, global health issues and, 89–90

Vata, in Ayurveda, 275, 275t, 277, 278t

Vedas, as Ayurveda source, 274b

Visualization *See also* Imagery
  defined, 106

Vital force, holism and, 38

Vitalism, lineage of, 192b
  mechanism *versus,* 39, 187
  Therapeutic Touch and, 173

Vitality, in naturopathy, 186

Vitamin supplements, antioxidant, 131, 131t
  in nutrition, 128–129, 129t

Vithoulkas, views of, 34–35

Watson, theory of, 42

Wegman, anthroposophism of, 214b

Wellness movement, holistic perspective
    and, 11b
Wesley, on herbs, 137
Western medicine, Chinese medicine *versus*,
    83, 84f
  other alternatives *versus*, 4
  See also Biomedicine; Conventional
    medicine
Women, in osteopathy, 229b
Women's movement, holistic perspective
    and, 10b
Worldview, defined, 24
Worldview Hypotheses, 24–28, 25t

Yin and yang, in Chinese medicine, 263,
    265, 267

Yoga, 285–303
  breathing in, 290, 294
  case studies of, 300–303
  conventional exercise *versus*, 288–289
  defined, 286
  history of, 285–286
  meditation in, 294
  postures of, 287–288, 288f–289f, 290t,
    291f–293f
  research into, 294–298, 295f–296f, 298f
  sutras in, 286, 286t
  systems of, 286–287
  therapeutic use of Iyengar, 298–303, 299f,
    302f

Zen Buddhism, meditation in, 107